Rare Cardiovascular Diseases

Editors

GIUSEPPE LIMONGELLI
EMANUELE MONDA
MICHELE LIONCINO
EDUARDO BOSSONE

HEART FAILURE CLINICS

www.heartfailure.theclinics.com

Consulting Editor
EDUARDO BOSSONE

Founding Editor
JAGAT NARULA

January 2022 • Volume 18 • Number 1

ELSEVIER

1600 John F. Kennedy Boulevard ● Suite 1800 ● Philadelphia, Pennsylvania, 19103-2899

http://www.theclinics.com

HEART FAILURE CLINICS Volume 18, Number 1
January 2022 ISSN 1551-7136, ISBN-13: 978-0-323-91987-6

Editor: Joanna Collett
Developmental Editor: Jessica Cañaberal

Heart Failure Clinics (ISSN 1551-7136) is published quarterly by Elsevier Inc., 360 Park Avenue South, New York, NY 10010-1710. Months of publication are January, April, July, and October. Business and editorial offices: 1600 John F. Kennedy Boulevard, Suite 1800, Philadelphia, PA 19103-2899. Periodicals postage paid at New York, NY, and additional mailing offices. Subscription prices are USD 277.00 per year for US individuals, USD 681.00 per year for US institutions, USD 100.00 per year for US students and residents, USD 300.00 per year for Canadian individuals, USD 701.00 per year for Canadian institutions, USD 315.00 per year for international individuals, USD 701.00 per year for international institutions, and USD 100.00 per year for Canadian and foreign students/residents. To receive student and resident rate, orders must be accompanied by name of affiliated institution, date of term, and the *signature* of program/residency coordinator on institution letterhead. Orders will be billed at individual rate until proof of status is received. Foreign air speed delivery is included in all *Clinics* subscription prices. All prices are subject to change without notice. **POSTMASTER:** Send address changes to *Heart Failure Clinics*, Elsevier Health Sciences Division, Subscription Customer Service, 3251 Riverport Lane, Maryland Heights, MO 63043. **Customer Service: 1-800-654-2452 (US and Canada). From outside of the US and Canada, call 314-447-8871. Fax: 314-447-8029. For print support, E-mail: JournalsCustomerService-usa@elsevier.com. For online support, E-mail: JournalsOnlineSupport-usa@elsevier.com.**

Reprints. For copies of 100 or more of articles in this publication, please contact the Commercial Reprints Department, Elsevier Inc., 360 Park Avenue South, New York, NY 10010-1710. Tel.: 212-633-3874; Fax: 212-633-3820; E-mail: reprints@elsevier.com.

Heart Failure Clinics is covered in *MEDLINE/PubMed (Index Medicus)*.

Contributors

CONSULTING EDITOR

EDUARDO BOSSONE, MD, PhD, FCCP, FESC, FACC
Director, Division of Cardiology, AORN Antonio Cardarelli Hospital, Naples, Italy

EDITORS

GIUSEPPE LIMONGELLI, MD, PhD, FESC
Inherited and Rare Cardiovascular Disease Unit, Department of Translational Medical Sciences, University of Campania "Luigi Vanvitelli," AORN dei Colli, Monaldi Hospital, Naples, Italy; Division of Cardiology, A.O.R.N. "Sant'Anna and San Sebastiano," Caserta, Italy Institute of Cardiovascular Sciences, University College of London and St. Bartholomew's Hospital, London, United Kingdom

EMANUELE MONDA, MD
Inherited and Rare Cardiovascular Disease Unit, Department of Translational Medical

Sciences, University of Campania "Luigi Vanvitelli," AORN dei Colli, Monaldi Hospital, Naples, Italy

MICHELE LIONCINO, MD
Inherited and Rare Cardiovascular Disease Unit, Department of Translational Medical Sciences, University of Campania "Luigi Vanvitelli," Naples

EDUARDO BOSSONE, MD, PhD, FCCP, FESC, FACC
Director, Division of Cardiology, AORN Antonio Cardarelli Hospital, Naples, Italy

AUTHORS

YOSHIHIRO J. AKASHY, MD, PhD
Department of Internal Medicine, St Marianna University School of Medicine, Kawasaki, Kanagawa, Japan

LEO AKIOYAMEN, MD
Faculty of Medicine, University of Toronto, Toronto, Ontario, Canada

FEDERICA AMODIO, MD
Department of Translational Medical Sciences, University of Campania "Luigi Vanvitelli," Naples, Italy

MARCELLO ARCA, MD
Department of Translational and Precision Medicine "Sapienza" University of Rome, Azienda Ospedaliero-Universitaria Policlinico Umberto I, Ex III Clinica Medica, Rome, Italy

LUIGI ASCIONE, MD
Department of Cardiology, AORN Ospedali dei Colli, Monaldi Hospital, Naples, Italy

RAFFAELE ASCIONE, MD
Department of Advanced Biomedical Sciences, University of Naples Federico II, Naples, Italy

ANGELIKI ASIMAKI, BSc, PhD
Molecular and Clinical Sciences Research Institute, St George's University of London, United Kingdom

MAURIZIO AVERNA, MD
Internal Medicine and Medical Specialities, Department of Health Promotion Sciences Maternal and Infantile Care, University of Palermo, A.O.U.P 'Paolo Giaccone' Padiglione n. 10, Palermo, Italy

ANWAR BABAN, MD, PhD
Department of Pediatric Cardiology and
Cardiac Surgery, Pediatric Cardiology and
Arrhythmia/Syncope Units, Bambino Gesù
Children Hospital and Research Institute,
IRCCS, Rome, Italy

MICHELE BELLINO, MD,
A.O.U. San Giovanni di Dio e Ruggi d'Aragona,
Salerno, Italy

ELENA BIAGINI, MD, PhD
Cardiology Unit, St. Orsola Hospital, IRCCS
Azienda Ospedaliero-Universitaria di Bologna,
Bologna, Italy

NUNZIA BORRELLI, MD
Department of Translational Medical Sciences,
University of Campania "Luigi Vanvitelli,"
Naples, Italy

**EDUARDO BOSSONE, MD, PhD, FCCP,
FESC, FACC**
Director, Division of Cardiology, AORN Antonio
Cardarelli Hospital, Naples, Italy

MARTINA CAIAZZA, MD
Inherited and Rare Cardiovascular Disease
Unit, Department of Translational Medical
Sciences, University of Campania "Luigi
Vanvitelli," AORN dei Colli, Monaldi Hospital,
Naples, Italy

PAOLO CALABRÒ, MD, PhD
Department of Translational Medical Sciences,
University of Campania "Luigi Vanvitelli,"
Naples, Italy; Division of Cardiology, A.O.R.N.
"Sant'Anna e San Sebastiano," Edificio C –
Cardiologia Universitaria, Caserta, Italy

GIULIO CALCAGNI, MD, PhD
The European Reference Network for Rare,
Low Prevalence and Complex Diseases of the
Heart - ERN GUARD-Heart, Pediatric
Cardiology and Arrhythmia/Syncope Units,
Bambino Gesù Children's Hospital IRCSS,
Rome, Italy

VICTORIA L. CAMMANN, MD
Department of Cardiology, University Heart
Center, University Hospital Zurich, Zurich,
Switzerland

LAURA CAPODICASA, MD
Inherited and Rare Cardiovascular Diseases
Unit, Department of Translational Sciences,
University of Campania "Luigi Vanvitelli,"
Department of Nephrology, Monaldi Hospital,
Naples, Italy

CHIARA CAPPELLETTO, MD
Cardiovascular Department, Azienda Sanitaria
Universitaria Giuliano Isontina (ASUGI),
University of Trieste, Trieste, Italy

PIO CASO, MD
Department of Cardiology, AORN Ospedali dei
Colli, Monaldi Hospital, Naples, Italy

SILVIA CASTELLETTI, MD, PhD
Istituto Auxologico Italiano, IRCCS-Center for
Cardiac Arrhythmias of Genetic Origin, Milan,
Italy

MARA CATALANO, MD
Department of Nuclear Imaging, AORN
Cardarelli Hospital, Naples, Italy

GIUSEPPE CERCIELLO, MD
Clinical Assistant, Haematology Unit,
Department of Clinical Medicine and Surgery,
University of Naples Federico II, Naples, Italy

ARTURO CESARO, MD
Department of Translational Medical Sciences,
University of Campania "Luigi Vanvitelli,"
Naples, Italy; Division of Cardiology, A.O.R.N.
"Sant'Anna e San Sebastiano," Edificio C –
Cardiologia Universitaria, Caserta, Italy

FLAVIA CHIOSI, MD
Department of Ophthalmology, Azienda
Ospedaliera dei Colli AORN Monaldi, Monaldi
Hospital, Naples, Italy

ANNAPAOLA CIRILLO, MD, PhD
Inherited and Rare Cardiovascular Disease
Unit, Department of Translational Medical
Sciences, University of Campania "Luigi
Vanvitelli," Naples, Italy

EMILIA CIRILLO, MD, PhD
Department of Translational Medical Sciences,
Section of Pediatrics, University of Naples
Federico II, Naples, Italy

RODOLFO CITRO, MD, PhD
A.O.U. San Giovanni di Dio e Ruggi d'Aragona, Salerno, Italy

DIEGO COLONNA, MD
Department of Translational Medical Sciences, University of Campania "Luigi Vanvitelli," Naples, Italy

ANTONELLO CREDENDINO, MD
Department of Orthopaedics, AORN dei Colli, Monaldi Hospital, Naples, Italy

GIULIA D'AMATI, MD, PhD
Department of Radiological, Oncological and Pathological Sciences, Sapienza University of Rome, Rome, Italy

DAVIDE D'ARIENZO, MD
Department of Nuclear Medicine, AORN Ospedali dei Colli, Monaldi Hospital, Naples, Italy

LAURA D'ERASMO, MD, PhD
Department of Translational and Precision Medicine "Sapienza" University of Rome, Azienda Ospedaliero-Universitaria Policlinico Umberto I, Ex III Clinica Medica, Rome, Italy

BARBARA D'ONOFRIO, MD
Inherited and Rare Cardiovascular Disease Unit, Department of Translational Medical Sciences, University of Campania "Luigi Vanvitelli," AORN dei Colli, Monaldi Hospital, Naples, Italy

ANTONIO DE LUCA, MD
Cardiovascular Department, Azienda Sanitaria Universitaria Giuliano Isontina (ASUGI), University of Trieste, Trieste, Italy

MARIA LUISA DE RIMINI, MD
Department of Nuclear Medicine, AORN Ospedali dei Colli, Monaldi Hospital, Naples, Italy

ALESSANDRO DELLA CORTE, MD, PhD
Department of Translational Medical Sciences, University of Campania "Luigi Vanvitelli," Naples, Italy

FRANCESCO DI FRAIA, MD
Inherited and Rare Cardiovascular Diseases Unit, Department of Translational Sciences, University of Campania "Luigi Vanvitelli," Naples, Italy

MARIA CRISTINA DIGILIO, MD
Genetics and Rare Disease Research Division, Bambino Gesù Children's Hospital, IRCCS, Rome, Italy

FRANCESCA DONGIGLIO, MD
Inherited and Rare Cardiovascular Disease Unit, Department of Translational Medical Sciences, University of Campania "Luigi Vanvitelli," AORN dei Colli, Monaldi Hospital, Naples, Italy

FABRIZIO DRAGO, MD
The European Reference Network for Rare, Low Prevalence and Complex Diseases of the Heart - ERN GUARD-Heart, Pediatric Cardiology and Arrhythmia/Syncope Units, Department of Paediatric Cardiology and Cardiac Surgery, Bambino Gesù Children's Hospital and Research Institute, IRCSS, Rome, Italy

AUGUSTO ESPOSITO, MD
Inherited and Rare Cardiovascular Disease Unit, Department of Translational Medical Sciences, University of Campania "Luigi Vanvitelli," AORN dei Colli, Monaldi Hospital, Naples, Italy

SILVIA FAVILLI, MD, PhD
Department of Pediatric Cardiology, Cardiology Unit, Meyer Children's Hospital, Florence, Italy

MATTEO DAL FERRO, MD
Cardiovascular Department, Azienda Sanitaria Universitaria Giuliano Isontina (ASUGI), University of Trieste, Trieste, Italy

FABIO FIMIANI, BSc
Unit of Inherited and Rare Cardiovascular Diseases, A.O.R.N. Dei Colli "V. Monaldi," Pediatric Cardiology Unit, Monaldi Hospital, Department of Translational Medical Sciences, University of Campania "Luigi Vanvitelli," Naples, Italy

FIORELLA FRATTA, MD
Department of Translational Medical Sciences, University of Campania "Luigi Vanvitelli", Naples, Italy

GIULIA FRISSO, MD, PhD
Dipartimento di Medicina Molecolare e
Biotecnologie Mediche, Università di Napoli
Federico II, CEINGE Advanced
Biotechnologies, CEINGE Biotecnologie
Avanzate, Scarl, Naples, Italy

ADELAIDE FUSCO, MD
Inherited and Rare Cardiovascular Disease
Unit, Department of Translational Medical
Sciences, University of Campania "Luigi
Vanvitelli," Naples

BRUCE D. GELB, MD, PhD
Department of Pediatrics, Icahn School of
Medicine at Mount Sinai, New York, New York,
USA

DOMINIQUE P. GERMAIN, MD, PhD
French Referral Centre for Fabry Disease,
Division of Medical Genetics, Hôpital
Raymond-Poincare, AP-HP, Garches, France

JELENA R. GHADRI, MD
Department of Cardiology, University Heart
Center, University Hospital Zurich, Zurich,
Switzerland

GIULIANA GIARDINO, MD, PhD
Department of Translational Medical Sciences,
Section of Pediatrics, University of Naples
Federico II, Naples, Italy

MARTA GIGLI, MD
Cardiovascular Department, Azienda Sanitaria
Universitaria Giuliano Isontina (ASUGI),
University of Trieste, Trieste, Italy

FRANCESCA GIROLAMI, BSc, MD
Cardiology Unit, Department of Pediatric
Cardiology, Meyer Children's Hospital,
Florence, Italy

PAOLO GOLINO, MD, PhD
Vanvitelli Cardiology Unit, Monaldi Hospital,
Department of Translational Sciences,
Professor, Department of Cardiology,
University of Campania "Luigi Vanvitelli,"
Naples, Italy

FELICE GRAGNANO, MD
Department of Translational Medical Sciences,
University of Campania "Luigi Vanvitelli,"
Naples, Italy; Division of Cardiology, A.O.R.N.
"Sant'Anna e San Sebastiano," Edificio C –
Cardiologia Universitaria, Caserta, Italy

CHIARA GRANATO, MD, PhD
Grupo de Enfermedades Cardiovasculares,
Vall d'Hebron Institut de Recerca (VHIR),
Barcelona, Spain

GIULIA GRILLI, MD
Cardiovascular Department, Azienda Sanitaria
Universitaria Giuliano Isontina (ASUGI),
University of Trieste, Trieste, Italy

**JUAN PABLO KASKI, BSc (Hons), MBBS,
MRCPCH, MD(Res), FESC, FRCP**
Centre for Inherited Cardiovascular Diseases,
Great Ormond Street Hospital, Institute of
Cardiovascular Sciences, University College
London, London, United Kingdom

GIUSEPPE LIMONGELLI, MD, PhD, FESC
Inherited and Rare Cardiovascular Disease
Unit, Department of Translational Medical
Sciences, University of Campania "Luigi
Vanvitelli," AORN dei Colli, Monaldi Hospital,
Naples, Italy; Division of Cardiology, A.O.R.N.
"Sant'Anna and San Sebastiano," Caserta,
Italy Institute of Cardiovascular Sciences,
University College of London and St.
Bartholomew's Hospital, London, United
Kingdom

MICHELE LIONCINO, MD
Inherited and Rare Cardiovascular Disease
Unit, Department of Translational Medical
Sciences, University of Campania "Luigi
Vanvitelli," Naples, Italy

VALENTINA LODATO, MD
Pediatric Cardiology and Arrhythmia/Syncope
Units, Bambino Gesù Children Hospital and
Research Institute, IRCCS, Rome, Italy

FIORE MANGANELLI, MD, PhD
Professor, Department of Neuroscience,
Reproductive Sciences and
Odontostomatology, University of Naples
'Federico II,' Naples, Italy

ANNACHIARA MARATEA, MD
Inherited and Rare Cardiovascular Disease
Unit, Department of Translational Medical
Sciences, University of Campania "Luigi
Vanvitelli," Naples, Italy

BRUNO MARINO, MD, PhD
Department of Pediatrics, Sapienza University
of Rome, Rome, Italy

MARCO MASÉ, MD
Cardiovascular Department, Azienda Sanitaria
Universitaria Giuliano Isontina (ASUGI),
University of Trieste, Trieste, Italy

ALFREDO MAURIELLO, MD
Department of Translational Medical Sciences,
University of Campania "Luigi Vanvitelli,"
Naples, Italy

CIRO MAURO, MD
Division of Cardiology, A.O.R.N. Antonio
Cardarelli Hospital, Naples, Italy

CRISTINA MAZZACCARA, MD
Dipartimento di Medicina Molecolare e
Biotecnologie Mediche, Università di Napoli
Federico II, CEINGE Advanced
Biotechnologies, CEINGE Biotecnologie
Avanzate, Scarl, Naples, Italy

MARIALUISA MAZZELLA, MD
Department of Translational Medical Sciences,
University of Campania "Luigi Vanvitelli,"
Naples, Italy

MARCO MERLO, MD
Cardiovascular Department, Azienda Sanitaria
Universitaria Giuliano Isontina (ASUGI),
University of Trieste, Trieste, Italy

LUISA MESTRONI, MD, FACC, FAHA, FESC
Cardiovascular Institute and Adult Medical
Genetics Program, University of Colorado
Anschutz Medical Campus, Aurora, Colorado,
USA

EMANUELE MONDA, MD
Inherited and Rare Cardiovascular Disease
Unit, Department of Translational Medical
Sciences, University of Campania "Luigi
Vanvitelli," AORN dei Colli, Monaldi Hospital,
Naples, Italy

ELISABETTA MOSCARELLA, MD, PhD
Department of Translational Medical Sciences,
University of Campania "Luigi Vanvitelli,"
Naples, Italy; Division of Cardiology, A.O.R.N.
"Sant'Anna e San Sebastiano," Edificio C –
Cardiologia Universitaria, Caserta, Italy

FRANCESCO NATALE, MD, PhD
Department of Translational Medical Sciences,
University of Campania "Luigi Vanvitelli,"
Naples, Italy

GERARDO NIGRO, MD, PhD
Department of Medical Translational Sciences,
Division of Cardiology, Monaldi Hospital,
University of Campania "Luigi Vanvitelli,"
Naples, Italy

STEFANO NISTRI, MD, PhD
Cardiology Service, CMSR Veneto Medica,
Altavilla Vicentina, Italy

**GABRIELLE NORRISH, BMBCh, BA,
MRCPCH, PhD**
Centre for Inherited Cardiovascular Diseases,
Great Ormond Street Hospital, Institute of
Cardiovascular Sciences, University College
London, United Kingdom

HIROYUKY OKURA, MD, PhD
Department of Cardiology, Gifu University
Graduate School of Medicine, Gifu,
Japan

IACOPO OLIVOTTO, MD
Cardiomyopathy Unit, University of Florence,
Florence, Italy

PAOLO ORABONA, MD
Department of Ophthalmology, Monaldi
Hospital, Naples, Italy

GIUSEPPE PACILEO, MD
Heart Failure and Cardiac Rehabilitation Unit,
Department of Cardiology, AORN dei Colli,
Monaldi Hospital, Naples, Italy

ROBERTA PACILEO, MD
Department of Translational Medical Sciences,
University of Campania "Luigi Vanvitelli,"
Naples, Italy

ESZTER DALMA PALINKAS, MD
Division of Non-Invasive Cardiology,
Department of Internal Medicine, Albert Szent-
Györgyi Clinical Center, Doctoral School of
Clinical Medicine, University of Szeged,
Szeged, Hungary; Cardiomyopathy Unit,
University of Florence, Florence, Italy

GIUSEPPE PALMIERO, MD
Department of Cardiology,
AORN Ospedali dei Colli,
Monaldi Hospital, Inherited and Rare
Cardiovascular Diseases Unit, Professor,
Department of Translational Medical Sciences,

University of Campania "Luigi Vanvitelli,"
Naples, Italy

GIOVANNI PARLAPIANO, MD
Laboratory of Medical Genetics, Bambino
Gesù Children Hospital and Research Institute,
Rome, Italy

SILVIA PASSANTINO, MD
Cardiology Unit, Department of Pediatric
Cardiology, Meyer Children's Hospital,
Florence, Italy

ANNALISA PASSARIELLO, MD, PhD
Pediatric Cardiology Unit, Monaldi Hospital,
University "Luigi Vanvitelli," Naples, Italy

GUGLIELMINA PEPE, MD, PhD
Department of Experimental and Clinical
Medicine, University of Florence, CRR Tuscany
Marfan Center, Florence, Italy

MAURIZIO PIERONI, MD, PhD
Cardiovascular Department, San Donato
Hospital, Arezzo, Italy

CLAUDIO PIGNATA, MD, PhD
Department of Translational Medical Sciences,
Section of Pediatrics, University of Naples
Federico II, Naples, Italy

ANTONIO PISANI, MD, PhD
Chair of Nephrology, Department of Public
Health, University Federico II of Naples,
Naples, Italy

ALDOSTEFANO PORCARI, MD
Cardiovascular Department, Azienda Sanitaria
Universitaria Giuliano Isontina (ASUGI),
University of Trieste, Trieste, Italy

VICENZO POTA, MD, PhD
Department of Women, Child and General and
Specialized Surgery, University of Campania
"Luigi Vanvitelli," Naples, Italy

ALEXANDROS PROTONOTARIOS, MD
UCL Institute of Cardiovascular Science,
London, United Kingdom

IOANNIS PROTONOTARIOS, MD
Southampton General Hospital (University
Hospital Southampton NHS Foundation Trust),
United Kingdom

CAROLINA PUTOTTO, MD, PhD
Department of Pediatrics, Sapienza University
of Rome, Rome, Italy

ILARIA RADANO, MD
A.O.U. San Giovanni di Dio e Ruggi d'Aragona,
Salerno, Italy

AMY E. ROBERTS, MD, PhD
Department of Cardiology, Children's Hospital
Boston, Boston, Massachusetts, USA

MARTA RUBINO, MD
Inherited and Rare Cardiovascular Disease
Unit, Department of Translational Medical
Sciences, University of Campania "Luigi
Vanvitelli," AORN dei Colli, Monaldi Hospital,
Naples, Italy

LUCIA RUGGIERO, MD
Department of Neurosciences, Reproductive
Sciences and Odontostomatology, University
of Naples Federico II, Naples, Italy

MARIA GIOVANNA RUSSO, MD, PhD
Department of Translational Medical Sciences,
University of Campania "Luigi Vanvitelli,"
Department of Pediatric Cardiology, AORN dei
Colli, Monaldi Hospital, Naples, Italy

GEMMA SALERNO, MD
Vanvitelli Cardiology Unit, Monaldi Hospital,
Naples, Italy

SIMONE SAMPAOLO, MD
Second Division of Neurology, Department of
Advanced Medical and Surgical Sciences,
University of Campania Luigi Vanvitelli, Naples,
Italy

BERARDO SARUBBI, MD, PhD
Adult Congenital Heart Diseases Unit, AORN
dei Colli, Monaldi Hospital, Department of
Translational Medical Sciences, University of
Campania "Luigi Vanvitelli," Naples, Italy

GIOACCHINO SCARANO, MD, PhD
Inherited and Rare Cardiovascular Disease
Unit, Department of Translational Medical
Sciences, University of Campania "Luigi
Vanvitelli," Naples, Italy

ALESSANDRA SCHIAVO, MD
Department of Translational Medical Sciences,
University of Campania "Luigi Vanvitelli,"

Naples, Italy; Division of Cardiology, A.O.R.N. "Sant'Anna e San Sebastiano," Edificio C – Cardiologia Universitaria, Caserta, Italy

GIOVANNI SIGNORE, MD
Inherited and Rare Cardiovascular Disease Unit, Department of Translational Medical Sciences, University of Campania "Luigi Vanvitelli," Naples, Italy

VICENZO SIMONELLI, MD
Division of Neurology, AORN Dei Colli, Monaldi Hospital, Naples, Italy

GIANFRANCO SINAGRA, MD, FESC
Cardiovascular Department, Azienda Sanitaria Universitaria Giuliano Isontina (ASUGI), University of Trieste, Trieste, Italy

DAVIDE STOLFO, MD
Cardiovascular Department, Azienda Sanitaria Universitaria Giuliano Isontina (ASUGI), University of Trieste, Trieste, Italy

MARCO TARTAGLIA, PhD
Genetics and Rare Disease Research Division, Bambino Gesù Children's Hospital, IRCCS, Rome, Italy

CHRISTIAN TEMPLIN, MD, PhD, FESC
Professor of Cardiology, Director, Andreas Grüntzig Heart Catheterization Laboratories, Department of Cardiology, University Hospital Zurich, University Heart Center, Zurich, Switzerland

ADALENA TSATSOPOULOU, MD
Paediatric Clinic - Hora Naxos, Unit of Inherited and Rare Cardiovascular Diseases, Onassis Cardiac Surgery Centre, Athens, Greece

ANDREA VERGARA, MD
Department of Translational Medical Sciences, University of Campania "Luigi Vanvitelli,"

Naples, Italy; Division of Cardiology, A.O.R.N. "Sant'Anna e San Sebastiano," Edificio C – Cardiologia Universitaria, Caserta, Italy

FEDERICA VERRILLO, MD
Inherited and Rare Cardiovascular Disease Unit, Department of Translational Medical Sciences, University of Campania "Luigi Vanvitelli," AORN dei Colli, Monaldi Hospital, Naples, Italy

PAOLO VERSACCI, MD, PhD
Department of Pediatrics, Sapienza University of Rome, Rome, Italy

ERICA VETRANO, MD
Inherited and Rare Cardiovascular Disease Unit, Department of Translational Medical Sciences, University of Campania "Luigi Vanvitelli," AORN dei Colli, Monaldi Hospital, Internal Medicine Unit, Naples, Italy

MICHAEL WÜRDINGER, MD
Department of Cardiology, University Heart Center, University Hospital Zurich, Zurich, Switzerland

KARIM WAHBI, MD, PhD
APHP, Cochin Hospital, Cardiology Department, FILNEMUS, Paris-Descartes, Sorbonne Paris Cité University, Paris, France

ZAFEIRENIA XYLOURI, MD
Southampton General Hospital (University Hospital Southampton NHS FoundationTrust), United Kingdom

MASSIMO ZECCHIN, MD
Cardiovascular Department, Azienda Sanitaria Universitaria Giuliano Isontina (ASUGI), University of Trieste, Trieste, Italy

Contents

Genetic testing in children with hypertrophic cardiomyopathy (HCM) can modify clinical management and lifestyle counseling. However, predicting long-term outcome and response to management in individual patients remains challenging, because of the peculiar genetic heterogeneity of the disease in the pediatric age range. Children with HCM secondary to an inborn error of metabolism or malformation syndromes tend to have a worse outcome compared with those with the classic sarcomeric form. Among the latter, adverse genetic features are represented by the identification of a pathogenic variant in MYH7, often associated with severe hypertrophy, a complex genotype, or a de novo variant.

Sudden cardiac death (SCD) is the most common cause of death in childhood hypertrophic cardiomyopathy (HCM) and occurs more frequently than in adult patients. Risk stratification strategies have traditionally been extrapolated from adult practice, but newer evidence has highlighted important differences between childhood and adult cohorts, with the implication that pediatric-specific risk stratification strategies are required. Current guidelines use cumulative risk factor thresholds to recommend implantable cardioverter defibrillator (ICD) implantation but have been shown to have limited discriminatory ability. Newer pediatric models that allow clinicians to calculate individualized estimates of 5-year risk allowing, for the first time, personalization of ICD implantation decision-making have been developed. This article describes the pathophysiology, risk factors, and approach to risk stratification for SCD in childhood HCM and highlights unanswered questions.

RASopathies are multisystemic disorders caused by germline mutations in genes linked to the RAS/mitogen-activated protein kinase pathway. Diagnosis of RASopathy can be triggered by clinical clues ("red flags") which may direct the clinician toward a specific gene test. Compared with sarcomeric hypertrophic cardiomyopathy, hypertrophic cardiomyopathy in RASopathies (R-HCM) is associated with higher prevalence of congestive heart failure and shows increased prevalence and severity of left ventricular outflow tract obstruction. Biventricular involvement and the association with congenital heart disease, mainly pulmonary stenosis, have been commonly described in R-HCM. The aim of this review is to assess the prevalence and unique features of R-HCM and to define the available therapeutic options.

Friedreich ataxia (FRDA) is an autosomal recessive neurodegenerative disorder caused by a homozygous GAA triplet repeat expansion in the frataxin gene. Cardiac involvement, usually manifesting as hypertrophic cardiomyopathy, can range from asymptomatic cases to severe cardiomyopathy with progressive deterioration of the left ventricular ejection fraction and chronic heart failure. The management of cardiac involvement is directed to prevent disease progression and cardiovascular complications. However, direct-disease therapies are not currently available for FRDA. The present review aims to describe the current state of knowledge regarding cardiovascular involvement of FRDA, focusing on clinical-instrumental features and management of cardiac manifestation.

Fabry disease (FD, OMIM 301500) is an X-linked lysosomal storage disease caused by pathogenic variants in the GLA gene. Cardiac involvement is common in FD and is responsible for impaired quality of life and premature death. The classic cardiac involvement is a nonobstructive form of hypertrophic cardiomyopathy, usually manifesting as concentric left ventricular hypertrophy, with subsequent arrhythmogenic intramural fibrosis. Treatment of patients with FD should be directed to prevent the disease progression to irreversible organ damage and organ failure. The aim of this review is to describe the current state of knowledge regarding cardiovascular involvement in FD, focusing on clinical and instrumental features, cardiovascular management, and targeted therapy.

Mitochondrial diseases (MD) include an heterogenous group of systemic disorders caused by sporadic or inherited mutations in nuclear or mitochondrial DNA (mtDNA), causing impairment of oxidative phosphorylation system. Hypertrophic cardiomyopathy is the dominant pattern of cardiomyopathy in all forms of mtDNA disease, being observed in almost 40% of the patients. Dilated cardiomyopathy, left ventricular noncompaction, and conduction system disturbances have been also reported. In this article, the authors discuss the current clinical knowledge on MD, focusing on diagnosis and management of mitochondrial diseases caused by mtDNA mutations.

Giuseppe Palmiero, Erica Vetrano, Marta Rubino, Emanuele Monda, Francesca Dongiglio, Michele Lioncino, Francesco Di Fraia, Martina Caiazza, Federica Verrillo, Laura Capodicasa, Giuseppe Cerciello, Fiore Manganelli, Mara Catalano, Davide D'Arienzo, Maria Luisa De Rimini, Raffaele Ascione, Paolo Golino, Pio Caso, Luigi Ascione, and Giuseppe Limongelli

Cardiac amyloidosis is an infiltrative disorder caused by transthyretin or immunoglobulin free light-chain deposition, which determines clinical disease with similar phenotype but different time course, prognosis and therapy. Multimodality imaging is the cornerstone for disease diagnosis and management. Multimodality imaging has revolutionized the approach to the disease favoring its awareness and simplifying its diagnosis, especially in ATTR cardiac amyloidosis. This describes the different imaging tools, from the traditional to the more novel ones, and highlights the different approach in each different setting (prognosis, subtyping, prognosis, monitoring disease progression, and response to therapy).

Michele Lioncino, Emanuele Monda, Giuseppe Palmiero, Martina Caiazza, Erica Vetrano, Marta Rubino, Augusto Esposito, Gemma Salerno, Francesca Dongiglio, Barbara D'Onofrio, Federica Verrillo, Giuseppe Cerciello, Fiore Manganelli, Giuseppe Pacileo, Eduardo Bossone, Paolo Golino, Paolo Calabrò, and Giuseppe Limongelli

Transthyretin cardiac amyloidosis (ATTR-CA) is a systemic disorder resulting from the extracellular deposition of amyloid fibrils of misfolded transthyretin protein in the heart. ATTR-CA is a life-threatening disease, which can be caused by progressive deposition of wild type transthyretin (wtATTR) or by aggregation of an inherited mutated variant of transthyretin (mATTR). mATTR Is a rare condition transmitted in an autosomal dominant manner with incomplete penetrance, causing heterogenous phenotypes which can range from predominant neuropathic involvement, predominant cardiomyopathy, or mixed. Diagnosis of ATTR-CA is complex and requires integration of different imaging tools (echocardiography, bone scintigraphy, magnetic resonance) with genetics, clinical signs, laboratory tests, and histology. In recent years, new therapeutic agents have shown good efficacy and impact on survival and quality of life in this subset of patients, nevertheless patients affected by ATTR-CA may still carry an unfavorable prognosis, thus highlighting the need for new therapies. This review aims to assess cardiovascular involvement, diagnosis, and management of patients affected by ATTR-CA.

Ioannis Protonotarios, Angeliki Asimaki, Zafeirenia Xylouri, Alexandros Protonotarios, and Adalena Tsatsopoulou

Naxos disease is a recessively inherited pattern of arrhythmogenic cardiomyopathy with palmoplantar keratoderma and woolly hair. The causative mutation identified in plakoglobin protein gene indicated a potential role of the desmosomal protein complex as culprit for cardiomyopathy. In the context of a family, the early evident cutaneous features may serve as a clinical screening tool to spot arrhythmogenic cardiomyopathy in subclinical stage. "Myocarditis-like episodes" may step up the disease evolution or mark a transition from concealed to symptomatic cardiomyopathy phase. Arrhythmogenic cardiomyopathy in Naxos disease shows increased penetrance and phenotypic expression but its arrhythmic risk is analogous to dominant forms.

> In the wide phenotypic spectrum of cardiomyopathies, sudden cardiac death (SCD) has always been the most visible and devastating disease complication. The introduction of implantable cardioverter-defibrillators for SCD prevention by the late 1980s has moved the question from how to whom we should protect from SCD, leaving clinicians with a measure of uncertainty regarding the most reliable option to guide identification of the highest-risk patients. In this review, we will go through all the available evidence in the field of arrhythmic expression and arrhythmic risk stratification in the different phenotypes of cardiomyopathies to provide practical suggestions in daily clinical management.

> Sudden unexplained death (SUD) is a tragic event for both the family and community, particularly when it occurs in young individuals. Sudden cardiac death (SCD) represents the leading form of SUD and is defined as an unexpected event without an obvious extracardiac cause, occurring within 1 hour after the onset of symptoms. In children, the main causes of SCD are inherited cardiac disorders, whereas coronary artery diseases (congenital or acquired), congenital heart diseases, and myocarditis are rare. The present review examines the current state of knowledge regarding SCD in children, discussing the epidemiology, clinical causes, and prevention strategies.

> Takotsubo syndrome is an acute reversible heart failure syndrome, most frequently seen in postmenopausal women and precipitated generally by significant emotional stress or physical illness. A sudden sympathetic activation seems to play a key role in the pathophysiology, but growing evidence is emerging about the role of inflammation in the subacute and chronic phases. An incidence of life-threatening complications occurring in the acute phase and at long-term follow-up has been demonstrated, comparable with the acute coronary syndrome. Multimodality imaging could be useful to stratify in-hospital and long-term prognosis. The efficacy of specific medical treatments in long-term follow-up should be investigated.

> The genetic background of congenital heart diseases (CHDs) is extremely complex, heterogenous, and still majorly to be determined. CHDs can be sporadic or familial.

In this article we discuss in detail the phenotypic spectrum of selected genes including MYH7, GATA4, NKX2-5, TBX5, and TBX20. Our goal is to offer the clinician a general overview of the clinical spectrum of the analyzed topics that are traditionally known as causative for CHDs but we underline in this review the possible progressive functional (cardiomyopathy) and electric aspects (arrhythmias) caused by the genetic background.

Clinical Manifestations of 22q11.2 Deletion Syndrome

Annapaola Cirillo, Michele Lioncino, Annachiara Maratea, Annalisa Passariello, Adelaide Fusco, Fiorella Fratta, Emanuele Monda, Martina Caiazza, Giovanni Signore, Augusto Esposito, Anwar Baban, Paolo Versacci, Carolina Putotto, Bruno Marino, Claudio Pignata, Emilia Cirillo, Giuliana Giardino, Berardo Sarubbi, Giuseppe Limongelli, and Maria Giovanna Russo

DiGeorge syndrome (DGS), also known as "22q11.2 deletion syndrome" (22q11DS) (MIM # 192430 # 188400), is a genetic disorder caused by hemizygous microdeletion of the long arm of chromosome 22. In the last decades, the introduction of fluorescence in situ hybridization assays, and in selected cases the use of multiplex ligation-dependent probe amplification, has allowed the detection of chromosomal microdeletions that could not be previously identified using standard karyotype analysis. The aim of this review is to address cardiovascular and systemic involvement in children with DGS, provide genotype-phenotype correlations, and discuss their medical management and therapeutic options.

The Heart Muscle and Valve Involvement in Marfan Syndrome, Loeys-Dietz Syndromes, and Collagenopathies

Adelaide Fusco, Alfredo Mauriello, Michele Lioncino, Giuseppe Palmiero, Fiorella Fratta, Chiara Granato, Annapaola Cirillo, Martina Caiazza, Emanuele Monda, Antonello Credendino, Giovanni Signore, Francesco Natale, Flavia Chiosi, Gioacchino Scarano, Alessandro Della Corte, Stefano Nistri, Maria Giovanna Russo, Giuseppe Limongelli, and Guglielmina Pepe

The inherited connective tissue disorders (Marfan syndrome, Loeys-Dietz syndrome [LDS], and Ehlers-Danlos syndrome [EDS]) involve connective tissue of various organ systems. These pathologies share many common features, nonetheless compared to Marfan syndrome, LDS' cardiovascular manifestations tend to be more severe. In contrast, no association is reported between LDS and the presence of ectopia lentis. The EDS are currently classified into thirteen subtypes. There is substantial symptoms overlap between the EDS subtypes, and they are associated with an increased incidence of cardiovascular abnormalities, such as mitral valve prolapse and aortic dissection.

New Frontiers in the Treatment of Homozygous Familial Hypercholesterolemia

Arturo Cesaro, Fabio Fimiani, Felice Gragnano, Elisabetta Moscarella, Alessandra Schiavo, Andrea Vergara, Leo Akioyamen, Laura D'Erasmo, Maurizio Averna, Marcello Arca, and Paolo Calabrò

Homozygous familial hypercholesterolemia (HoFH) is a rare genetic disorder. The most common cause is a mutation in both alleles of the gene encoding for the low-density lipoprotein (LDL) receptor, although other causative mutations have been identified. Complications of atherosclerotic cardiovascular disease are common in these patients; therefore, reducing the elevated LDL-cholesterol burden is critical in their management. Conventionally, this is achieved by patients initiating lipid-lowering therapy, but this can present challenges in clinical practice. Fortunately, novel therapeutic strategies have enabled promising innovations in HoFH

treatment. This review highlights recent and ongoing studies examining new therapeutic options for patients with HoFH.

Michael Würdinger, Victoria L. Cammann, Jelena R. Ghadri, and Christian Templin

Spontaneous coronary artery dissection is an infrequent cause of acute coronary
syndrome with comparable clinical features. Previously considered a rare disease,
recent scientific interest has revealed spontaneous coronary artery dissection as
an important differential diagnosis of acute coronary syndrome, especially in young
women, during pregnancy or postpartum, and in patients with fibromuscular
dysplasia or other arteriopathies. However, there remain many uncertainties
regarding pathophysiology, risk factors, acute treatment, and optimal long-term
management. The aim of this review is to summarize current scientific evidence
on epidemiology, management, and outcomes.

HEART FAILURE CLINICS

SERIES OF RELATED INTEREST

Cardiology Clinics
http://www.cardiology.theclinics.com/
Cardiac Electrophysiology Clinics
https://www.cardiacep.theclinics.com/
Interventional Cardiology Clinics
https://www.interventional.theclinics.com/

THE CLINICS ARE AVAILABLE ONLINE!
Access your subscription at:
www.theclinics.com

Preface

Rare Cardiovascular Diseases: From Genetics to Personalized Medicine

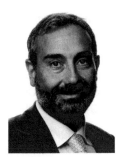
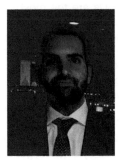
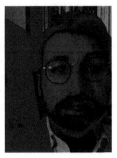
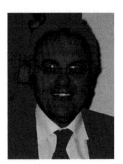

Giuseppe Limongelli, MD, PhD, FESC   Emanuele Monda, MD   Michele Lioncino, MD   Eduardo Bossone, MD, PhD, FCCP, FESC, FACC

Editors

Rare cardiovascular diseases represent a significant public health problem worldwide and, despite their low prevalence, have major effects on the quality of life of the affected patients and their families.

This issue of *Heart Failure Clinics* provides an overview of different rare cardiovascular diseases, focusing on different topics, such as epidemiology, cause, diagnostic strategies, pharmacologic therapies, prevention of complications, and future perspective.

The first part of the issue is dominated by cardiomyopathies (CMPs), defined as myocardial disorders in which the heart muscle is structurally and functionally abnormal, in the absence of coronary artery disease, hypertension, and valvular and congenital heart disease (CHD) sufficient to explain the observed phenotype.[1]

Hypertrophic cardiomyopathy (HCM) represents the most common CMP, with a prevalence estimated to be about 1:500 (0.2%) in adults[2]; however, it rarely occurs in the pediatric age group. Therefore, natural history, clinical course, and risk of adverse events in children with HCM are poorly understood. Girolami and colleagues discuss the role of genotype on the phenotype, clinical course, and risk of adverse events in children with HCM and emphasize genetic testing as an essential tool for the etiologic diagnosis and cascade screening in the proband's family member. Norrish and colleagues accurately describe the pathophysiology, risk factors, and approach to risk stratification for sudden cardiac death (SCD) in children with HCM and highlight major gaps in evidence and unmet needs that will require further studies.

The cause of HCM is extremely heterogeneous. Up to 10% of cases are caused by nonsarcomeric disorders, including inherited metabolic storage disorders, neuromuscular diseases, chromosome abnormalities, and malformation syndromes.[3-5] The age of onset of HCM represents an important diagnostic clue for specific causes.[3] Prevalence and clinical significance of cardiovascular involvement, particularly heart muscle disease, in systemic rare disease, including rasopathies (Lioncino and colleagues), Friedreich ataxia (Monda and colleagues), Fabry disease (Rubino and colleagues), and mitochondrial disease (Lioncino and colleagues), are the focus of the first part of this *Heart Failure Clinics* issue. Special attention has been offered to cardiac amyloidosis, an

Heart Failure Clin 18 (2022) xix–xxi
https://doi.org/10.1016/j.hfc.2021.10.001
1551-7136/22/© 2021 Published by Elsevier Inc.

emerging challenge in the field of heart failure and rare disease. Cardiac amyloidosis is the leading cause of HCM with restrictive physiology in elderly patients. It is an infiltrative disorder caused by myocardial deposition of misfolded aggregates of insoluble proteins, mainly represented by immunoglobulin light-chain or transthyretin (ATTR) amyloidosis. Multimodality imaging is essential to raise the suspicion of disease and is required to obtain an early diagnosis.[6] Palmiero and colleagues describe the role of multimodality imaging in cardiac amyloidosis and highlight the role of new imaging technologies in diagnosis, prognosis, monitoring disease progression, and response to therapy. Moreover, Lioncino and colleagues provide a comprehensive review on ATTR cardiac amyloidosis, aiming to assess cardiovascular involvement, diagnosis, and management of patients affected by ATTR cardiac amyloidosis.

Arrhythmogenic cardiomyopathy (ACM) is a myocardial disease characterized by progressive loss of ventricular myocardium and its replacement by fibrofatty tissue. Naxos disease is a rare disorder associating ACM with a cutaneous phenotype, characterized by palmoplantar keratoderma and peculiar wooly hair. Protonotarios and colleagues provide a comprehensive review on clinical and molecular aspects of Naxos disease, underlying the importance of the early identification of cutaneous features to detect ACM in subclinical stage, in the context of an affected family member.

SCD represents a significant issue in patients diagnosed with inherited cardiac disease.[7] Merlo and colleagues summarize the available evidence on the arrhythmic phenotype and risk stratification for SCD in the different CMPs and provide a valuable guide for the prevention and management of this terrible complication. On the other hand, Monda and colleagues examine the state of knowledge regarding SCD in children, discussing the epidemiology, clinical causes, and prevention strategies.

Stress CMP or Takotsubo syndrome is an acute cardiac syndrome characterized by an acute reversible myocardial injury characterized by transient regional systolic left ventricular dysfunction. Multimodality imaging plays a dominant role in risk stratification for in-hospital and long-term prognosis. Citro and colleagues review the epidemiology, pathogenesis, and clinical course of Takotsubo syndrome.

The second part of the issue focuses on rare diseases associated with CHDs, genetic syndromes, and rare coronary artery abnormalities.

CHDs are the most common type of birth defects, and their causes are generally classified as genetic and nongenetic categories. However, the role of the genetic background of CHDs is complex and poorly understood. Baban and colleagues provide an overview of the role of genetic variants on the pathogenesis of CHDs and underline the importance of genetic screening in CHDs in selected cases.

22q11.2 deletion syndrome is a genetic disorder caused by a hemizygous microdeletion of the long arm of chromosome 22 and represents the second leading chromosomal cause of CHD. Cirillo and colleagues aim to address cardiovascular and systemic involvement in children with 22q11.2 deletion syndrome, to provide genotype-phenotype correlation, and to discuss the therapeutic management of these patients.

Inherited thoracic aortopathies are a group of congenital conditions that predispose to disease of the thoracic aorta. Fusco and colleagues summarize the genetic and clinical features of patients with inherited aortopathies and outline current management strategies.

Homozygous familial hypercholesterolemia is a rare genetic disease, caused by a mutation in both alleles of the gene encoding the low-density lipoprotein cholesterol receptor. This condition leads to early and progressive atherosclerotic cardiovascular disease. In past years, different therapeutic targets for cholesterol-lowering therapy have been identified.[8,9] Cesaro and colleagues report the currently available treatments and emerging therapeutic strategies for homozygous familial hypercholesterolemia patients.

Spontaneous coronary artery dissection (SCAD) is defined as an epicardial coronary artery dissection that is not associated with atherosclerosis or trauma and is not iatrogenic. SCAD is considered an infrequent cause of acute coronary syndrome; however, it is assumed to be an underdiagnosed and underreported disease. Würdinger and colleagues present a comprehensive review on epidemiology, clinical presentation, predisposing factors, treatment, and outcome of SCAD.

In conclusion, the present issue of *Heart Failure Clinics* provides a comprehensive overview of different and mostly inherited and rare cardiovascular conditions, giving helpful information to clinicians for improving the diagnosis and clinical management of patients with rare diseases.

Giuseppe Limongelli, MD, PhD, FESC
Inherited and Rare Cardiovascular Diseases
Department of Translational Medical Sciences
University of Campania "Luigi Vanvitelli"
AO Colli–Monaldi Hospital
–ERN Guard Heart Member
Via L. Bianchi
80131 Naples, Italy

Emanuele Monda, MD
Department of Translational Medical Sciences
University of Campania "Luigi Vanvitelli"
Via L. Bianchi
80131 Naples, Italy

Michele Lioncino, MD
Department of Translational Medical Sciences
University of Campania "Luigi Vanvitelli"
Via L. Bianchi
80131 Naples, Italy

Eduardo Bossone, MD, PhD, FCCP, FESC, FACC
Division of Cardiology
AORN Antonio Cardarelli Hospital
Naples, Italy

E-mail addresses:
limongelligiuseppe@libero.it (G. Limongelli)
emanuelemonda@me.com (E. Monda)
michelelioncino@icloud.com (M. Lioncino)
ebossone@hotmail.com (E. Bossone)

REFERENCES

1. Elliott P, Andersson B, Arbustini E, et al. Classification of the cardiomyopathies: a position statement from the European Society of Cardiology Working Group on Myocardial and Pericardial Diseases. Eur Heart J 2008;29(2):270–6. https://doi.org/10.1093/eurheartj/ehm342.

2. Elliott PM, Anastasakis A, Borger MA, et al. 2014 ESC guidelines on diagnosis and management of hypertrophic cardiomyopathy: the Task Force for the Diagnosis and Management of Hypertrophic Cardiomyopathy of the European Society of Cardiology (ESC). Eur Heart J 2014;35(39):2733–79. https://doi.org/10.1093/eurheartj/ehu284.

3. Limongelli G, Monda E, Tramonte S, et al. Prevalence and clinical significance of red flags in patients with hypertrophic cardiomyopathy. Int J Cardiol 2020;299: 186–91. https://doi.org/10.1016/j.ijcard.2019.06.073.

4. Monda E, Rubino M, Lioncino M, et al. Hypertrophic cardiomyopathy in children: pathophysiology, diagnosis, and treatment of non-sarcomeric causes. Front Pediatr 2021;9:632293. https://doi.org/10.3389/fped.2021.632293.

5. Caiazza M, Rubino M, Monda E, et al. Combined PTPN11 and MYBPC3 gene mutations in an adult patient with Noonan syndrome and hypertrophic cardiomyopathy. Genes (Basel) 2020;11(8):947. https://doi.org/10.3390/genes11080947.

6. Monda E, Palmiero G, Lioncino M, et al. External validation of the increased wall thickness score for the diagnosis of cardiac amyloidosis. Int J Cardiol 2021; 339:99–101. https://doi.org/10.1016/j.ijcard.2021.07.035.

7. Monda E, Sarubbi B, Russo MG, et al. Unexplained sudden cardiac arrest in children: clinical and genetic characteristics of survivors [published online ahead of print 2020 Jul 28]. Eur J Prev Cardiol 2020. https://doi.org/10.1177/2047487320940863. 2047487320940863.

8. Cesaro A, Bianconi V, Gragnano F, et al. Beyond cholesterol metabolism: the pleiotropic effects of proprotein convertase subtilisin/kexin type 9 (PCSK9). Genetics, mutations, expression, and perspective for long-term inhibition. Biofactors 2020;46(3):367–80. https://doi.org/10.1002/biof.1619.

9. Cesaro A, Schiavo A, Moscarella E, et al. Lipoprotein(a): a genetic marker for cardiovascular disease and target for emerging therapies. J Cardiovasc Med (Hagerstown) 2021;22(3):151–61. https://doi.org/10.2459/JCM.0000000000001077.

The Influence of Genotype on the Phenotype, Clinical Course, and Risk of Adverse Events in Children with Hypertrophic Cardiomyopathy

Francesca Girolami, BSc[a],[*],[1], Silvia Passantino, MD[a],[1], Federica Verrillo, MD[b], Eszter Dalma Palinkas, MD[c],[d],[e], Giuseppe Limongelli, MD, PhD[b], Silvia Favilli, MD[a], Iacopo Olivotto, MD[e]

KEYWORDS

- Cardiomyopathies in children • Genetic analysis • Genotype • Phenotype • Prognosis

KEY POINTS

- Predicting long-term outcome, risk of adverse events, and response to treatment in children with HCM is challenging.
- Genetic testing in pediatric HCM is an essential step in establishing a diagnosis and may, in selected cases, dictate clinical management.
- Secondary forms of HCM caused by inborn errors of metabolism (IEMs), syndromes such as RA-Sopathies, or neuromuscular disorders are generally associated with worse clinical outcome.
- In children with sarcomeric HCM, the identification of a complex genotype or a *de novo* variant may imply worse prognosis.
- Pathogenic variants in thin filament genes are associated with mild degrees of hypertrophy but greater arrhythmic propensity in children.

Hypertrophic cardiomyopathy (HCM) in children is rare and may present at any age, but preferentially clusters in the first year of life, with a frequency 3 times higher than in older age groups, due to the prevalence of peculiar genetic causes.[1] The disease is characterized by a pathologic increase in myocardial thickness, with a nondilated left ventricular (LV) chamber, unexplained by pressure overload (eg, due to systemic hypertension or aortic stenosis). Pediatric HCM may be the cause of heart failure and, infrequently, of sudden cardiac death, both of which may occur at any age.[1–3]

The genetic basis of HCM is heterogeneous in children, often associated with rare, family-specific ("private") mutations, not infrequently de novo. Even though most cases are caused by variants in genes coding for components of the sarcomere or the cytoskeleton, pediatric HCM is much more diverse compared with adult cohorts, due to a high prevalence of syndromic conditions,

The authors have nothing to disclose.
[a] Cardiology Unit, Meyer Children's Hospital, Viale Pieraccini 24, 50139 Florence, Italy; [b] Department of Translational Medical Sciences, Inherited & Rare Cardiovascular Diseases, University of Campania 'Luigi Vanvitelli', Monaldi Hospital, Naples, Italy; [c] Division of Non-Invasive Cardiology, Department of Internal Medicine, Albert Szent-Györgyi Clinical Center, University of Szeged, Szeged, Hungary; [d] Doctoral School of Clinical Medicine, University of Szeged, Szeged, Hungary; [e] Cardiomyopathy Unit, University of Florence, Florence, Italy
[1] Contributed equally.
* Corresponding author.
E-mail address: girolami.fra@gmail.com

Heart Failure Clin 18 (2022) 1–8
https://doi.org/10.1016/j.hfc.2021.07.013
1551-7136/22/© 2021 Elsevier Inc. All rights reserved.

neuromuscular disorders, and inborn errors of metabolism.[4] In addition, secondary causes should be considered, including maternal diabetes, congenital insulin-producing tumors, and congenital heart disease.[4–6] Thus, the detection of an HCM phenotype represents a mere starting point in the diagnostic process: similar echocardiographic findings may result from classic sarcomeric HCM, RASopathies such as Noonan syndrome, glycogen storage disorders such as Danon disease, or a mitochondrial cardiomyopathy such as mitochondrial encephalopathy, lactic acidosis, and stroke-like episodes (MELAS) (**Fig. 1**).[7] Genetic testing, guided by appropriate clinical red flags (**Table 1**) is an essential step of the diagnostic process in children with HCM, more so than in adults, providing decisive information for clinical management and lifestyle counseling[8]

CLINICAL FEATURES AND DIAGNOSIS

In children younger than 1 year, the most common clues to the diagnosis of HCM are a heart murmur detected during pediatric consultation or symptoms of congestive heart failure such as feeding difficulties, impaired growth, and sweating, whereas older children and adolescents may be asymptomatic or present with the typical features seen in adults, such as palpitations, chest pain, syncope, and exercise limitation. Cardiac arrest is a tragic but rare presentation. Of note, extracardiac red flags are prevalent and more often decisive for a correct diagnosis, compared with adult patients.[1,3]

At echocardiographic examination, concentric LV hypertrophy (LVH) is the most common phenotype in syndromic HCM, whereas asymmetric septal hypertrophy is typical of the sarcomeric form, followed by apical hypertrophy, right ventricular hypertrophy, and isolated posterior wall hypertrophy. LV outflow tract obstruction is present at

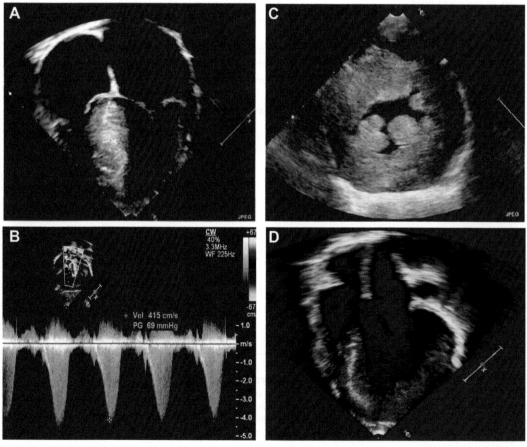

Fig. 1. Central illustration. Genetic testing is key to individualized management in pediatric HCM. (*A, B*) Sarcomeric and obstructive HCM requiring medical therapy and eventually myectomy. (*C*) HCM in Pompe disease requiring enzyme replacement therapies. (*D*) HCM in Danon disease requiring more aggressive treatment, for example, early transplant.

Table 1
Red flags for clinical differential diagnosis in children with hypertrophic cardiomyopathy

Sarcomeric HCM	IEMs	Syndromic HCM
Asymmetric hypertrophy	Concentric hypertrophy	Concentric or biventricular hypertrophy
LV outflow obstruction, abnormal implantation of papillary muscles, mitral regurgitation, arrhythmias	Arrhythmias	LV outflow tract obstruction, congenital heart disease (pulmonary stenosis/dysplasia, peripheral pulmonary arteries stenosis, atrial septal defect, atrioventricular septal defect)
	Learning disability and cognitive defects, seizures, neurosensorial deafness, blindness, stroke, dystonia	Mental retardation, neurosensorial deafness
	Short stature, peripheral muscle weakness, renal failure, hepatosplenomegaly	Short stature, webbed neck, cryptorchidism, coagulation defects
	Macrocephaly, large anterior fontanelle, coarsened facial features, retinal abnormalities, strabismus	Characteristic facies (broad forehead, down slanting palpebral fissures, hypertelorism, and low-set ears)
MYH7, MYBPC3, TNNT2, TNNI3, TPM1, ACTC1, MYL2, MYL3, PLN, ACTN2, CSRP3, JPH2	*PRKAG2, LAMP2, GAA, GLA, TMEM70, ELAC2, mt-DNA (MELAS, MERF, mitochondrial disease genes)*	*PTPN11, SOS1, HRAS, BRAF*

Abbreviations: IEMs inborn error of metabolism; LV, left ventricular.

rest in 25% to 40% of children with HCM; concomitant right ventricular outflow tract obstruction is often a feature of syndromic HCM. Cardiac magnetic resonance allows the identification of myocardial fibrosis by late gadolinium enhancement and is useful in monitoring disease progression. The most common electrocardiographic (ECG) findings in children are voltage criteria for LVH, ST-T abnormalities, and pathologic Q waves.[6,7]

GENETIC BASIS OF NONSYNDROMIC HYPERTROPHIC CARDIOMYOPATHY

Classic, nonsyndromic HCM is an autosomal dominant disease, with incomplete penetrance and variable expressivity. Over 3 decades ago, a missense mutation in the β-myosin heavy chain gene, *MYH7*, was first identified as causal for HCM in a large Canadian family. In subsequent years, numerous genes coding for proteins of sarcomere, Z-disc, or intracellular calcium modulators have been associated with the disease, and HCM has therefore been defined as a "disease of the sarcomere."[9] Overall, more than 1500 HCM-

associated, largely "private" variants have been described, and pathogenic variants are found in 50% to 60% of familial forms of HCM. The most prevalent include 3 genes coding for thick filament proteins: *MYH7-β*, myosin heavy chain; *MYL2*, regulatory myosin light chain; and *MYL3*, essential myosin light chain; 4 coding for components of the thin filament: *TPM1*, α tropomyosin; *TNNT2*, cardiac troponin T; TNNI3, cardiac troponin I; and *ACTC1*, cardiac actin; and an assembly protein: *MYBPC3*, cardiac myosin-binding protein C. *MYH7* and *MYBPC3* have the highest prevalence and, combined, account for 30% to 40% of diagnoses both in children and in adults. Haploinsufficiency due to loss-of-function alleles is the disease mechanism behind *MYBPC3*-related HCM, whereas a negative dominance model is the basis of other sarcomeric genes such as *MYH7*. In addition, rare variants have been reported in genes coding for protein of the Z-disc, such as *MYH6*, α myosin heavy chain, *TCAP*, and telethonin, and in genes involved in calcium homeostasis pathways, such as *VCL*, vinculin, and *JPH2*, junctophilin 2.[4,5,8] To date, several papers suggest that most variants identified in nonsarcomeric genes implicated in HCM are not associated with the condition.[10] For this reason, diagnostic screening of genes only with definitive association with HCM should be included in next-generation sequencing (NGS) targeted panels.[11] Finally, "complex genotypes," characterized by the co-occurrence of more than one pathogenetic variant in a single patient, represent a small but important patient subset, characterized by early disease onset, severe phenotype, and adverse outcome including enhanced risk of sudden cardiac death.[9]

Inborn Errors of Metabolism

Most cases of HCM caused by inborn errors of metabolism (IEMs) are due to glycogen storage disorders (Pompe disease, gene *GAA*; Danon disease, gene *LAMP2* or *PRKAG2* disease gene), lysosomal storage disorders (mucopolysaccharidoses [MPS] and Anderson Fabry disease), and mitochondrial diseases (MELAS, MERRF, *TMEM70,* and *ELAC2*).[1,4,7,12] The X-linked Anderson Fabry disorder is due to alpha-galactosidase deficiency: even though an HCM phenotype only develops in the third decades in males, extracardiac features such as acroparestesias may present early during childhood. The infantile (autosomal recessive) form of Pompe disease results from a complete deficiency of acid alpha-glucosidase and presents in newborns with severe HCM, respiratory failure, hypotonia, impaired growth, and macroglossia. Signs of heart failure usually develop between 2 and 6 months of age and include cyanosis, dyspnea, tachycardia, and susceptibility to respiratory infections. Echocardiography shows massive and diffuse LVH. A less severe, juvenile form of Pompe, characterized by reduced (but not abolished) levels of alpha-glucosidase activity, presents in the first decade of life with a mild or absent cardiac involvement.[13,14] Danon disease is an X-linked form presenting with the clinical triad of cardiomyopathy, intellectual disability, and skeletal myopathy. Cardiac manifestations include left or biventricular hypertrophy and ECG anomalies such as the Wolf-Parkinson-White syndrome.[15] *PRKAG2* syndrome, another glycogen storage disorder, is characterized by severe and progressive cardiac hypertrophy, arrhythmias, short PR, and conduction defects leading to juvenile atrioventricular block. MPS are a large group of lysosomal storage diseases characterized by glycosaminoglycan accumulation with cardiac features such as LVH, mitral and aortic regurgitation, mitral annulus calcification, and coronary artery narrowing. Finally,

mitochondrial cardiomyopathy has most often matrilinear transmission pattern with LVH, left ventricular noncompaction, and arrhythmias secondary to genetic defects involving the mitochondrial respiratory chain (see **Table 1**). Patients have a unique constellation of skeletal myopathy with exercise intolerance, neurosensory deafness, diabetes, and low stature. However, not all the mitochondrial cardiomyopathies have a matrilinear transmission pattern. These cardiomyopathies can also be inherited with autosomal dominant, recessive, or X-linked pattern.

Hypertrophic cardiomyopathy in RASopathies

The most common malformation syndromes associated with an HCM phenotype are the RASopathies, a heterogeneous group of diseases caused by mutations in genes of the RAS-MAPK cascade, including *PTPN11, BRAF, RAF1, SOS1 HRAS,* and *KRAS*. This group comprises conditions as diverse as Noonan, LEOPARD, cardio-facio-cutaneous, and Costello syndromes, characterized by short stature, facial dimorphisms, neurodevelopmental delay, and ectodermal abnormalities. These syndromes are typically inherited in an autosomal dominant pattern with variable expression. Heart involvement is a dominating feature, present in up to 80% of affected patients, and can be more rapidly progressive than the sarcomeric form.[16] HCM represents the most frequent cardiac phenotype, often accompanied by dynamic LV outflow tract obstruction (except for LEOPARD syndrome in which pulmonary stenosis is the predominant feature). However, besides hypertrophy, pulmonary stenosis, atrial septal defects, and valvular anomalies are also common findings in all RASopathies.

NEUROMUSCULAR DISEASES

Neuromuscular diseases represent a rare cause of HCM. The most common is Friedreich ataxia, an autosomal recessive condition caused by homozygous or compound heterozygous mutations in the gene encoding frataxin (*FXN*).[1] Frataxin is a nuclear-encoded mitochondrial iron chaperone involved in iron-sulfur biogenesis and heme biosynthesis. Some studies have also suggested that frataxin functions as an iron storage molecule, an antioxidant, and a tumor suppressor. Most patients with Friedreich ataxia have a GAA repeat expansion in the *FXN* gene. In addition, about 2% of cases of Friedreich ataxia are due to point mutations, the other 98% being due to expansion of a GAA trinucleotide repeat in intron 1. Syndromic and metabolic forms of HCM occur in infancy or early childhood, whereas neuromuscular forms are more commonly diagnosed in adolescence in view of their progressive clinical course.[17]

STRATEGIES FOR GENETIC TESTING

Genetic testing is essential in the diagnostic algorithm of pediatric HCM (**Fig. 2**), to differentiate primary sarcomeric forms from IEMs and syndromic contexts, as well as to expand performing cascade screening in the proband's family members.[18] In addition, identifying genes responsible for the disease can help to define recurrence risk for future pregnancies.

Patient counseling, gene sequencing, and variant interpretation along with metabolic screening should be performed in centers with specific expertise in cardiogenetics reflecting a multidisciplinary approach.[19–21]

NGS offers several benefits such as high throughput, speed, and sensitivity in variant detection, compared with Sanger-based techniques, and represents the standard in most laboratories. However, for children younger than 1 year, especially when extracardiac features are present, NGS panels can be insufficient to identify the causative variant. On the contrary the whole-exome sequencing (WES) analysis, has the huge advantage of identifying novel genes, typically causative of childhood cardiomyopathies, and as knowledge evolves, it allows also the periodic reanalysis of the NGS data.[22–25] Furthermore, to detect de novo variants, more common in infants, WES is the most powerful tool. Certainly, this novel technique has its known limitations; however, this concern can be managed through genetic counseling and the sharing of the informed consent.[22,24,26]

In conclusion, we assume that in children older than 1 year with nonsyndromic HCM, including adolescents, targeted NGS HCM gene panels should be preferred, whereas in infants to reach early diagnosis and to avoid long, costly, and distressing "diagnostic odysseys," WES analysis represents the best strategy for genetic testing.

CLINICAL COURSE AND RISK OF ADVERSE EVENTS

The clinical trajectories, long-term outcome, and response to treatment of HCM in children are difficult to predict.[26–28] Although the increasing number of studies assessing genotype-phenotype relationships contributes to our accuracy in risk stratification, it is important to remember that individual variability in clinical expression remains a major challenge in prognostication, particularly in children, even among individuals of the same family.[1] As previously discussed, the first step requires an accurate genetic diagnosis to distinguish sarcomeric HCM from its IEM or syndromic phenocopies, because of the considerable differences in natural history and management strategies.[4] For example, mutations in *LAMP2* causing Danon disease are usually associated with rapid disease

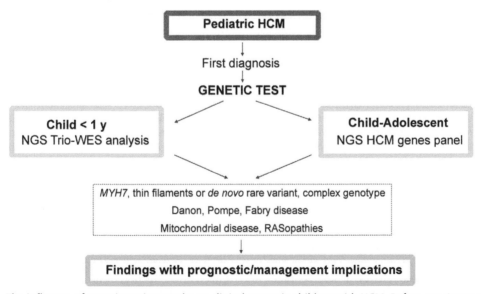

Fig. 2. The influence of genetic testing results on clinical course in children with HCM. Before age 1 year a next-generation sequencing (NGS)-Trio-whole-exome sequencing (WES)-based approach is the best strategy to screen patients with HCM; in children, adolescents, or when there is a clear clinical diagnosis of an isolated, nonsyndromic form of HCM, NGS genes panel approach should be preferred.

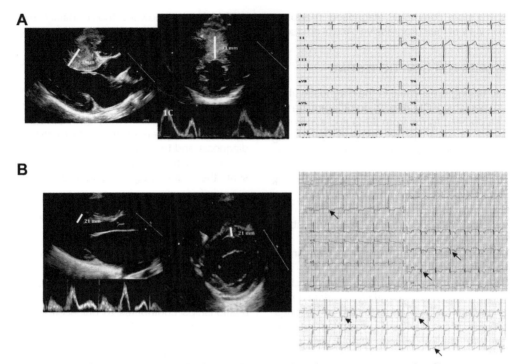

Fig. 3. The degree of LV hypertrophy in children with HCM with pathogenic variants in thin filament genes is not predictive of the risk of adverse events. (*A*) Child with a massive hypertrophy (septal maximal wall thickness = 33 mm) without events and negative genetic test. (*B*) A 9-year-old child with a mild hypertrophy (septal maximal wall thickness = 21 mm) presented a cardiac arrest (aborted) and a pathogenic variant in *TNNI3* gene.

progression and refractory heart failure in males, requiring early consideration for heart transplant.[29] Compared with sarcomeric HCM, Noonan-related cardiomyopathy presents with earlier onset and increased risk of heart failure and early mortality. Long-term prognosis is frequently poor, especially in the presence of biventricular obstruction and in carriers of *PTPN11* and *RIT1* pathogenic variants.[30] Among patients with *PRKAG2* mutations, both ventricular arrhythmia and juvenile AV blocks are common, calling for early prophylaxis with a pacemaker- implantable cardioverter-defibrillator; however, subcutaneous devices, without pacing capabilities, should be avoided in this context.

Among children with sarcomeric HCM, the identification of a complex genotype (2 mutations in the same or different sarcomeric genes) is usually associated with early onset and adverse clinical outcomes, as in adult patients.[31,32] Recently the presence of de novo variants has been shown to correlate with a higher risk of adverse events. Notably, de novo variants occur in up to 29% of pediatric HCM, seem to be linked to paternal age, and their identification is important both for the proband and counseling regarding risk of recurrence in subsequent pregnancies. Indeed, the proband's siblings will not share a genetic

predisposition to develop HCM, with the exception of extremely rare germinal mosaicisms.[33]

Thin filament gene mutations seem to play an important role in children with HCM. Homozygous variants in *TNNI3* genes, recently identified in infants with HCM, represent a rare cause associated with a severe outcome.[34] In a recent report by our group[35] children with mutations in *TNNT2* or in other thin filament genes exhibited a relatively small degree of hypertrophy but were exposed to increased risk of rhythm disturbances and a high incidence of sudden death (**Fig. 3**). These data are in agreement with those of previous studies by the London group, showing an increased risk of adverse outcome due to sudden death and progression toward restrictive end-stage disease in young patients with HCM with thin filament mutations.[36]

SUMMARY

Childhood HCM is typically caused by rare, family-specific mutations, commonly de novo. Investigating the genotype of HCM in children is extremely important, because it may help guide management more decisively and more often than in adults. Despite expanding knowledge, genotype-phenotype correlations in this young patient subset remain elusive, calling for broader, international studies in the field.

CLINICS CARE POINTS

- Consider "red flag" approach when evaluating children with HCM to provide lucid guide for clinical management and lifestyle advices.
- When suspecting HCM in a child always perform genetic counseling and metabolic screening.
- Less than age 1 year always use NGS Trio-WES analysis to identify complex genotypes and de novo rare variants.
- Plan a closer follow-up in patients with de novo rare variants or complex genotypes.
- Genotype early to distinguish between classical sarcomeric HCM and phenocopies and advise proper pharmacologic and invasive therapy.
- Detect Danon disease and provide early personalized care to the children and its family.
- In the presence of thin filament pathogenic variants in children evaluate the arrhythmic burden and initiate early adequate treatment to prevent end-stage disease phase.

CONFLICT OF INTEREST

The authors have no conflicts of interest relevant to this article to disclose.

AUTHOR CONTRIBUTIONS

All authors approved the final manuscript as submitted and agree to be accountable for all aspects of the work.

DATA AVAILABILITY STATEMENT

Data sharing is not applicable to this article as no datasets were generated or analyzed in this study.

REFERENCES

1. Lipshultz SE, Law YM, Asante-Korang A, et al. Cardiomyopathy in children: classification and diagnosis: a scientific statement from the American Heart Association. Circulation 2019;140(1):e9–68.
2. Colan SD, Lipshultz SE, Lowe AM, et al. Epidemiology and cause-specific prognosis of hypertrophic cardiomyopathy in children: findings from the Pediatric Cardiomyopathy Registry. Circulation 2007; 115(6):773–81.
3. Limongelli G, Monda E, Tramonte S, et al. Prevalence and clinical significance of red flags in patients with hypertrophic cardiomyopathy. Int J Cardiol 2020;299:186–91.
4. Girolami F, Morrone A, Brambilla A, et al. Genetic testing in pediatric cardiomyopathies: implications for diagnosis and management. Prog Pediatr Cardiol 2018;51:24–30.
5. Lee TM, Hsu DT, Kantor P, et al. Pediatric cardiomyopathies. Circ Res 2017;121(7):855–73.
6. Norrish G, Cantarutti N, Pissaridou E, et al. Risk factors for sudden cardiac death in childhood hypertrophic cardiomyopathy: a systematic review and meta-analysis. Eur J Prev Cardiol 2017;24(11): 1220–30.
7. Lipshultz SE, Orav EJ, Wilkinson JD, et al, Pediatric Cardiomyopathy Registry Study Group. Risk stratification at diagnosis for children with hypertrophic cardiomyopathy: an analysis of data from the Pediatric Cardiomyopathy Registry. Lancet 2013; 382(9908):1889–97.
8. Ware SM, Wilkinson JD, Tariq M, et al. Genetic causes of cardiomyopathy in children: first results from the pediatric cardiomyopathy genes study. J Am Heart Assoc 2021;10(9):e017731. https://doi. org/10.1161/JAHA.120.017731.
9. Ho CY, Day SM, Ashley EA, et al. Genotype and lifetime burden of disease in hypertrophic cardiomyopathy: Insights from the Sarcomeric Human Cardiomyopathy Registry (SHaRe). Circulation 2018;138(14):1387–98.
10. Mazzarotto F, Girolami F, Boschi B, et al. Defining the diagnostic effectiveness of genes for inclusion in panels: the experience of two decades of genetic testing for hypertrophic cardiomyopathy at a single center. Genet Med 2019;21(2):284–92.
11. Ingles J, Goldstein J, Thaxton C, et al. Evaluating the clinical validity of hypertrophic cardiomyopathy genes. Circ Genom Precis Med 2019;12(2): e002460.
12. Moak JP, Kaski JP. Hypertrophic cardiomyopathy in children. Heart 2012;98(14):1044–54. https://doi. org/10.1136/heartjnl-2011-300531.
13. Tunca Sahin G, Ozgur S, Kafali HC, et al. Clinical characteristics of hypertrophic cardiomyopathy in children: An 8-year single center experience. Pediatr Int 2021;63(1):37–45.
14. Monda E, Rubino M, Lioncino M, et al. Hypertrophic cardiomyopathy in children: pathophysiology, diagnosis, and treatment of non-sarcomeric causes. Front Pediatr 2021;9:632293.
15. Arad M, Maron BJ, Gorham JM, et al. Glycogen storage diseases presenting as hypertrophic cardiomyopathy. N Engl J Med 2005;352(4):362–72.

16. Pierpont ME, Digilio MC. Cardiovascular disease in Noonan syndrome. Curr Opin Pediatr 2018;30(5):601–60.

17. Rupp S, Felimban M, Schänzer A, et al. Genetic basis of hypertrophic cardiomyopathy in children. Clin Res Cardiol 2019;108(3):282–9.

18. Girolami F, Frisso G, Benelli M, et al. Contemporary genetic testing in inherited cardiac disease: tools, ethical issues, and clinical applications. J Cardiovasc Med (Hagerstown) 2018;19:1–11.

19. Hershberger RE, Givertz M, Ho CY, et al. Genetic evaluation of cardiomyopathy: a clinical practice resource of the American College of Medical Genetics and Genomics (ACMG). Genet Med 2018;20(9):899–909.

20. Chung WK, Ho C, Lee T, et al. Genetics of pediatric cardiomyopathies. Prog Pediatr Cardiol 2018;49:18–9.

21. Ackerman MJ, Priori SG, Willems S, et al. HRS/EHRA expert consensus statement on the state of genetic testing for the channelopathies and cardiomyopathies this document was developed as a partnership between the Heart Rhythm Society (HRS) and the European Heart Rhythm Association (EHRA). Heart Rhythm 2011;8:1308–1339.20.

22. Mazzarotto F, Olivotto I, Walsh R. Advantages and perils of clinical whole-exome and whole-genome sequencing in cardiomyopathy review. Cardiovasc Drugs Ther 2020;34(2):241–53.

23. Charron P, Arad M, Arbustini E, et al. Genetic counselling and testing in cardiomyopathies: a position statement of the European Society of Cardiology Working Group on Myocardial and Pericardial Diseases. Eur Heart J 2010;31:2715–26.

24. Rojnueangnit K, Sirichongkolthong B, Wongwandee R, et al. Identification of gene mutations in primary pediatric cardiomyopathy by whole exome sequencing. Pediatr Cardiol 2020;41:165–74.

25. Quiat D, Witkowski L, Zouk H, et al. Retrospective analysis of clinical genetic testing in pediatric primary dilated cardiomyopathy: testing prognosis and the effects of variant reclassification. Am Heart J 2020;9(11).

26. Vasilescu C, Ojala TH, Brilhante V, et al. Genetic basis of severe childhood-onset cardiomyopathies. J Am Coll Cardiol 2018;72(19):2324–38.

27. Mathew L, Zahavich, Lafreniere-Roula M, et al. Utility of genetics for risk stratification in pediatric hypertrophic cardiomyopathy. Clin Cenetics 2018;93(2):310–9. https://doi.org/10.1111/cge.13157.

28. Norrish G, Ding T, Field E, et al. A validation study of the European Society of Cardiology guidelines for risk stratification of sudden cardiac death in childhood hypertrophic cardiomyopathy. Europace 2019;21(10):1559–65.

29. Lotan D, Salazar-Mendiguchía J, Mogensen J, et al. Clinical profile of cardiac involvement in danon disease: a multicenter European Registry. Circ Genom Precis Med 2020;13(6):e003117.

30. Aly SA, Boyer KM, Muller B-AA, et al. Complicated ventricular arrhythmia and hematologic myeloproliferative disorder in RIT1-associated Noonan syndrome: expanding the phenotype and review of the literature. Mol Genet Genomic Med 2020;8:e1253.

31. Ware SM, Wilkinson JD, Tariq M, et al. Genetic causes of cardiomyopathy in children: first results from the pediatric cardiomyopathy genes study. J Am Heart Assoc 2021;10(9):e017731.

32. Mathew J, Zahavich L, Lafreniere-Roula M, et al. Utility of genetics for risk stratification in pediatric hypertrophic cardiomyopathy. Clin Genet 2018;93(2):310–9.

33. Parrott A, Khoury PR, Shikany AR, et al. Investigation of de novo variation in pediatric cardiomyopathy. Am J Med Genet C Semin Med Genet 2020;184(1):116–23.

34. Kühnisch J, Herbst C, Al-Wakeel-Marquard S, et al. Targeted panel sequencing in pediatric primary cardiomyopathy supports a critical role of TNNI3. Clin Genet 2019;96(6):549–59.

35. Maurizi N, Passantino S, Spaziani G, et al. Long-term prognosis of pediatric-onset hypertrophic cardiomyopathy and age-specific risk factors for lethal arrhythmic events. JAMA Cardiol 2018;3:520–5.

36. Kaski JP, Syrris P, Burch M, et al. Idiopathic restrictive cardiomyopathy in children is caused by mutations in cardiac sarcomere protein genes. Heart 2008;94(11):1478–84.

The Risk of Sudden Death in Children with Hypertrophic Cardiomyopathy

Gabrielle Norrish, BMBCh, BA, MRCPCH, PhD[a,b],
Juan Pablo Kaski, BSc (Hons), MBBS, MRCPCH, MD(Res), FESC, FRCP[a,b],*

KEYWORDS

- Sudden death • Children • Hypertrophic cardiomyopathy • Risk models

KEY POINTS

- Sudden cardiac death (SCD) is the most common cause of death in childhood hypertrophic cardiomyopathy and occurs more frequently than in adult patients.
- Important differences between childhood and adult cohort have been described with the implication that the pediatric-specific risk stratification methods are needed.
- Current guidelines using cumulative risk factors to guide implantable cardioverter defibrillator implantation have been shown to have limited discrimination.
- New pediatric models have been developed to allow clinicians to calculate individualized estimates of 5-year risk of SCD.

INTRODUCTION

Hypertrophic cardiomyopathy (HCM) is defined as left ventricular hypertrophy (LVH) in the absence of abnormal loading conditions.[1] The prevalence of HCM during childhood is estimated at 3 in 100,000[2] births, with a reported annual incidence of less than 0.5/100,000[2–4] from population registry studies, making it the second most common cardiomyopathy presenting during childhood. The underlying etiology is heterogeneous and includes inborn errors of metabolism (IEM), RASopathy syndromes, and neuromuscular disease, but most cases of childhood-onset HCM, even in very young children, are caused by variants in sarcomere protein genes.[5–9] The natural history and overall outcome of childhood HCM is highly variable and largely dependent on the underlying etiology and age of presentation. Children with presumed sarcomeric HCM have a relatively good prognosis, with an estimated 5-year survival more than 80%, but patients with syndromic disease (IEM or RASopathy syndromes) or infantile onset (in the first year of life) are recognized to have a worse overall prognosis.[5,7,8] The majority of deaths occurring in infancy are heart failure related, but sudden cardiac death (SCD) is the most common cause of death during childhood.[5,10] Identifying those at highest risk of malignant ventricular arrhythmias is therefore an important part of clinical care. This article describes the pathophysiology, risk factors, and approach to risk stratification for SCD in childhood HCM.

PATHOPHYSIOLOGY OF SUDDEN DEATH IN HYPERTROPHIC CARDIOMYOPATHY

The hallmark macroscopic and histologic features of HCM include myocyte disarray, fibrosis, and small-vessel disease. The extent of myocyte disarray was associated with SCD in a postmortem study of HCM,[11] but the mechanism by which this proarrhythmic substrate translates into an

[a] Centre for Inherited Cardiovascular Diseases, Great Ormond Street Hospital, London, UK; [b] Institute of Cardiovascular Sciences University College London, UK
* Corresponding author. Centre for Inherited Cardiovascular Diseases, Great Ormond Street Hospital, London WC1N 3JH, UK.
E-mail address: j.kaski@ucl.ac.uk

Heart Failure Clin 18 (2022) 9–18
https://doi.org/10.1016/j.hfc.2021.07.012

increased risk of ventricular arrhythmias is incompletely understood. It is likely that the pathophysiology is multifactorial, with LVH causing dispersion of repolarization, myocardial disarray disrupting cell alignment, and areas of fibrosis creating a localized conduction block and altered calcium sensitivity.[12,13] The observation that the overall incidence of SCD in HCM is low[14,15] despite these universal underlying structural and biochemical abnormalities suggests that transient electrical (such as premature ventricular ectopics, supraventricular tachycardias) or structural changes (such as ischemia or dynamic outflow tract obstruction) in the context of a proarrhythmic substrate are the trigger for ventricular arrhythmias. The primary underlying arrhythmia resulting in SCD is usually ventricular fibrillation (VF) or ventricular tachycardia (VT) in most cases.

RISK OF SUDDEN CARDIAC DEATH IN PEDIATRIC HYPERTROPHIC CARDIOMYOPATHY

Early studies in small, highly selected patient groups from tertiary centers reported a high incidence of SCD during childhood of up to 7% per year.[16,17] Over time, data from larger, more representative population cohort studies have suggested much lower SCD incidence rates, with current estimates between 0.8% and 2% per year.[10,14,15] Outside of infancy, SCD is the most common cause of death in pediatric HCM, and recent population studies have reported that arrhythmic events are responsible for more than 50% of adverse events occurring within 10 years of diagnosis, with a cumulative incidence of 8.8%.[10] A single study has described a higher incidence of SCD in the preadolescent and early adolescent years (9–14 yrs), but this has not been confirmed in other populations.[18] It is clear, however, that the incidence of SCD reported in pediatric population studies is substantially higher than that seen in similar-sized adult cohorts (<0.8%),[19,20] with the result that children are considered to be at higher risk of arrhythmic events. This perception has recently been confirmed using longitudinal datasets from the Sarcomeric Human Cardiomyopathy Registry (SHaRE), in which patients with pediatric-onset HCM (aged 1–18 years) were 36% more likely to experience an arrhythmic event during follow-up than those diagnosed in adulthood.[10]

SUDDEN CARDIAC DEATH PREVENTION

No medical treatment is currently recommended as preventative therapy for SCD in HCM. High-dose beta-blockade (up to 23 mg/kg propranolol daily) has been described to reduce the risk of SCD in a single-center study,[21] but these results have not been independently confirmed in either pediatric or adult populations. The mainstay of preventative therapy is the implantable cardioverter defibrillator (ICD), which has been shown to be effective at terminating malignant ventricular arrhythmias in children and adults with HCM.[22,23] Children who have previously experienced a malignant arrhythmia are widely accepted to be at high risk of future arrhythmic events and are recommended for a secondary prevention ICD implantation as a class I indication.[1,24] In a recent national cohort study of children with HCM and an ICD from the United Kingdom (UK), almost two-thirds of patients with a secondary prevention device received an appropriate ICD therapy for a ventricular tachyarrhythmia within 5 years of follow-up.[25] However, this is at the expense of an increased risk of device-related complications (including lead fracture or migration, infective endocarditis, or venous occlusion) and inappropriate therapies compared with adult patients. Retrospective population studies have reported that, over a relatively short follow-up time (mean 5–7 years), ICD-related complications occur in up to 30% of childhood cohorts, most commonly system infection, lead fracture/failure, or need for lead repositioning/replacement due to somatic growth.[23,25] Historically, this group of patients have been considered to be at high risk of inappropriate therapies, which have been reported to occur in up to one-third of patients from population series.[22,23,26,27] More recent data from the UK suggest that this risk may not be as high as previously thought and comparable with adult patients (≈8%).[25,28] However, as this younger group of patients has an ongoing lifetime exposure to these risks and no device or programming strategies have been identified to reduce this risk,[25] the balance between benefit and harm for primary prevention ICD implantation is particularly important. In this context, it is essential to accurately identify those children at highest risk who would benefit most from ICD implantation.

RISK FACTORS FOR SUDDEN CARDIAC DEATH IN PEDIATRIC HYPERTROPHIC CARDIOMYOPATHY

Until recently, our understanding of the clinical risk factors for SCD events in childhood HCM was limited and largely extrapolated from adult literature. The first systematic review and meta-analysis of risk factors in childhood disease was performed in 2017 and identified four major clinical risk factors associated with SCD events in two or more univariable analyses: previous VF or sustained VT, unexplained syncope, nonsustained ventricular tachycardia (NSVT), and extreme LVH [defined as a left ventricular (LV) maximal wall thickness ≥30 mm or Z score ≥6.[29] The number of studies available for inclusion in this meta-analysis was small (n = 23), and individual studies reported small, often heterogeneous, patient cohorts (all but 3 had <150 participants). Nonetheless, this provided the first pediatric-specific systematic assessment of risk factors for SCD events. This study also suggested important differences between adult and pediatric risk factors. In particular, although there is robust evidence to support the use of family history of SCD in adult patients, there is insufficient evidence to support its use during childhood. Only one study reported a significant association in a small cohort of patients with an ICD who had *a priori* been determined to be at high risk of malignant arrhythmias by treating clinicians.[26] Possible explanations for this include a higher prevalence of *de novo* variants in childhood HCM, low proportion of sarcomeric disease in the included cohorts, or incomplete reporting of family history. Recent multicenter collaborative population studies (including HCM Risk-Kids,[14] PRiMACY,[15] and SHaRE[10]) have provided further evidence and novel insights into the risk factors identified by this meta-analysis, as well as evidence for additional risk factors, such as left atrial diameter and left ventricular outflow tract obstruction (LVOTO). A brief description of the main risk factors for SCD in childhood HCM can be found later in discussion and in **Table 1**.

Left Ventricular Hypertrophy

Recent large pediatric cohort studies have confirmed the importance of LVH for risk stratification, but the most appropriate measure of LVH is unknown as published studies vary widely in their definition and measure [including interventricular septal thickness (IVST), LV posterior wall thickness (LVPWT), septal thickness/cavity ratio, Body surface area-corrected measurements, and absolute maximal left ventricular wall thickness (MLVWT)[14,15,30,34]]. Extreme LVH (defined as MLVWT ≥ 30 mm or Z score ≥6) is recommended as a threshold for ICD implantation decisions in current North American and European risk stratification guidelines.[1,24] The evidence for using this particular threshold is limited, and the interpretation of all z score thresholds is inherently hampered by the use of different normative population data, each of which will provide a different z score for the same individual. The meta-analysis identified extreme LVH as a major risk factor with a combined hazard ratio of 1.8 [95% confidence interval (CI) = 0.75–4.32], although this did not reach threshold for significance (*P* value = 0.19). Nonetheless, the implication of using a threshold is that risk increases linearly with increasing LVH. Recent publications from large population studies (HCM Risk-Kids[14] and PRIMaCY[15]) have challenged this view, showing that a nonlinear relationship exists between measures of LVH and SCD risk, with the result that beyond a particular threshold, risk plateaus or starts to fall. The mechanism behind these observations is unknown, but it is in keeping with the relationship between MLVWT and SCD risk in a large adult HCM study.[42]

Nonsustained Ventricular Tachycardia

NSVT is defined as ≥3 consecutive ventricular beats occurring at a rate greater than 120 bpm lasting less than 30 seconds.[1] The true prevalence of NSVT in childhood HCM is unknown, with estimates from retrospective cohorts between 8% and 30%.[14,15,23,30,43] It was identified as a major risk factor in the meta-analysis with a pooled hazard ratio of 2.13 (95% CI = 1.21–3.74, *P* value = 0.0009).[29] No study has assessed the importance of frequency, rate, or length of NSVT detected on ambulatory electrocardiograph (ECG) in childhood, and the significance of exercise-induced arrhythmias is also unknown.

Unexplained Syncope

Unexplained syncope, presumed secondary to malignant arrhythmias, has been identified as a risk factor for SCD in childhood HCM with a pooled odds ratio of 2.64 (95% CI = 1.21–5.79, *P* value = 0.02). The timing of a syncopal event has been shown to be important in adult HCM cohorts (recent syncope (within 6 months) associated with a 5-fold increased risk[44]) but has not been explored in pediatric cohorts.

TRADITIONAL APPROACH TO RISK STRATIFICATION

The traditional approach to risk stratification in childhood HCM is based on conventionally accepted risk factors largely extrapolated from adult practice (extreme LVH, unexplained syncope, NSVT, and family history of SCD).[1,24] As has been discussed earlier, some of these traditional risk factors have insufficient evidence to support their use in childhood disease. Reflecting the finding in adult cohorts that coexistence of

Table 1
Risk factors for sudden cardiac death in childhood HCM

Major Risk Factor	Clinical Risk Factor	Comment
Major risk factors	Previous VF/VT	Pooled HR = 5.4 (95% CI = 3.67–7.95, P value <.001). Pooled OR = 5.06 (95% CI = 2.11–12.17, P value <.001)
	Unexplained syncope	Pooled HR = 1.89 (95% CI = 0.69–5.16, P value = 0.22). Pooled OR = 2.64 (95% CI = 1.21–5.79, P value = 0.02)
	NSVT	Pooled HR = 2.13 (95% CI = 1.21–3.74, P value = 0.0009). Pooled OR = 2.05 (95% CI = 0.98–4.28, P value = 0.06).
	Extreme LVH	Pooled HR = 1.8 (95% CI = 0.75–4.32, P value = 0.19). Pooled OR = 1.70 (95% CI = 0.85–3.40, P value = 0.13). The most useful measure of LVH for risk stratification is unknown.
Other putative risk factors	LA dilatation	Left atrial size was not included as a major risk factor in the meta-analysis, but a significant association has subsequently been reported in four studies.[14,15,30,31]
	LVOT gradient	The definition of LVOT obstruction varies in the literature. Increasing LVOT gradient has been linked to SCD,[30,32] and two large studies have described an inverse relationship between LVOT gradient and risk in childhood.[14,15]
	Family history of SCD	Only 1/10 studies reported a significant association between a family history of SCD and SCD event.[26] There is limited evidence to support its use as a risk factor during childhood.
	Age	The role of age in SCD is not fully understood. SCD risk has been reported to be increased in preadolescent years (9–14 yrs),[18] and children presenting in infancy are believed to be at lower risk.[7,33]
	12-lead ECG	Proposed 12-lead ECG features include measures of LVH[34] and abnormal repolarisation,[35] but a recent large study showed no association between individual ECG parameters and risk.[36] An ECG risk score has been developed by Ostman-Smith et al,[35] but this was shown to have only moderate discriminatory ability in an external validation study.[36]
	LGE on CMRI	LGE has been shown to increase during childhood and is associated with left ventricular hypertrophy.[37] It is unclear if LGE is an independent risk factor for SCD.[38,39]
	Genotype	The role of genotype in SCD risk during childhood is not fully understood. In small cohorts, the presence of a pathogenic sarcomeric mutation has been described to be associated with worse prognosis[40] and certain genotypes associated with higher arrhythmic risk.[41]

Abbreviations: CI, confidence interval; HR, hazard ratio; LGE, late gadolinium enhancement; OR, odds ratio.

Adapted from Norrish G, Cantarutti N, Pissaridou E, Ridout DA, Limongelli G, Elliott PM, Kaski JP. Risk factors for sudden cardiac death in childhood hypertrophic cardiomyopathy: A systematic review and meta-analysis. Eur J Prev Cardiol. 2017 Jul;24(11):1220-1230.

multiple risk factors was associated with an increased risk of SCD,[45] cumulative risk factor thresholds are recommended in current guidelines to guide ICD implantation decisions. This approach to risk stratification provides relative rather than absolute estimates of risk and has been shown in an external validation study from the UK to have only moderate discriminatory ability [c-0.62 (95% CI = 0.55–0.70)], leading to unnecessary ICD implantation in many.[46] Current risk stratification guidelines continue to recommend this practice although the number of risk factors required to meet the threshold for considering ICD implantation differs (≥1 risk factor in the American Heart Association [AHA]/American College of Cardiology [ACC] guideline[24] and ≥2 risk factors in the European Society of Cardiology [ESC] guidelines[1]). The newer North American guidelines published in 2020 suggest that additional risk factors, including the presence of late gadolinium enhancement (LGE) on cardiac magnetic resonance imaging (CMRI) and LV systolic function, could also be helpful in select pediatric patients. **Table 2** shows the current guidelines for risk stratification in childhood disease.

PERSONALIZED APPROACH TO RISK STRATIFICATION FOR CHILDHOOD HYPERTROPHIC CARDIOMYOPATHY

The limited ability of current guidelines to discriminate between high- and low-risk patients has led to interest in developing a more personalized approach to risk stratification for these patients. Current risk stratification practice for adults with HCM has moved away from the traditional approach of using cumulative risk factors in favor of using a validated risk prediction model that provides individualized estimates of risk. The HCM Risk-SCD model uses readily available clinical risk factors to calculate individualized estimated for 5-year SCD risk to guide implantation decisions, but is not validated for use in pediatric populations (<16 years of age).[20] External validation of the adult risk model in a childhood cohort showed it to have poor correlation between predicted and observed

risk (underestimated for all risk groups), confirming that its use should not be extrapolated to childhood patients.[14] In 2019, the first validated pediatric-specific risk model for SCD was developed and published (HCM Risk-Kids) in a large (n = 1024), international cohort of children with nonsyndromic HCM.[14] The new pediatric model uses 5 readily available clinical predictors preselected from over 3 decades of published literature (MLVWT Z score, LA Z score, maximal LVOT gradient, NSVT, and unexplained syncope) assessed at the time of baseline clinical evaluation to calculate personalized estimates of 5-year SCD risk. Age was not included as a predictor variable in the model as, outside of infancy, its role in prognosis remains unclear.[10,18] However, the effect of age may have been mitigated by accounting for somatic growth using body surface area corrected, rather than absolute 2D, echocardiographic measurements. Internal validation of HCM Risk-Kids showed that the model had better discrimination between high- and low-risk patients than current pediatric guidelines with good calibration between the expected and observed risk (**Fig. 1**). The performance is similar to that reported in adult cohorts for the adult HCM Risk-SCD model (C-index 0.69 vs 0.70).[19] The HCM Risk-Kids model is available online (https://hcmriskkids.org)/) allowing clinicians to calculate individualized estimates of risk for the first time, and external validation studies have been completed to confirm the superior performance of this model in an independent study population.

Following the publication of HCM Risk-Kids, an alternative pediatric-specific risk model (PRIMaCY) was developed and published using a largely North American cohort (n = 572).[15] The final models are similar despite differences in their approaches to risk factor selection, with the exception that

Table 2
Risk stratification guidelines for SCD for childhood HCM

	Recommendations	Class
ACCF/AHA	An ICD is recommended if prior event (SCD, VF, sustained VT)	1
	An ICD is reasonable if one or more risk factors (family history SCD, massive hypertrophy, unexplained syncope, apical aneurysm, ejection fraction ≤50%, NSVT	2a
	An ICD may be considered if extensive LGE on CMR	2b
ESC	An ICD is recommended if prior cardiac arrest or sustained VT	1
	An ICD should be considered in children with two or more major paediatric risk factors (extreme LVH, unexplained syncope, NSVT, Family history of SCD)	2a
	An ICD may be considered in children with a single major paediatric risk factor if overall considered to be a net benefit from ICD therapy	2b

Data from American College of Cardiology Foundation/American Heart Association (2020) b) European Society of Cardiology (2014).

PRIMaCY includes two measures of LVH (IVST and LVPWT) and age as an independent predictor. External validation of this model in a small cohort of 285 patients from the SHaRe consortium confirmed that the performance of the model was superior to current guidelines (C-statistic 0.707) and similar to the HCM Risk-Kids model. No direct comparison of the two models has been performed, although given their similarities, it is plausible that their performance will be similar. A comparison of the two models is shown in **Table 3**.

A final alternative model that has been proposed for use in childhood HCM is the ECG risk score, which comprises 8 parameters (deviation in QRS axis, pathologic T wave inversion in the limb or precordial leads, ST-segment depression, dominant S wave inV4, limb-lead amplitude sum, 12-lead amplitude duration product, and QTc). The 12-lead ECG provides valuable quantitative and qualitative information about a patient's phenotype, and the ECG risk score has been described to predict arrhythmic events with a high negative and positive predictive value (99% and 45% respectively).[35] Until recently, these findings had not been confirmed or refuted in an external validation study. However, a recent external validation study in 356 children from HCM Risk-Kids cohort showed the ECG risk score had only moderate discriminatory ability (similar to the current guidelines but lower than HCM Risk-Kids or PRIMaCY) to predict 5-year SCD events with a low positive predictive value (10%).[36] Despite most patients having ECG abnormalities, no individual or combined ECG score was associated with arrhythmic events in this independent population. This suggests that the ability of the 12-lead ECG to improve risk stratification in childhood HCM is limited.

FUTURE DIRECTIONS

In the past 5 years, the development of pediatric-specific risk models has allowed clinicians to calculate individualized estimates of risk for the first time and deliver personalized care. This represents a significant advance for risk stratification of childhood disease and patient management. These models have not yet been adopted by clinical guidelines, and further validation studies are required to assess performance in real-world clinical practice, which will be facilitated by the availability of both models on freely available public Web sites. Such studies would also help determine if a 5-year risk threshold is appropriate for recommending ICD implantation in childhood HCM analogous to that seen in the adult guidelines.

Although both models outperform current risk stratification guidelines, they remain imperfect and additional risk factors are likely to be important for prognosis. LGE on CMRI is a marker of fibrosis and has been shown to be a risk factor for SCD in adult cohorts independently of traditional clinical risk factors with an apparent linear association between risk and proportion of LGE.[47] In childhood disease, LGE has been shown

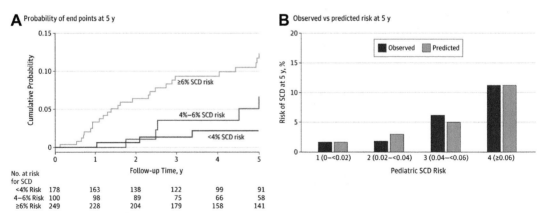

Fig. 1. Performance of HCM Risk-Kids model (*A*) Kaplan–Meier curve showing cumulative probability of meeting SCD end point within 5 years by estimated clinical risk group (*B*) Comparison of observed and predicted risk by clinical risk group. (*From* Norrish G, Ding T, Field E, Ziółkowska L, Olivotto I, Limongelli G, Anastasakis A, Weintraub R, Biagini E, Ragni L, Prendiville T, Duignan S, McLeod K, Ilina M, Fernández A, Bökenkamp R, Baban A, Kubuš P, Daubeney PEF, Sarquella-Brugada G, Cesar S, Marrone C, Bhole V, Medrano C, Uzun O, Brown E, Gran F, Castro FJ, Stuart G, Vignati G, Barriales-Villa R, Guereta LG, Adwani S, Linter K, Bharucha T, Garcia-Pavia P, Rasmussen TB, Calcagnino MM, Jones CB, De Wilde H, Toru-Kubo J, Felice T, Mogensen J, Mathur S, Reinhardt Z, O'Mahony C, Elliott PM, Omar RZ, Kaski JP. Development of a Novel Risk Prediction Model for Sudden Cardiac Death in Childhood Hypertrophic Cardiomyopathy (HCM Risk-Kids). JAMA Cardiol. 2019 Sep 1;4(9):918-927; with permission.)

Table 3
Comparison of personalized risk models for SCD risk stratification in childhood HCM

Model characteristic	HCM Risk-Kids	PRiMACY
Development cohort		
Sample size	1024	572
Age	≤ 16	≤ 18
Number of SCD events		
Predictor variables		
LVMWT Z score	X	
IVST Z score		X
LVPWT Z score		X
LA Z score	X	X
Maximal LVOT gradient (mmHg)	X	X
NSVT	X	X
Unexplained syncope	X	X
Age		X
Model validation		
Internal	0.69 (95% CI = 0.66–0.72)	0.75 (CI not provided)
External	Ongoing	0.71 (CI not provided)
Model website	https://hcmriskkids.org/	https://primacycalculator.com/

Abbreviation: CI, confidence interval; LVMWT, left ventricular maximal wall thickness.
Data from Refs.[14,15]

to be associated with the degree of LVH and to increase during follow-up.[37,38] Its role as an independent risk factor has not clearly been established, but a single-center study has reported improved discriminatory performance of both the current guidelines and the HCM Risk-Kids model with the addition of LGE as either a binary or a continuous variable.[48] Future multicentre studies are required to investigate the role of LGE in pediatric risk stratification.

The role of genotype in risk stratification for childhood HCM remains unclear, with studies reporting conflicting findings. Although patients with a disease-causing sarcomeric variant have been reported to have a higher cumulative lifetime risk of adverse events,[49] recent data, including more than 1000 children with HCM, from the SHaRE registry did not find a higher lifetime risk of arrhythmic events for genotype positive patients.[10] Inclusion of genotype status (positive or negative) in the PRIMaCY model did not significantly improve model predictions.[15] Efforts to explore genotype–phenotype correlations in HCM have been limited by significant genetic heterogeneity and variable or incomplete age-related penetrance, but insufficient evidence currently exists to support the use of genotype at the level of the gene or gene region in risk stratification for childhood disease. As yet-unidentified genetic and epigenetic modifiers are likely to play an important role in the expression of sarcomeric disease, and a variant specific approach, including assessment of the contribution of common genetic variants, is likely to be needed.[50] Such analysis will be limited by small numbers of patients with individual variants and will require multicentre collaborative efforts.

Finally, work to date has focused on patients with HCM secondary to sarcomeric protein variants and little is known about risk stratification in patients with nonsyndromic disease (eg, RAS-opathy or IEM). This group of patients is traditionally considered to be at lower risk for arrhythmic events, although population studies have reported SCD events in an important minority.[5,51,52] Future studies are required to determine if risk stratification methods developed in sarcomeric disease can be extrapolated to nonsyndromic patients and identify disease-specific risk factors.

SUMMARY

SCD is the most common cause of death outside of infancy in childhood HCM and occurs more frequently than in adult patients. Systematic evaluation of individual risk factors has revealed important differences between childhood- and adult-onset disease and led to the development of pediatric-specific risk models. These models allow clinicians to calculate individualized estimates of 5-year risk for the first time and are an important tool for shared ICD implantation decision-making. Future studies are required to investigate additional risk factors and provide real-life validation to further improve risk stratification for childhood HCM.

DISCLOSURES

This work was supported by the British Heart Foundation (grant number FS/16/72/32270) to GN and JPK. JPK is supported by Max's Foundation and Great Ormond Street Hospital Children's Charity. JPK is supported by a Medical Research Council Clinical (MRC)-National Institute for Health Research (NIHR) Clinical Academic Research Partnership (CARP) award. This work is (partly) funded by the NIHR GOSH BRC.

CLINICS CARE POINTS

- Ensure systematic risk stratification for SCD events is performed for all childhood patients with HCM
- Risk stratification for childhood HCM should be systematic and include assessment of left ventricular hypertrophy, left atrial diameter, LV outflow tract gradient, presence of malignant arrhythmias on ambulatory ECG monitoring, and unexplained syncope.
- Consider using a pediatric-specific risk model (HCM Risk-Kids or PRiMACY) to calculate individualized estimates of 5-year SCD risk.

REFERENCES

1. Elliott PM, Anastasakis A, Borger MA, et al. 2014 ESC Guidelines on diagnosis and management of hypertrophic cardiomyopathy: the Task Force for the Diagnosis and Management of Hypertrophic Cardiomyopathy of the European Society of Cardiology (ESC). Eur Heart J 2014;35(39):2733–79.
2. Arola A, Jokinen E, Ruuskanen O, et al. Epidemiology of idiopathic cardiomyopathies in children and adolescents. A nationwide study in Finland. Am J Epidemiol 1997;146(5):385–93.
3. Nugent AW, Daubeney PE, Chondros P, et al. The epidemiology of childhood cardiomyopathy in Australia. N Engl J Med 2003;348(17):1639–46.
4. Lipshultz SE, Sleeper LA, Towbin JA, et al. The incidence of pediatric cardiomyopathy in two regions of the United States. N Engl J Med 2003;348(17):1647–55.
5. Norrish G, Field E, McLeod K, et al. Clinical presentation and survival of childhood hypertrophic cardiomyopathy: a retrospective study in United Kingdom. Eur Heart J 2019;40(12):986–93.
6. Kaski JP, Syrris P, Esteban MT, et al. Prevalence of sarcomere protein gene mutations in preadolescent children with hypertrophic cardiomyopathy. Circ Cardiovasc Genet 2009;2(5):436–41.
7. Nugent AW, Daubeney PE, Chondros P, et al. Clinical features and outcomes of childhood hypertrophic cardiomyopathy: results from a national population-based study. Circulation 2005;112(9):1332–8.
8. Colan SD, Lipshultz SE, Lowe AM, et al. Epidemiology and cause-specific outcome of hypertrophic cardiomyopathy in children: findings from the Pediatric Cardiomyopathy Registry. Circulation 2007;115(6):773–81.
9. Morita H, Rehm HL, Menesses A, et al. Shared genetic causes of cardiac hypertrophy in children and adults. N Engl J Med 2008;358(18):1899–908.
10. Marston NA, Han L, Olivotto I, et al. Clinical characteristics and outcomes in childhood-onset hypertrophic cardiomyopathy. Eur Heart J 2021;42(20):1988–96.
11. Varnava AM, Elliott PM, Mahon N, et al. Relation between myocyte disarray and outcome in hypertrophic cardiomyopathy. Am J Cardiol 2001;88(3):275–9.
12. Wang L, Kim K, Parikh S, et al. Hypertrophic cardiomyopathy-linked mutation in troponin T causes myofibrillar disarray and pro-arrhythmic action potential changes in human iPSC cardiomyocytes. J Mol Cell Cardiol 2018;114:320–7.
13. Saumarez RC, Heald S, Gill J, et al. Primary ventricular fibrillation is associated with increased paced right ventricular electrogram fractionation. Circulation 1995;92(9):2565–71.
14. Norrish G, Ding T, Field E, et al. Development of a Novel Risk Prediction Model for Sudden Cardiac Death in Childhood Hypertrophic Cardiomyopathy (HCM Risk-Kids). JAMA Cardiol 2019;4(9):918–27.
15. Miron A, Lafreniere-Roula M, Fan CS, et al. A Validated Model for Sudden Cardiac Death Risk Prediction in Pediatric Hypertrophic Cardiomyopathy. Circulation 2020;142(3):217–29.
16. McKenna WJ, Franklin RC, Nihoyannopoulos P, et al. Arrhythmia and prognosis in infants, children and adolescents with hypertrophic cardiomyopathy. J Am Coll Cardiol 1988;11(1):147–53.
17. McKenna WJ, Deanfield JE. Hypertrophic cardiomyopathy: an important cause of sudden death. Arch Dis Child 1984;59(10):971–5.

18. Ostman-Smith I, Wettrell G, Keeton B, et al. Age- and gender-specific mortality rates in childhood hypertrophic cardiomyopathy. Eur Heart J 2008;29(9): 1160–7.

19. O'Mahony C, Jichi F, Ommen SR, et al. International External Validation Study of the 2014 European Society of Cardiology Guidelines on Sudden Cardiac Death Prevention in Hypertrophic Cardiomyopathy (EVIDENCE-HCM). Circulation 2018;137(10): 1015–23.

20. O'Mahony C, Jichi F, Pavlou M, et al. A novel clinical risk prediction model for sudden cardiac death in hypertrophic cardiomyopathy (HCM risk-SCD). Eur Heart J 2014;35(30):2010–20.

21. Ostman-Smith I, Wettrell G, Riesenfeld T. A cohort study of childhood hypertrophic cardiomyopathy: improved survival following high-dose beta-adrenoceptor antagonist treatment. J Am Coll Cardiol 1999;34(6):1813–22.

22. Kaski JP, Tome Esteban MT, Lowe M, et al. Outcomes after implantable cardioverter-defibrillator treatment in children with hypertrophic cardiomyopathy. Heart 2007;93(3):372–4.

23. Maron BJ, Spirito P, Ackerman MJ, et al. Prevention of sudden cardiac death with implantable cardioverter-defibrillators in children and adolescents with hypertrophic cardiomyopathy. J Am Coll Cardiol 2013;61(14):1527–35.

24. Ommen SR, Mital S, Burke MA, et al. 2020 AHA/ACC Guideline for the Diagnosis and Treatment of Patients With Hypertrophic Cardiomyopathy: Executive Summary: A Report of the American College of Cardiology/American Heart Association Joint Committee on Clinical Practice Guidelines. Circulation 2020;142(25):e533–57.

25. Norrish G, Chubb H, Field E, et al. Clinical outcomes and programming strategies of implantable cardioverter-defibrillator devices in paediatric hypertrophic cardiomyopathy: a UK National Cohort Study. Europace 2020;23(3):400–8.

26. Kamp AN, Von Bergen NH, Henrikson CA, et al. Implanted defibrillators in young hypertrophic cardiomyopathy patients: a multicenter study. Pediatr Cardiol 2013;34(7):1620–7.

27. Dechert BE, Bradley DJ, Serwer GA, et al. Implantable Cardioverter Defibrillator Outcomes in Pediatric and Congenital Heart Disease: Time to System Revision. Pacing Clin Electrophysiol 2016;39(7):703–8.

28. O'Mahony C, Lambiase PD, Quarta G, et al. The long-term survival and the risks and benefits of implantable cardioverter defibrillators in patients with hypertrophic cardiomyopathy. Heart 2012; 98(2):116–25.

29. Norrish G, Cantarutti N, Pissaridou E, et al. Risk factors for sudden cardiac death in childhood hypertrophic cardiomyopathy: A systematic review and meta-analysis. Eur J Prev Cardiol 2017;24(11):1220–30.

30. Ziolkowska L, Turska-Kmiec A, Petryka J, et al. Predictors of Long-Term Outcome in Children with Hypertrophic Cardiomyopathy. Pediatr Cardiol 2016; 37(3):448–58.

31. Maskatia SA, Decker JA, Spinner JA, et al. Restrictive physiology is associated with poor outcomes in children with hypertrophic cardiomyopathy. Pediatr Cardiol 2012;33(1):141–9.

32. Balaji S, DiLorenzo MP, Fish FA, et al. Risk factors for lethal arrhythmic events in children and adolescents with hypertrophic cardiomyopathy and an implantable defibrillator: An international multicenter study. Heart Rhythm 2019;16(10):1462–7.

33. Alexander PMA, Nugent AW, Daubeney PEF, et al. Long-Term Outcomes of Hypertrophic Cardiomyopathy Diagnosed During Childhood: Results From a National Population-Based Study. Circulation 2018; 138(1):29–36.

34. Ostman-Smith I, Wettrell G, Keeton B, et al. Echocardiographic and electrocardiographic identification of those children with hypertrophic cardiomyopathy who should be considered at high-risk of dying suddenly. Cardiol Young 2005;15(6):632–42.

35. Ostman-Smith I, Sjoberg G, Rydberg A, et al. Predictors of risk for sudden death in childhood hypertrophic cardiomyopathy: the importance of the ECG risk score. Open Heart 2017;4(2):e000658.

36. Norrish G, Topriceanu C, Qu C, et al. The role of the electrocardiographic phenotype in risk stratification for sudden cardiac death in childhood hypertrophic cardiomyopathy. Eur J Prev Cardiol 2021. https://doi.org/10.1093/eurjpc/zwab046.

37. Axelsson Raja A, Farhad H, Valente AM, et al. Prevalence and Progression of Late Gadolinium Enhancement in Children and Adolescents with Hypertrophic Cardiomyopathy. Circulation 2018; 138(8):782–92.

38. Windram JD, Benson LN, Dragelescu A, et al. Distribution of Hypertrophy and Late Gadolinium Enhancement in Children and Adolescents with Hypertrophic Cardiomyopathy. Congenit Heart Dis 2015;10(6):E258–67.

39. Smith BM, Dorfman AL, Yu S, et al. Clinical significance of late gadolinium enhancement in patients<20 years of age with hypertrophic cardiomyopathy. Am J Cardiol 2014;113(7):1234–9.

40. Mathew J, Zahavich L, Lafreniere-Roula M, et al. Utility of genetics for risk stratification in pediatric hypertrophic cardiomyopathy. Clin Genet 2018;93(2):310–9.

41. Maurizi N, Passantino S, Spaziani G, et al. Long-term Outcomes of Pediatric-Onset Hypertrophic Cardiomyopathy and Age-Specific Risk Factors for Lethal Arrhythmic Events. JAMA Cardiol 2018;3(6): 520–5.

42. O'Mahony C, Jichi F, Monserrat L, et al. Inverted U-shaped relation between the risk of sudden cardiac death and maximal left ventricular wall

thickness in hypertrophic cardiomyopathy. Circ Arrhythm Electrophysiol 2016;9(6):e003818.

43. Yetman AT, Hamilton RM, Benson LN, et al. Long-term outcome and prognostic determinants in children with hypertrophic cardiomyopathy. J Am Coll Cardiol 1998;32(7):1943–50.

44. Spirito P, Autore C, Rapezzi C, et al. Syncope and risk of sudden death in hypertrophic cardiomyopathy. Circulation 2009;119(13):1703–10.

45. Elliott PM, Poloniecki J, Dickie S, et al. Sudden death in hypertrophic cardiomyopathy: identification of high risk patients. J Am Coll Cardiol 2000;36(7):2212–8.

46. Norrish G, Ding T, Field E, et al. A validation study of the European Society of Cardiology guidelines for risk stratification of sudden cardiac death in childhood hypertrophic cardiomyopathy. Europace 2019;21(10):1559–65.

47. Weng Z, Yao J, Chan RH, et al. Prognostic Value of LGE-CMR in HCM: A Meta-Analysis. JACC Cardiovasc Imaging 2016;9(12):1392–402.

48. Petryka-Mazurkiewicz J, Ziolkowska L, Kowalczyk-Domagala M, et al. LGE for Risk Stratification in Primary Prevention in Children With HCM. JACC Cardiovasc Imaging 2020;13(12):2684–6.

49. Ho CY, Day SM, Ashley EA, et al. Genotype and Lifetime Burden of Disease in Hypertrophic Cardiomyopathy: Insights from the Sarcomeric Human Cardiomyopathy Registry (SHaRe). Circulation 2018;138(14):1387–98.

50. Harper AR, Goel A, Grace C, et al. Common genetic variants and modifiable risk factors underpin hypertrophic cardiomyopathy susceptibility and expressivity. Nat Genet 2021;53(2):135–42.

51. Calcagni G, Limongelli G, D'Ambrosio A, et al. Cardiac defects, morbidity and mortality in patients affected by RASopathies. CARNET study results. Int J Cardiol 2017;245:92–8.

52. Limongelli G, Sarkozy A, Pacileo G, et al. Genotype-phenotype analysis and natural history of left ventricular hypertrophy in LEOPARD syndrome. Am J Med Genet A 2008;146A(5):620–8.

Hypertrophic Cardiomyopathy in RASopathies
Diagnosis, Clinical Characteristics, Prognostic Implications, and Management

Michele Lioncino, MD[a], Emanuele Monda, MD[a], Federica Verrillo, MD[a],
Elisabetta Moscarella, MD, PhD[a,b], Giulio Calcagni, MD, PhD[c,d],
Fabrizio Drago, MD[c,d], Bruno Marino, MD, PhD[e], Maria Cristina Digilio, MD[f],
Carolina Putotto, MD, PhD[e], Paolo Calabrò, MD, PhD[a,b],
Maria Giovanna Russo, MD, PhD[a,g], Amy E. Roberts, MD, PhD[h],
Bruce D. Gelb, MD, PhD[i], Marco Tartaglia, PhD[f],
Giuseppe Limongelli, MD, PhD[a,b],*

KEYWORDS

- RASopathies • Noonan • Hypertrophic cardiomyopathy • Costello • Cardio-facio.cutaneous
- LEOPARD

KEY POINTS

- RASopathies are developmental multisystemic disorders caused by germline mutation in genes linked to the RAS/mitogen-activated protein kinase pathway.
- Hypertrophic cardiomyopathy is the second most common cardiovascular manifestation in RASopathies and exhibits unique features such as the coexistence of congenital heart disease and early-onset congestive heart failure and accounts for significant mortality rates.
- Diagnosis of a RASopathy could be suggested by clinical clues ("red flags"), which could raise the suspicion of an underlying malformation syndrome and direct the clinician toward a specific genetic test.

INTRODUCTION

RASopathies are a group of developmental multisystemic disorders caused by germline mutations in genes encoding signal transducers and regulatory proteins functionally linked to the RAS/mitogen-activated protein kinase (MAPK) pathway. Collectively, these disorders have an estimated prevalence of 1 in 1000 to 1 in 2500[1] among live births.

According to a large clinical registry,[2] RASopathies may represent the underlying diagnosis in ~18% of childhood hypertrophic cardiomyopathy

[a] Department of Translational Medical Sciences, University of Campania "Luigi Vanvitelli", Naples; [b] Division of Cardiology, A.O.R.N. "Sant'Anna & San Sebastiano", Caserta I-81100, Italy; [c] The European Reference Network for Rare, Low Prevalence and Complex Diseases of the Heart - ERN GUARD-Heart; [d] Pediatric Cardiology and Arrhythmia/Syncope Units, Bambino Gesù Children's Hospital IRCSS, Rome, Italy; [e] Department of Pediatrics, Sapienza University of Rome, Rome, Italy; [f] Genetics and Rare Disease Research Division, Bambino Gesù Children's Hospital, IRCCS, Rome, Italy; [g] Department of Pediatric Cardiology, AORN dei Colli, Monaldi Hospital, Naples; [h] Department of Cardiology, Children's Hospital Boston, Boston, MA, USA; [i] Department of Pediatrics, Icahn School of Medicine at Mount Sinai, New York, NY, USA
* Corresponding author. Department of Translational Medical Sciences, University of Campania "Luigi Vanvitelli", Naples.
E-mail address: limongelligiuseppe@libero.it

Heart Failure Clin 18 (2022) 19–29
https://doi.org/10.1016/j.hfc.2021.07.004
1551-7136/22/© 2021 Elsevier Inc. All rights reserved.

Table 1
Clinical red flags for RASopathies

Facial features	NS: broad forehead, down slanting palpebral fissures, hypertelorism, low set ears, pterygium colli, epicanthal folds, short and depressed nasal root CS: hypertelorism, down slanting palpebral fissures. Facial features are coarser. Feeding and suction difficulties are more prevalent. CFCS: macrocephaly, bitemporal narrowing, coarse facial features, small curly friable hair with sparse eyebrows with hyperkeratosis (ulerythema ophryogenes), broad nasal base, wide labial philtrum. Coarser than NS
Cardiovascular	Pulmonary valve stenosis, hypertrophic cardiomyopathy, mitral valve dysplasia, atrial septal defect, ventricular septal defect, atrioventricular septal defect, aortic coarctation, coronary arteries abnormalities
Electrocardiography	Extreme right-axis deviation (north west axis), left or right bundle branch block (NSML), prolonged QT (NSML), repolarization abnormalities, multifocal atrial tachyarrhythmia (CS)
Musculoskeletal	Short stature, hypotonia (CFCS), Pes planus (CFCS), scoliosis, pectus deformity, hip dysplasia, osteopenia/osteoporosis
Dermatologic	Cafè-au-lait spots, papillomas (CS), palmar keratoderma, acanthosis nigricans, keratosis pilaris (CFC), ulerythema ophryogenes (CFC), lentigines (NSML), multiple pigmented nevi
Genitourinary	Cryptorchidism, transitional cell carcinoma of the urinary bladder (CS)
Hematopoietic	Easy bruising, von Willebrand disease, coagulation defects, thrombocytopenia, NS/myeloproliferative disease (leukocytosis with monocytosis, thrombocytopenia, and hepatosplenomegaly)
Gastrointestinal	Failure to thrive, gastroesophageal reflux, intestinal malrotation, pyloric stenosis
Sensorineural	Hearing loss, laryngomalacia, cataract, strabismus
Neurologic	Seizures, infantile spasms, hydrocephalus, Chiari I malformation, intellectual disability
Endocrine	Growth hormone deficiency, hypoglycemia, delayed puberal spurt, short stature
Oncology	Juvenile myelomonocytic leukemia, lymphedema

Abbreviations: CFCS, cardiofaciocutaneous syndrome; CS, Costello syndrome; HCM, hypertrophic cardiomyopathy; NS, Noonan syndrome.

(HCM), particularly among infants younger than 1 year, where they account for ~42% of the cases.

The disorders constituting the RASopathies include Noonan syndrome (NS), NS with multiple lentigines (NSML, previously known as LEOPARD syndrome), cardiofaciocutaneous syndrome (CFCS), Mazzanti syndrome (also known as NS-like disorder with loose anagen hair), Costello syndrome (CS), type 1 neurofibromatosis, and Legius syndrome which are well recognized and clinically characterized[3]; however, other clinically related conditions are emerging.[4]

Although each RASopathy exhibits a unique clinical phenotype, these syndromes share many overlapping characteristics, including growth retardation, craniofacial features, cryptorchidism, cognitive deficits, renal malformations, bleeding disorders, variable predisposition to certain cancers, and congenital heart disease (CHD).[5–8] Diagnosis of a RASopathy could be suggested by clinical clues ("red flags"),[9] which could raise the suspicion of an underlying malformation syndrome and direct the clinician toward a specific genetic test (**Table 1**).

It should be noted that the extent of clinical variability characterizing each RASopathy is strictly related to the extent of molecular variability and heterogeneity of these disorders. For example, NS, which is the most common disorder among the RASopathies. This disease is caused by mutations in more than 10 genes (ie, *PTPN11*, *SOS1*, *SOS2*, *NRAS*, *KRAS*, *MRAS*, *RRAS2*, *RIT1*, *LZTR1*, *RAF1*, *MAP2K1*), which are preferentially associated with certain features, including proper growth and cognition (*SOS1*, *SOS2*), high prevalence of pulmonary stenosis (PS) (*PTPN11*), or HCM (eg, *RAF1*, *MRAS*, and *RIT1*).[4,10–15] On the contrary, other RASopathies are relatively homogeneous, being caused by a narrow spectrum of mutations in single genes, as in the case of CS and Mazzanti syndrome, which are caused by a bunch of mutations in *HRAS* and *SHOC2*, respectively.[3]

HYPERTROPHIC CARDIOMYOPATHY IN RASopathies

After CHD, HCM is the second most common cardiovascular abnormality observed in RASopathies,[2,16–22] with worse clinical outcomes when associated with early onset presentation.

Compared with sarcomeric forms (S-HCM), HCM in RASopathies (R-HCM) shows increased prevalence and severity of left ventricular outflow tract obstruction (LVOTO)[17,19,20,23] and higher rates of hospitalizations for heart failure or need for septal myectomy during childhood.[23] R-HCM presents earlier in infancy, with a mean age at diagnosis of 6 months, whereas S-HCM mostly presents during adolescence.[24] Congestive heart failure (CHF) is significantly more common in R-HCM (24% vs 9%)[25] and accounts for a substantial early mortality. Patients affected by RASopathies are more likely to require heart failure hospitalizations or cardiovascular interventions,[23] mainly septal myectomies and pulmonary valvuloplasties.[26–28]

In 5% to 10% of the cases, R-HCM is associated to a severe clinical presentation, particularly for infants with signs of heart failure, with a 70% one-year mortality. With the exception of these cases, clinical status tends to improve over time, and progression of left ventricular hypertrophy (LVH), described in S-HCM, seems uncommon in R-HCM.[23,29] On the contrary, left ventricular reverse remodeling with regression of myocardial wall thickness z-scores over time on serial echocardiography has been reported in many clinical studies.[23,26,28]

LVOTO is common among patients with RASopathies, and its prevalence may be due to the contribution of other cardiovascular abnormalities such as displacement of papillary muscles, anomalous insertion of mitral chordae, or fibrous tissue causing midventricular obstruction.[7,30,31] Mitral valve disease has been considered a marker of complexity in patients with HCM and may carry a negative prognosis, being associated with reintervention and mortality.[32] In particular, compared with age- and sex-matched healthy controls, the length of the anterior leaflet of mitral valve is significantly increased in patients with R-HCM[30]; moreover, anterior displacement of the papillary muscles may cause distortion of the subvalvular apparatus.

Biventricular hypertrophy may represent a useful clinical clue ("red flag") for the suspicion of

R-HCM,[33] and its presence may indicate the co-occurrence of right ventricular outflow tract obstruction. The prevalence of PS ranges between ~25% and 70% in this subgroup of patients: The pulmonary valve is often dysplastic and shows signs of commissural fusion.[27,34] In particular, PS is severe in ~30% of the cases and moderate in ~10%. Patients with mild PS are unlikely to require intervention, and their natural history is similar to that of patients without PS.[28,35] In contrast, patients with moderate-to-severe PS often require percutaneous balloon valvuloplasty, but due to valvular dysplasia, the outcomes may be unfavorable, with high rates of reintervention.[26,36]

Beyond PS, which is observed in up to 65% of the patients, other CHDs commonly occur among patients with RASopathies: "Secundum atrial septal defect" (ASD) has been observed in ~8% to 30% of the cases,[11,26–28,31,37–39] as well as ventricular septal defect (VSD) (~5%–10%)[19,26,27,31,40] and atrioventricular canal defect (AVCD) (up to 15% of the cases). The association with AVCD is of pivotal importance: Mitral valve abnormalities (such as double orifice and parachute mitral valves) have a significant association with AVCD. Moreover, cranial displacement of the aortic valve anulus relative to the ventricular apex, which determines the so-called "gooseneck" deformity, may contribute to LVOTO.[39,41,42] Complete AVCD is uncommon in RASopathies, and morphologic data are insufficient to define whether a specific AVC subtype, according to the Rastelli classification, is more prevalent.

Left-sided obstructive lesions are rare in RASopathies, although aortic stenosis, coarctation of the aorta, and isolated MV stenosis have been reported in the setting of NS.[43–45]

Coronary artery abnormalities are a relevant finding in RASopathies and may contribute to cause myocardial ischemia and worsen the imbalance between myocardial oxygen supply and demand. According to a registry,[31] aneurysms in coronary arteries have been identified in ~15% of the cases, invariably involving left coronary artery but independently from a specific pathogenic variant.[46] Long-term outcomes of coronary dilatation are not completely understood: As coronary artery aneurysms have been associated to atherothrombosis, the role of antiplatelet drugs in primary prevention of myocardial infarction is debated, and no specific recommendation can be made.[47]

Although HCM, AVCD, and PS have been considered classic cardiovascular defects in the setting of RASopathies, recent data coming from a multicenter retrospective study seem to report

Table 2
Clinical manifestations, mutated genes, and classical heart defects with their relative prevalence among RASopathies and relative prevalence of hypertrophic cardiomyopathy

Gene	Clinical Features	HCM
Noonan syndrome		
PTPN11	PVS (65%), atrioventricular septal defects (18%), ASD (10%), VSD (9%), PDA (6%), mitral valve abnormalities (2.5%), Tetralogy of Fallot (<1%), aortic coarctation (<1%)	HCM (20%)
SOS1	PVS (70%), ASD (14.5%), mitral valve abnormalities (4%)	HCM (18%)
RAF1	PVS (21%), ASD (20%), mitral valve abnormalities (13%), Tetralogy of Fallot (2.8%), aortic coarctation (1.8%)	HCM (65%)
RIT1	PVS (74%), ASD (30%), PDA (7%), mitral valve abnormalities (13%), biventricular obstruction (<1%)	HCM (36%)
SHOC2	PVS (32%), ASD (32%), mitral valve abnormalities (27%), VSD (13%)	HCM (30%)
NRAS	PVS (14%)	HCM (39%)
CBL	PVS (50%), ASD (10%), mitral valve abnormalities (10%)	HCM (10%)
Noonan syndrome with multiple lentigines		
PTPN11	Biventricular hypertrophy (46%), LVOTO (40%), ventricular tachycardia, conduction abnormalities, mitral valve abnormalities (42%), PVS (21%), ASD (6%), atrioventricular septal defects, coronary artery abnormalities	HCM (85%)
RAF1	Mitral valve abnormalities (100%), PVS (40%), high risk of SCD	HCM (100%)
BRAF	-	HCM (60%–85%)
Costello syndrome		
HRAS	Atrial tachycardia (56%), PVS	HCM (65%)
Cardiofaciocutaneous syndrome		
BRAF1	PVS (45%), ASD (30%), VSD (8%). Tetralogy of Fallot (7%)	HCM (40%)
MAP2K1-MAP2K2	PVS (65%–100%), septal defects (15%)	HCM (40%)
KRAS	PVS (40%), mitral valve abnormalities (26%), ASD (20%), VSD (13%)	HCM (20%)

Abbreviations: ASD, atrial septal defect; HCM, hypertrophic cardiomyopathy; PDA, patent ductus arteriosus; PVS, pulmonary valve stenosis; VSD, ventricular septal defect.

a high prevalence of primary mitral regurgitation (24%, 4%) and aortic insufficiency (25%) or structural abnormalities of the ascending aorta, including kinking and aortic root dilatation.[31]

The summary of cardiovascular manifestations, involved genes, and their relative prevalence among RASopathies is shown in **Table 2**. The proposed algorithm for the diagnosis and management of R-HCM is shown in **Fig. 1**.

Hypertrophic Cardiomyopathy in Noonan Syndrome with Multiple Lentigines

HCM is present in ~85% of the patients affected by NSML, among the highest rate among RASopathies. LVOTO may be associated to NSML in up to 40% of the cases, and biventricular hypertrophy is reported in nearly half of the patients. HCM is often diagnosed in early infancy, and the clinical phenotype almost invariably manifests before the appearance of the lentigines.[19] Interestingly, patients with severe biventricular involvement often show high mortality rates, compared with mild asymptomatic cases, who have relatively benign clinical outcomes and frequent regression of LVH.[27,48] Electrocardiographic abnormalities and progressive conduction abnormalities often coexist with HCM: In particular, a superiorly oriented QRS axis even in the absence of biventricular involvement, pseudo-infarction q waves, and prolonged corrected QT interval have been observed among NSML patients.[19] A possible limitation in the existing study outcomes among

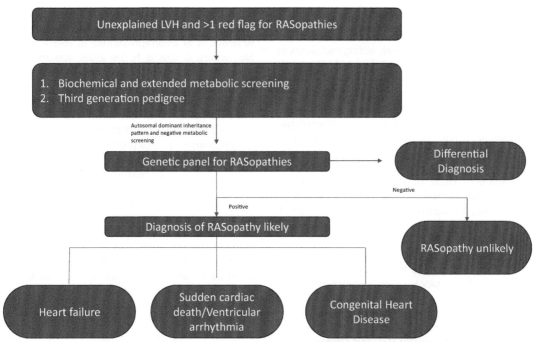

Fig. 1. Proposed algorithm for the diagnosis and management of RASopathy-associated HCM (R-HCM).

patients with NSML is that, in some studies, diagnosis is based on clinical criteria without genotype corroboration. Of note, differentiating NSML from NS can be challenging, particularly in infants, for whom the prevalence of cutaneous manifestations is incomplete, and lentigines are not present.[24] NSML is caused by a narrow spectrum of dominantly acting mutations in *PTPN11*. Many clinically relevant genotype-phenotype correlations should be considered: Patients harboring missense RASopathy variants in *BRAF*, *LZTR1*, *RAF1*, and *RIT1* show an increased prevalence of LVH compared with carriers of *PTPN11* pathogenic variants. In addition, some authors have reported worse HF and arrhythmic outcomes in a subgroup of patients harboring the missense Gln510Glu allele (*PTPN11*, exon 13).[16] Interestingly, the molecular spectrum of NSML-causing *PTPN11* mutations does not overlap the pattern of mutations observed in NS, and the biochemical behavior of these two classes of mutations is completely different, with the former impairing the catalytic activity of SHP2, the protein encoded by *PTPN11*, and the latter promoting enhanced activation of the phosphatase[49–51]

Hypertrophic Cardiomyopathy in Costello Syndrome

Among patients diagnosed with CS, approximately 65% fulfills diagnostic criteria for HCM: In this subgroup, the coexistence with CHD is reported in ~40% of the cases, and 60% may have LVOTO. Most patients seem to show subaortic septal thickening, although other patterns, such as biventricular or concentric hypertrophy, have been reported.[52] The natural history of HCM in CS is variable, with a documented rate of progression in ~40% of the cases. Of note, a significant number of patients with severe HCM underwent septal myectomy (25%). Regression of LVH has been reported in 10% of the patients, although data reported do not allow the establishment of genotype-phenotype correlations.[18,24,52,53] The comparison between the two commonest alleles for the *HRAS* gene (pG12S and pG13 C) with a pathogenic role in CS has shown no significant difference in the prevalence of HCM.[54] Severe cardiomyopathy, associated with pleural and pericardial effusion as well as lung abnormalities has been observed in carriers of G12 C and G12D alleles.[55] Atrial tachyarrhythmias are seen in more than 50% of the patients affected by CS, particularly non-reentrant atrial tachycardia and multifocal or ectopic atrial tachycardia.[56] The natural history of atrial arrhythmias is usually benign in CS, with spontaneous regression within the first year of life and responsiveness to medical therapy, whereas ventricular arrhythmias are rare. Later-onset atrial fibrillation and atrial flutter have been reported, but their prognostic significance is unknown.[57]

Hypertrophic Cardiomyopathy in Cardiofaciocutaneous Syndrome

CFCS is caused by dominantly acting mutations in *BRAF*, *MAP2K1*, and *MAP2K2*. Nearly 75% of children with CFC have cardiovascular involvement, mainly PS, which can be diagnosed in 45% of the cases. HCM can be identified in ~40% of patients during infancy,[6] with a variable phenotype, sometimes rapidly progressive and resulting in heart transplantation or death and, in other cases, with a mild phenotypic expression.[6] Of note, the prevalence of HCM is not significantly different among patients who carry *BRAF* pathogenic variant mutation compared with carriers of MEK1 or MEK2 alleles.[58,59] The most common coexisting forms of CHD are ASD (8%–18%) and VSD (11%–22%).[60,61] Although uncommon in CFCS, arrhythmias can include ventricular preexcitation, atrioventricular block, or supraventricular tachycardia.[59]

Hypertrophic Cardiomyopathy in Noonan Syndrome and Clinically Related Disorders

Among RASopathies, HCM seems less common in NS, with a reported prevalence of ~20% among affected individuals. Interestingly patients with Mazzanti syndrome and harboring a recurrent missense substitution in *SHOC2* seem to have a slightly higher prevalence of HCM (25%).[62] Three independent studies reported that germline variants in *CBL* underlie a clinical syndrome with many overlapping features with NS, although HCM seems not to be associated to this condition.[63–65] Among children with NS and HCM, asymmetrical septal hypertrophy is the most common presentation (75.6%), whereas apical involvement is rare.[66] A 12-lead electrocardiogram can show extreme right heart deviation ("north west axis"), reflecting biventricular involvement.[33] Genotype characterization can offer useful diagnostic clues in the management of NS-associated HCM. In particular, among patients harboring *PTPN11* variants, the prevalence of HCM is low, whereas individuals affected by NS with causal variants in *RAF1* and *RIT1* are more likely to develop HCM.[24]

PATHOPHYSIOLOGY OF HYPERTROPHIC CARDIOMYOPATHY IN RASopathies

Different signaling pathways seem to be involved in the molecular pathogenesis of HCM in RASopathies. Almost 50% of the cases of NS are caused by missense gain-of-function mutations in *PTPN11*, which typically cluster around the phosphotyrosine phosphatase domains of SHP2, causing constitutive activation of the protein.[67]

Interestingly, HCM is underrepresented in patients harboring missense changes in *PTPN11* or *SOS1*, whereas it is overrepresented is *RAF1*-mutated NS, where it seems to be allele-specific.[14,68] A distinct class of variants in *PTPN11* was associated to NSML, which carries a higher lifetime risk of HCM.[49] While NS-causing variants may promote upregulation of RAS/MAPK cascade, alleles involved in NSML should be considered as dominant negative mutants promoting enhanced signal flow through the PI3K-AKT-mTOR pathway. In a murine model of NS bearing the p.L613 V mutation in the *Raf1* gene, increased RAS/MAPK signaling was observed both in fibroblasts and in neonatal cardiomyocytes. Consistent with that observation, treatment with an MEK inhibitor seemed to induce positive reverse remodeling in *Raf1*[L613V] mice.[69] Treatment with trametinib, an MEK inhibitor, has been associated to reversal of LVH and LVOTO in two cases of *RIT1*-mutated NS within 4 months after initiation of the therapy. Remodeling was associated with a favorable clinical response and a catch-up in somatic growth, which may be attributable to recovery from severe HF.[70] In contrast, a mouse model of NSML bearing the p.Y279 C mutation in the *Ptpn11* gene showed impaired ligand-evoked ERK phosphorylation and increased signal flow through the PI3K-AKT-mTOR pathway. Treatment with rapamycin, an mTOR inhibitor, rescued the cardiac phenotype in *Ptpn11*[Y279C] mice.[71] In the last years, everolimus was used to prevent CHF in patients with severe HCM, but regression of LVH was not documented.[48]

PROGNOSTIC IMPLICATIONS OF HYPERTROPHIC CARDIOMYOPATHY IN RASopathies

The diagnosis of HCM significantly affects the outcome in patients affected by NS: Long-term studies have demonstrated that severity of cardiovascular involvement is associated with a lower survival rate, with higher risk of death in patients younger than 2 years and adolescents. Specific risk factors for early mortality include evidence of HF during the first 6 months of life, low cardiac output, significant diastolic disfunction, and several cardiac interventions.[7,25]

Taken together, the outcomes of children affected by R-HCM seem to reflect a distinct disease course compared with carriers of sarcomere pathogenic variants: Patients with R-HCM can be severely affected during the perinatal and infancy periods, are more likely to require septal myectomy or pulmonary balloon valvuloplasty, and lack the typical progression of LVH during adolescence and young age.[23,28]

Histopathologic studies have demonstrated that patients with R-HCM had a similar amount of quantified fibrosis compared with nonsyndromic familial HCM caused by sarcomere protein mutations. Of note, fibrotic changes are already present in an early phase of disease, in contrast to S-HCM, in which myocardial disarray and fibrosis develop over time.[23]

Apical aneurysms have been described in R-HCM, nonetheless their overall prevalence and clinical significance have not been assessed yet.[72]

HCM is the main cause of sudden cardiac death (SCD) among adolescents and young adults.[73] Among patients with R-HCM, sustained ventricular tachycardia (VT) is frequent and related to the risk of SCD.[74–76] Although the overall risk of SCD appears lower than that in HCM caused by sarcomere mutations, disease-specific risk factors are currently an area of debate.[23,28] A previous history of VT or cardiac arrest, unexplained syncope, nonsustained VT, or massive LVH has been associated with higher risk of SCD and may require Implantable cardioverter defibrillator implantation.[73] However, the weight of isolated risk factors, irrespective of their magnitude (ie, massive LVH), is not clear, and the risk could be higher when many risk factors coexist in the same patient. Interestingly, other conventional risk factors such as age, family history of SCD, and left atrial z score should be evaluated carefully in children, whereas LVOT gradient seems not associated to SCD.[77] Recently, two scores have been validated for risk stratification in pediatric patients.[77,78]

MANAGEMENT AND FUTURE PERSPECTIVES

Medical therapy remains the first-line option in patients with R-HCM. Nonvasodilating beta blockers should be titrated to the maximum tolerated dose in patients, and diuretic dose should be accurately set to reduce congestive status and HF symptoms, while avoiding hypovolemia, which could increase LVOTO. When beta blockers are ineffective or not tolerated, nonvasodilating calcium channel blockers could be administered in children older than 6 months. Of note, there are several reports of severe bradycardia and HF worsening in infants with LVOT gradients greater than 100 mm Hg, suggesting that verapamil could be harmful in this clinical setting.[79,80]

In patients who remain symptomatic despite beta-blockers, disopyramide could be a therapeutic option to reduce obstruction. Recently, mavacamten has shown to improve functional status in S-HCM, nevertheless further studies are needed to assess its role in nonsarcomeric variants. Surgical myectomy may be considered in patients who remain symptomatic for significant LVOTO despite maximal medical therapy and should be performed in specialized centers with high-volume experience.[81,82] Orthotopic heart transplantation (OHT) is rarely performed in patients with NS,[83] although it should be considered in patients with severe HF symptoms with evidence of refractoriness to medical therapy, intractable ventricular arrhythmias, cardiogenic shock requiring inotropes, and in case of severe diastolic dysfunction.[84,85] Early multiorgan damage should not be considered a contraindication for heart transplantation, but careful evaluation of absolute contraindication is required, to exclude the risk of futility in case of moderate or severe end organ dysfunction.[86] According to the Pediatric Cardiomyopathy Registry,[87,88] cumulative waitlist mortality was significantly high in infants affected by HCM, suggesting a malignant course of disease and the presence of comorbidities in critically ill infants. Poorer outcomes were observed in patients listed for priority in status 1 or younger than 1 year than in older children and patients listed in status 2.[89] Therefore, OHT should be considered as early as possible and before clinical deterioration in patients with R-HCM.

Proof of concept that inhibition of the RAS/MAPK cascade could induce regression of LVH and cardiac remodeling in patients affected by RASopathies has been achieved by clinical evaluation of trametinib, an MEK inhibitor, in two patients with RIT1-induced NS, with significant regression of LVH within 4 months after initiation of treatment.[70] On the contrary, among children with NSML with germline loss-of-function variation in PTPN11, the overactivation in PI3K-AKT-mTOR pathway was partially reversed with the use of rapamycin.[48,71] The design of therapeutic trials is challenging in patients with RASopathies because of the rarity of disease, patient variability in disease progression and regression, and the heterogeneity of molecular mechanisms.[90] Possible future treatment candidates may include farnesil transferase inhibitors, pan-RAF inhibitors, SHP2 inhibitors, and, because copper is required for catalytic activity of MEK kinases, chelation with ammonium tetrathiomolybdate.

CLINICS CARE POINTS

- RASopathy should be suspected in infants (<1 year) with new-onset HCM and clinical red flags.
- Patients affected by RASopathies are more likely to require HF hospitalizations or cardiovascular interventions.

- In 5% to 10% of the cases, R-HCM is associated to a severe clinical presentation, particularly for infants with signs of heart failure.
- The prevalence of pulmonary stenosis (PS) ranges between ~25% and 70% in this subgroup of patients.
- Other CHDs commonly occur among patients with RASopathies: "secundum atrial septal defect", as well as ventricular septal defect, atrioventricular canal defect (AVCD), mitral valve abnormalities, coronary arteries abnormalities, and left-sided obstructive lesions.
- In selected cases, rapamycin or MEK1 inhibitors may promote regression of left ventricular hypertrophy and should be considered as a therapeutic option.

ACKNOWLEDGMENTS

The authors would like to acknowledge Michela Piscopo, Daniela Lafera, and Ciro De Prisco who made possible our research and clinical activity.

DISCLOSURE

The authors declare that they have no conflict of interest.

REFERENCES

1. Mendez HMM, Opitz JM. Noonan syndrome: A review. Am J Med Genet 1985;21(3):493–506.
2. Norrish G, Field E, Mcleod K, et al. Clinical presentation and survival of childhood hypertrophic cardiomyopathy: a retrospective study in United Kingdom. Eur Heart J 2019;40(12):986–93.
3. Tartaglia M, Gelb BD, Zenker M. Noonan syndrome and clinically related disorders. Best Pract Res Clin Endocrinol Metab 2011;25(1):161–79.
4. Motta M, Pannone L, Pantaleoni F, et al. Enhanced MAPK1 Function Causes a Neurodevelopmental Disorder within the RASopathy Clinical Spectrum. Am J Hum Genet 2020;107(3):499–513.
5. Hennekam RCM. Costello syndrome: An overview. Am J Med Genet C Semin Med Genet 2003;117 C(1):42–8.
6. Pierpont MEM, Magoulas PL, Adi S, et al. Cardio-facio-cutaneous syndrome: clinical features, diagnosis, and management guidelines. Pediatrics 2014;134(4):e1149–62.
7. Calcagni G, Limongelli G, D'Ambrosio A, et al. Cardiac defects, morbidity and mortality in patients affected by RASopathies. CARNET study results. Int J Cardiol 2017;245:92–8.
8. Roberts AE, Allanson JE, Tartaglia M, et al. Noonan syndrome. Lancet 2013;381(9863):333–42.
9. Limongelli G, Monda E, Tramonte S, et al. Prevalence and clinical significance of red flags in patients with hypertrophic cardiomyopathy. Int J Cardiol 2020;299:186–91.
10. Tartaglia M, Pennacchio LA, Zhao C, et al. Gain-of-function SOS1 mutations cause a distinctive form of Noonan syndrome. Nat Genet 2007;39(1):75–9.
11. Tartaglia M, Kalidas K, Shaw A, et al. PTPN11 mutations in noonan syndrome: Molecular spectrum, genotype-phenotype correlation, and phenotypic heterogeneity. Am J Hum Genet 2002;70(6):1555–63.
12. Lepri F, De Luca A, Stella L, et al. SOS1 mutations in Noonan syndrome: Molecular spectrum, structural insights on pathogenic effects, and genotype-phenotype correlations. Hum Mutat 2011;32(7):760–72.
13. Cordeddu V, Yin JC, Gunnarsson C, et al. Activating Mutations Affecting the Dbl Homology Domain of SOS2 Cause Noonan Syndrome. Hum Mutat 2015;36(11):1080–7.
14. Pandit B, Sarkozy A, Pennacchio LA, et al. Gain-of-function RAF1 mutations cause Noonan and LEOPARD syndromes with hypertrophic cardiomyopathy. Nat Genet 2007;39(8):1007–12.
15. Yaoita M, Niihori T, Mizuno S, et al. Spectrum of mutations and genotype–phenotype analysis in Noonan syndrome patients with RIT1 mutations. Hum Genet 2016;135(2):209–22.
16. Limongelli G, Sarkozy A, Pacileo G, et al. Genotype-phenotype analysis and natural history of left ventricular hypertrophy in LEOPARD syndrome. Am J Med Genet A 2008;146(5):620–8.
17. Cerrato F, Pacileo G, Limongelli G, et al. A standard echocardiographic and tissue Doppler study of morphological and functional findings in children with hypertrophic cardiomyopathy compared to those with left ventricular hypertrophy in the setting of Noonan and LEOPARD syndromes. Cardiol Young 2008;18(6):575–80.
18. Gripp KW, Lin AE. Costello syndrome: A Ras/mitogen activated protein kinase pathway syndrome (rasopathy) resulting from HRAS germline mutations. Genet Med 2012;14(3):285–92.
19. Sarkozy A, Digilio MC, Dallapiccola B. Leopard syndrome. Orphanet J Rare Dis 2008;3(1). https://doi.org/10.1186/1750-1172-3-13.
20. Calcagni G, Adorisio R, Martinelli S, et al. Clinical Presentation and Natural History of Hypertrophic Cardiomyopathy in RASopathies. Heart Fail Clin 2018;14(2):225–35.
21. Monda E, Rubino M, Lioncino M, et al. Hypertrophic Cardiomyopathy in Children: Pathophysiology, Diagnosis, and Treatment of Non-sarcomeric Causes. Front Pediatr 2021;9:632293.
22. Caiazza M, Rubino M, Monda E, et al. Combined ptpn11 and mybpc3 gene mutations in an adult

patient with noonan syndrome and hypertrophic cardiomyopathy. Genes (Basel) 2020;11(8):1–6.

23. Kaltenecker E, Schleihauf J, Meierhofer C, et al. Long-term outcomes of childhood onset Noonan compared to sarcomere hypertrophic cardiomyopathy. Cardiovasc Diagn Ther 2019;9(S2):S299–309.

24. Gelb BD, Roberts AE, Tartaglia M. Cardiomyopathies in Noonan syndrome and the other RASopathies. Prog Pediatr Cardiol 2015;39(1):13–9.

25. Wilkinson JD, Lowe AM, Salbert BA, et al. Outcomes in children with Noonan syndrome and hypertrophic cardiomyopathy: A study from the Pediatric Cardiomyopathy Registry. Am Heart J 2012;164(3):442–8.

26. Prendiville TW, Gauvreau K, Tworog-Dube E, et al. Cardiovascular disease in Noonan syndrome. Arch Dis Child 2014;99(7):629–34.

27. Linglart L, Gelb BD. Congenital heart defects in Noonan syndrome: Diagnosis, management, and treatment. Am J Med Genet C Semin Med Genet 2020;184(1):73–80.

28. Colquitt JL, Noonan JA. Cardiac Findings in Noonan Syndrome on Long-term Follow-up. Congenit Heart Dis 2014;9(2):144–50.

29. Maron BJ, Tajik AJ, Ruttenberg HD, et al. Hypertrophic cardiomyopathy in infants: Clinical features and natural history. Circulation 1982;65(1 I):7–17.

30. Maron MS, Olivotto I, Harrigan C, et al. Mitral valve abnormalities identified by cardiovascular magnetic resonance represent a primary phenotypic expression of hypertrophic cardiomyopathy. Circulation 2011;124(1):40–7.

31. Calcagni G, Gagliostro G, Limongelli G, et al. Atypical cardiac defects in patients with RASopathies: Updated data on CARNET study. Birth Defects Res 2020;112(10):725–31.

32. Marino B, Gagliardi MG, Digilio MC, et al. Noonan syndrome: Structural abnormalities of the mitral valve causing subaortic obstruction. Eur J Pediatr 1995;154(12):949–52.

33. Rapezzi C, Arbustini E, Caforio ALP, et al. Diagnostic work-up in cardiomyopathies: bridging the gap between clinical phenotypes and final diagnosis. A position statement from the ESC Working Group on Myocardial and Pericardial Diseases. Eur Heart J 2013;34(19):1448–58.

34. Pierpont ME, Digilio MC. Cardiovascular disease in Noonan syndrome. Curr Opin Pediatr 2018;30(5):601–8.

35. Shaw AC, Kalidas K, Crosby AH, et al. The natural history of Noonan syndrome: A long-term follow-up study. Arch Dis Child 2007;92(2):128–32.

36. Holzmann J, Tibby SM, Rosenthal E, et al. Results of balloon pulmonary valvoplasty in children with Noonan's syndrome. Cardiol Young 2018;28(5):647–52.

37. Ishizawa A, Oho SI, Dodo H, et al. Cardiovascular abnormalities in Noonan syndrome: The clinical findings and treatments. Pediatr Int 1996;38(1):84–90.

38. Bertola DR, Sugayama SM, Albano LM, et al. Noonan syndrome: a clinical and genetic study of 31 patients. Rev Hosp Clin Fac Med Sao Paulo 1999;54(5):147–50.

39. Marino B, Digilio MC, Toscano A, et al. Congenital heart diseases in children with Noonan syndrome: An expanded cardiac spectrum with high prevalence of atrioventricular canal. J Pediatr 1999;135(6):703–6.

40. Zenker M, Buheitel G, Rauch R, et al. Genotype-phenotype correlations in Noonan syndrome. J Pediatr 2004;144(3):368–74.

41. Digilio MC, Romana Lepri F, Lisa Dentici M, et al. Atrioventricular canal defect in patients with RASopathies. Eur J Hum Genet 2013;21(2):200–4.

42. Pradhan AK, Pandey S, Usman K, et al. Noonan syndrome with complete atrioventricular canal defect with pulmonary stenosis. J Am Coll Cardiol 2013;62(20):1905.

43. Zmolikova M, Puchmajerova A, Hecht P, et al. Coarctation of the aorta in Noonan-like syndrome with loose anagen hair. Am J Med Genet Part A 2014;164(5):1218–21.

44. Lam J, Corno A, Oorthuys HWE, et al. Unusual combination of congenital heart lesions in a child with Noonan's syndrome. Pediatr Cardiol 1982;3(1):23–6.

45. Digilio MC, Marino B, Giannotti A, et al. Noonan syndrome with cardiac left-sided obstructive lesions. Hum Genet 1997;99(2):289.

46. Calcagni G, Baban A, De Luca E, et al. Coronary artery ectasia in Noonan syndrome: Report of an individual with SOS1 mutation and literature review. Am J Med Genet Part A 2016;170(3):665–9.

47. Kawsara A, Núñez Gil IJ, Alqahtani F, et al. Management of Coronary Artery Aneurysms. JACC Cardiovasc Interv 2018;11(13):1211–23.

48. Hahn A, Lauriol J, Thul J, et al. Rapidly progressive hypertrophic cardiomyopathy in an infant with Noonan syndrome with multiple lentigines: Palliative treatment with a rapamycin analog. Am J Med Genet Part A 2015;167(4):744–51.

49. Calcagni G, Digilio MC, Marino B, et al. Pediatric patients with RASopathy-associated hypertrophic cardiomyopathy: The multifaceted consequences of PTPN11 mutations. Orphanet J Rare Dis 2019;14(1):163.

50. Tartaglia M, Martinelli S, Stella L, et al. Diversity and functional consequences of germline and somatic PTPN11 mutations in human disease. Am J Hum Genet 2006;78(2):279–90.

51. Hanna N, Montagner A, Lee WH, et al. Reduced phosphatase activity of SHP-2 in LEOPARD syndrome: Consequences for PI3K binding on Gab1. FEBS Lett 2006;580(10):2477–82.

52. Lin AE, Alexander ME, Colan SD, et al. Clinical, pathological, and molecular analyses of cardiovascular abnormalities in Costello syndrome: A Ras/

MAPK pathway syndrome. Am J Med Genet Part A 2011;155(3):486–507.

53. Gripp KW, Rauen KA. Costello Syndrome. 1993. Available at: http://www.ncbi.nlm.nih.gov/pubmed/20301680. Accessed September 5, 2020.

54. Gripp KW, Hopkins E, Sol-Church K, et al. Phenotypic analysis of individuals with Costello syndrome due to HRAS p.G13C. Am J Med Genet Part A 2011;155(4):706–16.

55. Kerr B, Delrue MA, Sigaudy S, et al. Genotype-phenotype correlation in Costello syndrome: HRAS mutation analysis in 43 cases. J Med Genet 2006; 43(5):401–5.

56. Levin MD, Saitta SC, Gripp KW, et al. Nonreentrant atrial tachycardia occurs independently of hypertrophic cardiomyopathy in RASopathy patients. Am J Med Genet Part A 2018;176(8):1711–22.

57. Gripp KW, Morse LA, Axelrad M, et al. Costello syndrome: Clinical phenotype, genotype, and management guidelines. Am J Med Genet Part A 2019; 179(9):1725–44.

58. Abe Y, Aoki Y, Kuriyama S, et al. Prevalence and clinical features of Costello syndrome and cardio-facio-cutaneous syndrome in Japan: Findings from a nationwide epidemiological survey. Am J Med Genet Part A 2012;158 A(5):1083–94.

59. Allanson JE, Annerén G, Aoki Y, et al. Cardio-facio-cutaneous syndrome: Does genotype predict phenotype? Am J Med Genet C Semin Med Genet 2011;157(2):129–35.

60. Kavamura MI, Peres CA, Alchorne MMA, et al. CFC index for the diagnosis of cardiofaciocutaneous syndrome. Am J Med Genet 2002;112(1):12–6.

61. Armour CM, Allanson JE. Further delineation of cardio-facio-cutaneous syndrome: Clinical features of 38 individuals with proven mutations. J Med Genet 2008;45(4):249–54.

62. Mazzanti L, Cacciari E, Cicognani A, et al. Noonan-like syndrome with loose anagen hair: A new syndrome? Am J Med Genet 2003;118 A(3):279–86.

63. Martinelli S, De Luca A, Stellacci E, et al. Heterozygous germline mutations in the CBL tumor-suppressor gene cause a noonan syndrome-like phenotype. Am J Hum Genet 2010;87(2):250–7.

64. Niemeyer CM, Kang MW, Shin DH, et al. Germline CBL mutations cause developmental abnormalities and predispose to juvenile myelomonocytic Leukemia. Nat Genet 2010;42(9):641.

65. Pérez B, Mechinaud F, Galambrun C, et al. Germline mutations of the CBL gene define a new genetic syndrome with predisposition to juvenile myelomonocytic leukaemia. J Med Genet 2010;47(10): 686–91.

66. Nishikawa T, Ishiyama S, Shimojo T, et al. Hypertrophic cardiomyopathy in Noonan syndrome. Pediatr Int 1996;38(1):91–8.

67. Tartaglia M, Mehler EL, Goldberg R, et al. Mutations in PTPN11, encoding the protein tyrosine phosphatase SHP-2, cause Noonan syndrome. Nat Genet 2001;29(4):465–8.

68. Tartaglia M, Gelb BD. Disorders of dysregulated signal traffic through the RAS-MAPK pathway: Phenotypic spectrum and molecular mechanisms. Ann N Y Acad Sci 2010;1214(1):99–121.

69. Wu X, Simpson J, Hong JH, et al. MEK-ERK pathway modulation ameliorates disease phenotypes in a mouse model of Noonan syndrome associated with the Raf1L613V mutation. J Clin Invest 2011;121(3): 1009–25.

70. Andelfinger G, Marquis C, Raboisson MJ, et al. Hypertrophic Cardiomyopathy in Noonan Syndrome Treated by MEK-Inhibition. J Am Coll Cardiol 2019; 73(17):2237–9.

71. Marin TM, Keith K, Davies B, et al. Rapamycin reverses hypertrophic cardiomyopathy in a mouse model of LEOPARD syndrome-associated PTPN11 mutation. J Clin Invest 2011;121(3):1026–43.

72. Hudsmith LE, Petersen SE, Francis JM, et al. Hypertrophic cardiomyopathy in Noonan syndrome closely mimics familial hypertrophic cardiomyopathy due to sarcomeric mutations. Int J Cardiovasc Imaging 2006;22(3–4):493–5.

73. Ommen SR, Mital S, Burke MA, et al. 2020 AHA/ACC Guideline for the Diagnosis and Treatment of Patients With Hypertrophic Cardiomyopathy. Circulation 2020. https://doi.org/10.1161/cir.0000000000000937.

74. Petrin Z, Soffer B, Daniels SJ. Sudden cardiac arrest in the field in an 18-year-old male athlete with Noonan syndrome: Case presentation and 5-year follow-up. Cardiol Young 2019;29(9):1214–6.

75. Aydin A, Yilmazer MS, Gurol T. Sudden death in a patient with Noonan syndrome. Cardiol Young 2011;21(2):233–4.

76. Eichhorn C, Voges I, Daubeney PEF. Out-of-hospital cardiac arrest and survival in a patient with Noonan syndrome and multiple lentigines: A case report. J Med Case Rep 2019;13(1). https://doi.org/10.1186/s13256-019-2096-6.

77. Miron A, Lafreniere-Roula M, Steve Fan CP, et al. A validated model for sudden cardiac death risk prediction in pediatric hypertrophic cardiomyopathy. Circulation 2020;142(3):217–29.

78. Kaski JP, Norrish G, Ding T, et al. Development of a Novel Risk Prediction Model for Sudden Cardiac Death in Childhood Hypertrophic Cardiomyopathy (HCM Risk-Kids). JAMA Cardiol 2019;4(9):918–27.

79. Moran AM, Colan SD. Verapamil therapy in infants with hypertrophic cardiomyopathy. Cardiol Young 1998;8(3):310–9.

80. Spicer RL, Rocchini AP, Crowley DC, et al. Hemodynamic effects of verapamil in children and

adolescents with hypertrophic cardiomyopathy. Circulation 1983;67(2):413–20.

81. Poterucha JT, Johnson JN, O'Leary PW, et al. Surgical Ventricular Septal Myectomy for Patients with Noonan Syndrome and Symptomatic Left Ventricular Outflow Tract Obstruction. Am J Cardiol 2015; 116(7):1116–21.

82. Hemmati P, Dearani JA, Daly RC, et al. Early Outcomes of Cardiac Surgery in Patients with Noonan Syndrome. Semin Thorac Cardiovasc Surg 2019. https://doi.org/10.1053/j.semtcvs.2018.12.004.

83. McCallen LM, Ameduri RK, Denfield SW, et al. Cardiac transplantation in children with Noonan syndrome. Pediatr Transplant 2019;23(6). https://doi.org/10.1111/petr.13535.

84. Mehra MR, Canter CE, Hannan MM, et al. The 2016 International Society for Heart Lung Transplantation listing criteria for heart transplantation: A 10-year update. J Heart Lung Transplant 2016;35(1):1–23.

85. Rossano JW, Cherikh WS, Chambers DC, et al. The Registry of the International Society for Heart and Lung Transplantation: Twentieth Pediatric Heart Transplantation Report-2017; Focus Theme: Allograft ischemic time. J Heart Lung Transplant 2017. https://doi.org/10.1016/j.healun.2017.07.018.

86. Topilsky Y, Pereira NL, Shah DK, et al. Left ventricular assist device therapy in patients with restrictive and hypertrophic cardiomyopathy. Circ Hear Fail 2011;4(3):266–75.

87. Lipshultz SE, Sleeper LA, Towbin JA, et al. The Incidence of Pediatric Cardiomyopathy in Two Regions of the United States. N Engl J Med 2003;348(17):1647–55.

88. Colan SD, Lipshultz SE, Lowe AM, et al. Epidemiology and cause-specific outcome of hypertrophic cardiomyopathy in children: Findings from the Pediatric Cardiomyopathy Registry. Circulation 2007; 115(6):773–81.

89. Gajarski R, Naftel DC, Pahl E, et al. Outcomes of Pediatric Patients With Hypertrophic Cardiomyopathy Listed for Transplant. J Heart Lung Transplant 2009;28(12):1329–34.

90. Gross AM, Frone M, Gripp KW, et al. Advancing RAS/RASopathy therapies: An NCI-sponsored intramural and extramural collaboration for the study of RASopathies. Am J Med Genet Part A 2020; 182(4):866–76.

Diagnosis and Management of Cardiovascular Involvement in Friedreich Ataxia

Emanuele Monda, MD[a], Michele Lioncino, MD[a], Marta Rubino, MD[a],
Silvia Passantino, MD[b], Federica Verrillo, MD[a], Martina Caiazza, MD[a],
Annapaola Cirillo, MD[a], Adelaide Fusco, MD[a], Francesco Di Fraia, MD[a],
Fabio Fimiani, MD[a], Federica Amodio, MD[a], Nunzia Borrelli, MD[a],
Alfredo Mauriello, MD[a], Francesco Natale, MD, PhD[a],
Gioacchino Scarano, MD, PhD[a], Francesca Girolami, MD[b],
Silvia Favilli, MD, PhD[b], Giuseppe Limongelli, MD, PhD[a,c],*

KEYWORDS

- Friedreich ataxia • Left ventricular hypertrophy • Hypertrophic cardiomyopathy • Diagnosis
- Therapy

KEY POINTS

- Friedreich ataxia is an autosomal recessive neurodegenerative disorder that principally affects the heart and the nervous system.
- Cardiac involvement represents a common disorder in Friedreich ataxia and is responsible for premature death, particularly in early-onset cases.
- No specific treatments are available for Friedreich ataxia cardiomyopathy. However, gene therapy and stem cells–based therapy might be available as future therapeutic options.

FRIEDREICH ATAXIA
Introduction, Epidemiology, Pathophysiology, Clinical Features

Friedreich ataxia (FRDA) is an autosomal recessive neurodegenerative disorder that principally affects the heart and the nervous system, caused by a homozygous GAA triplet repeat expansion in the frataxin (FTX) gene.[1] Frataxin is a highly conserved protein that acts as an iron chaperone protein and is essential to energy metabolism.[2] It is expressed throughout the body and is positively correlated to tissue with high requirements of energy metabolism.[3] The dysregulation in frataxin protein owing to the accumulation of GAA repeat expansions localized to the first intron of the FXN locus results in cardiac muscle cells and neuron involvement.[4] The pathologic onset is associated with 40 to 60 repeats that can increase to more than 1700 repeats, and the number of repeats is positively correlated with earlier onset and disease severity.[4] The typical age of disease onset in FRDA is in the second decade of life; however, late-onset

[a] Department of Translational Medical Sciences, University of Campania "Luigi Vanvitelli", Via L. Bianchi, 80131 Naples, Italy; [b] Department of Pediatric Cardiology, Meyer Children's Hospital, Viale Gaetano Pieraccini, 24, 50139 Florence, Italy; [c] Institute of Cardiovascular Sciences, University College of London and St. Bartholomew's Hospital, Grower Street, London WC1E 6DD, UK
* Corresponding author. Inherited and Rare Cardiovascular Diseases, Department of Translational Medical Sciences, University of Campania "Luigi Vanvitelli", AO Colli–Monaldi Hospital–ERN Guard Heart Member, 80131 Naples, Italy.
E-mail address: limongelligiuseppe@libero.it

Heart Failure Clin 18 (2022) 31–37
https://doi.org/10.1016/j.hfc.2021.07.001
1551-7136/22/© 2021 Elsevier Inc. All rights reserved.

and very late-onset, with the disease onset after 25 and 40 years, respectively, are atypical phenotypes and show slower disease progression.[5–15]

Patients with FRDA developed several progressive neuromuscular symptoms and nonneurologic manifestations, including hypertrophic cardiomyopathy (HCM) and diabetes mellitus.[5,16,17] The first symptoms usually appear in the second decade, or more rarely in infancy or adulthood,[18] and gait instability is the typical presenting symptom. Subsequently, other neurologic features, such as dysarthria, sensory loss, areflexia, and pyramidal signs, can appear.[18]

Diagnosis of Friedreich Ataxia

FRDA is a multisystemic disorder that can affect several organs and tissue, resulting in neurologic, cardiac, musculoskeletal, and endocrinologic manifestations[18] (**Table 1**). Several diagnostic criteria have been proposed to clinically suspect the diagnosis of FRDA.[18,19] However, genetic testing with the identification of the biallelic expansion of the GAA repeats in the first intron of the FTX gene or the compound heterozygotes of the GAA expansion and a point mutation or a gene/intragenic deletion is required for diagnosis.[20,21]

Diagnosis of Cardiovascular Involvement in Friedreich Ataxia

Cardiac involvement is observed in most patients with FRDA[4] and can contribute to disability and cause premature death, particularly in early-onset cases. Of note, FRDA is among the most important nonsarcomeric causes of HCM in children and adolescents,[22–25] and early onset of FRDA predicts cardiac severity, worse left ventricular hypertrophy and function, and mortality.[26]

Cardiac involvement, usually manifesting as HCM, can range from asymptomatic cases with mild expression to severe cardiomyopathy with progressive deterioration of the left ventricular ejection fraction and chronic heart failure, which may result in premature death.[27–30] The hypertrophic phase seems to derive from the striking proliferation of mitochondria within the cardiomyocytes, whereas the evolution to the hypokinetic phase is due to the increased sensitivity to oxidative stress and the respiratory chain defects caused by the deficiency of the inner mitochondrial membrane protein frataxin, and to the progressive iron accumulation, fibrosis, and loss of contractile fibers.[31–34]

There appears to be no specific relationship between the degree of neurologic deficit and cardiac involvement.[35] Left ventricular outflow tract obstruction is very rare in FRDA. Dilated cardiomyopathy represents often a disease progression from the hypertrophic form,[29] and patients who develop a dilated cardiomyopathy have a poor prognosis with progressive cardiac deterioration leading to refractory heart failure and death.[4] Moreover, arrhythmias may occur and are represented principally by supraventricular arrhythmias and atrial fibrillation; ventricular arrhythmias are rarely reported.[36] Patients with FRDA have an impaired myocardial perfusion reserve index, which is associated with microvascular disease and fibrosis, and occur also in absence of significant hypertrophy and before clinical heart failure.[37] Myocardial infarction is rare, and coronary lesions have been principally associated with long-standing diabetes.

A systematic approach for the detection of cardiovascular involvement in FRDA patients is mandatory and requires electrocardiography and Holter monitoring, for the assessment of electrical depolarization, repolarization, and arrhythmias, echocardiography and cardiac magnetic resonance (CMR), for the evaluation of cardiac chamber dimensions, wall thickness, systolic and diastolic function, and tissue characterization, and biomarkers, for myocyte decay. Different staging systems for HCM in FRDA have been proposed (**Table 2**).[30,38] The Mitochondrial Protection with Idebenone in Cardiac or Neurological Outcome study group[30] suggested a classification into no, mild, intermediate, and severe cardiomyopathy based on left ventricular wall thickness and left ventricular ejection fraction. In particular,

Table 1
Clinical manifestation of Friedreich ataxia

Neurologic	Cardiac	Orthopedic	Endocrinological
Ataxia	Hypertrophic cardiomyopathy	Scoliosis	Insulin resistance
Dysarthria	Progressive left ventricular	Pes cavus	Diabetes mellitus
Lower limb areflexia	dilation and heart failure		
Lower limb muscle weakness			
Auditory neuropathy			
Reduced visual acuity			

Table 2
Proposed staging systems for hypertrophic cardiomyopathy in Friedreich ataxia

Grading	MICONOS Study[30]	Weidemann et al[38]
0	No FRDA-CM: Normal echo-IVSTd and MRI EF $\geq$50%	No FRDA-CM: No ECG, Echo, CRM, or biochemical abnormalities
1	Mild FRDA-CM: echo-IVSTd exceeding the predicted normal echo-IVSTd by <18% and MRI EF $\geq$50%	Mild FRDA-CM: T-wave inversion at ECG LVPWT <11 mm No myocardial fibrosis at CMR EF $\geq$55% Normal hsTNT
2	Intermediate FRDA-CM: echo-IVSTd exceeding the predicted normal echo-IVSTd by $\geq$18% and MRI EF $\geq$50%	Mild FRDA-CM: T-wave inversion at ECG LVPWT $\geq$11 mm No myocardial fibrosis at CMR EF $\geq$55% Normal hsTNT
3	Severe FRDA-CM: MRI EF <50%	Severe FRDA-CM: Myocardial fibrosis at CMR Elevated hsTNT
4	—	End-stage FRDA-CM: EF <55%

Abbreviations: EF, ejection fraction; FRDA-CM, Friedreich ataxia cardiomyopathy; IVSTd, end-diastolic interventricular septal wall thickness; LVPWT, left ventricular end-diastolic posterior wall thickness; MICONOS, mitochondrial protection with idebenone in cardiac or neurologic outcome.

patients with an end-diastolic interventricular septum wall thickness into the normal range, exceeding the predicted normal by less than 18% or $\geq$18%, were classified as having no, mild, and intermediate cardiomyopathy, respectively. On the other hand, patients with ejection fraction less than 50% were classified as having severe cardiomyopathy.

Weidemann and colleagues[38] have proposed a novel staging system for myocardial involvement in FRDA, based on the presence of T-wave inversion on electrocardiography, left ventricular ejection fraction less than 55%, left ventricular end-diastolic posterior wall thickness $\geq$11, fibrosis on CMR, and high-sensitive troponin T (hsTNT). Using these parameters, they proposed the following staging: mild cardiomyopathy (only T-wave inversion); intermediate cardiomyopathy (T-wave inversion and echocardiographic evidence of left ventricular hypertrophy but without fibrosis on CMR); severe cardiomyopathy (fibrosis on CMR and raised hsTNT); end-stage cardiomyopathy (left ventricular ejection fraction <55%). However, both the staging systems suffer from limitation, principally because of the absence of evidence of their prognostic usefulness.

Electrocardiography

Negative T waves, especially in inferolateral leads, are present in virtually all patients with FRDA

cardiomyopathy and represent the earliest signs of a cardiomyopathy, followed by signs of LVH, left axis deviation, and other repolarization abnormalities.[39,40] About 10% to 30% of patients show conduction disturbance, supraventricular ectopic beats, and/or atrial fibrillation,[30,38] as the result of the progressive fibrotic replacement.

Ambulatory electrocardiogram monitoring

Patients with FRDA may have an increased risk for paroxysmal supraventricular tachycardia or atrial fibrillation. Thus, 24- to 48-hour electrocardiogram (ECG) Holter monitoring is recommended in patients with cardiac involvement.

Echocardiography

Echocardiography is required for diagnosis and monitoring patients with FRDA and cardiovascular involvement. It manifests as concentric LVH with an end-diastolic wall thickness usually less than 15 mm, with preserved left ventricular ejection fraction and without left ventricular outflow tract obstruction.[41] Asymmetric LVH has been identified in a few cases,[42] and left ventricular dilatation and left ventricular dysfunction are evidenced in the advanced cases in the setting of dilated cardiomyopathy.[29] The diastolic function can be normal or mildly impaired in patients with FRDA cardiomyopathy.[43] Global longitudinal strain is reduced in patients with LVH with a significant reduction in those that progress to hypokinetic dilated cardiomyopathy.[43] Moreover, it has been identified as an early marker of systolic dysfunction.[44]

Cardiac magnetic resonance

CMR represents the gold standard for measuring ventricular dimensions, wall thicknesses, LV mass, and systolic function. Myocardial fibrosis, as late gadolinium enhancement, is present in nearly all patients with end-stage (dilatative phase) or severe cardiomyopathy. Generally, fibrosis is patchy and irregular, affecting different left ventricular wall segments with the typical localization in the midwall, and no predominant region in the left ventricle for the occurrence of late gadolinium is described.[40] In FRDA patients, reduced native T1 values can be observed, and this reduction may be explained by a mild cardiac iron accumulation.[45]

Laboratory tests

High-sensitivity troponin levels have been observed in FRDA patients with advanced cardiomyopathy with myocardial fibrosis at CMR.[38]

Management of Cardiac Involvement in Friedreich Ataxia

Hypertrophic cardiomyopathy

General management of HCM in FRDA is based on the current clinical practice guidelines.[46,47] However, beta-blockers and calcium antagonists should be monitored carefully because of their potential harm, given the loss of contractile fibers in the myocardium.[31–34] Asymmetrical LVH with left ventricular outflow tract obstruction is rare, and the need for myectomy to manage obstruction is exceptional.[48]

Arrhythmias and conduction disorders

As described before, patients with FRDA have an increased risk for paroxysmal supraventricular tachycardia or atrial fibrillation. The risk of embolic stroke associated with atrial fibrillation cannot be evaluated with the current scoring system; thus, patients with FRDA and HCM should receive oral anticoagulation irrespective of other risk factors.[46,47,49]

Moreover, because of the progressive fibrosis and scarring, they can develop progressive atrioventricular blocks and bradyarrhythmias.[30,38] On the other hand, the risk for ventricular arrhythmias is low,[26,50,51] and sudden cardiac death represents a rare cause of death in FRDA. Permanent cardiac pacing should be considered to manage symptomatic bradyarrhythmias according to the current clinical practice guidelines.[52,53]

Heart failure

Heart failure represents the major cause of death in patients with FRDA.[26] A recent long-term follow-up study[26] showed that among 133 patients, 15 died at a mean age of 39 years after a mean follow-up of 10.5 years. Among these, 8 patients died of cardiovascular causes: 6 patients died of progressive heart failure; 2 patients had atrial fibrillation and progressive heart failure and died after cardioembolic stroke. The investigators found that longer GAA repeats, earlier age at onset, higher septal wall thickness and left ventricular mass index, and lower left ventricular ejection fraction were independent predictors of mortality. A progressive regression of left ventricular hypertrophy over time, an increase in left ventricular diameters, and a reduction of left ventricular ejection fraction, resulting in dilated and hypokinetic cardiomyopathy and clinical heart failure, were observed.

Thus, cardiac follow-up in FRDA is required to identify early systolic dysfunction and start appropriate management.[54–56]

Disease-direct therapy

No specific treatments are available for FRDA cardiomyopathy. Different therapeutic strategies with the aim of reducing oxidative stress have been proposed, focused on increasing FXN levels and/or alleviating the consequences of frataxin loss.[57–67]

Idebenone, a coenzyme Q_{10} analogue that has been shown to have antioxidant activity and to facilitate mitochondrial phosphorylation as an electron carrier, has shown the potential to benefit hypertrophy in terms of left ventricular mass in open-label studies, but randomized controlled trials have not shown any clear benefit.[68] Specifically, although the first preliminary study showed promising improvement of the cardiac outcomes in FRDA patients,[69] 4 randomized placebo-controlled phase III clinical trials evidenced no significant effects on the neurologic or cardiac function in different groups of FRDA patients.[70–73]

On the other hand, gene therapy and stem cells–based therapy might be future therapeutic options for patients with FRDA.[74,75] Perdomini and colleagues[74] tested the efficacy of adeno-associated virus rh10 vector expressing FXN in a mouse model of FRDA and showed that gene therapy prevents the onset of cardiac disease and, if administer after the onset of heart failure, was able to completely reverse the cardiomyopathy at the cellular, molecular, and functional level within a few days.

SUMMARY

Cardiac involvement is among the most common cause of death in FRDA and is responsible for impaired quality of life. HCM is the most common form of cardiac involvement in FRDA, and a comprehensive clinical and instrumental evaluation is required to early detect and properly manage its manifestations and prevent complications.

CLINICS CARE POINTS

- Genetic testing with the identification of the biallelic expansion of the GAA repeats in the first intron of the FTX gene or the compound heterozygotes of the GAA expansion and a point mutation or a gene/intragenic deletion is required for the diagnosis of Friedreich ataxia.

- A systematic approach for the detection of cardiovascular involvement in Friedreich ataxia patients is mandatory and requires electrocardiography and Holter monitoring, for the assessment of electrical depolarization, repolarization, and arrhythmias, echocardiography and cardiac magnetic resonance, for the evaluation of cardiac chamber dimensions, wall thickness, systolic and diastolic function, and tissue characterization, and biomarkers, for myocyte decay.

- Friedreich ataxia is among the most important nonsarcomeric causes of hypertrophic cardiomyopathy in children and adolescents, and early onset of Friedreich ataxia predicts cardiac severity, worse left ventricular hypertrophy and function, and mortality.

ACKNOWLEDGMENTS

The authors would like to acknowledge Michela Piscopo, Daniela Lafera, and Ciro De Prisco who made possible our research and clinical activity.

REFERENCES

1. Campuzano V, Montermini L, Moltò MD, et al. Friedreich's ataxia: autosomal recessive disease caused by an intronic GAA triplet repeat expansion. Science 1996;271(5254):1423–7.
2. Cai K, Frederick RO, Tonelli M, et al. Interactions of iron-bound frataxin with ISCU and ferredoxin on the cysteine desulfurase complex leading to Fe-S cluster assembly. J Inorg Biochem 2018;183: 107–16.
3. Babcock M, de Silva D, Oaks R, et al. Regulation of mitochondrial iron accumulation by Yfh1p, a putative homolog of frataxin. Science 1997;276(5319): 1709–12.
4. Dürr A, Cossee M, Agid Y, et al. Clinical and genetic abnormalities in patients with Friedreich's ataxia. N Engl J Med 1996;335(16):1169–75.
5. Delatycki MB, Paris DB, Gardner RJ, et al. Clinical and genetic study of Friedreich ataxia in an Australian population. Am J Med Genet 1999;87(2):168–74.
6. Lecocq C, Charles P, Azulay JP, et al. Delayed-onset Friedreich's ataxia revisited. Mov Disord 2016;31(1): 62–9.
7. Tsou AY, Paulsen EK, Lagedrost SJ, et al. Mortality in Friedreich ataxia. J Neurol Sci 2011;307(1–2):46–9.
8. Delatycki MB, Corben LA. Clinical features of Friedreich ataxia. J Child Neurol 2012;27(9):1133–7.
9. Koeppen AH, Mazurkiewicz JE. Friedreich ataxia: neuropathology revised. J Neuropathol Exp Neurol 2013;72(2):78–90.
10. Ackroyd RS, Finnegan JA, Green SH. Friedreich's ataxia. A clinical review with neurophysiological and echocardiographic findings. Arch Dis Child 1984;59(3):217–21.
11. Morral JA, Davis AN, Qian J, et al. Pathology and pathogenesis of sensory neuropathy in Friedreich's ataxia. Acta Neuropathol 2010;120(1):97–108.
12. Koeppen AH, Ramirez RL, Becker AB, et al. Dorsal root ganglia in Friedreich ataxia: satellite cell proliferation and inflammation. Acta Neuropathol Commun 2016;4(1):46.
13. Nachbauer W, Boesch S, Reindl M, et al. Skeletal muscle involvement in Friedreich ataxia and potential effects of recombinant human erythropoietin administration on muscle regeneration and neovascularization. J Neuropathol Exp Neurol 2012;71(8):708–15.
14. França MC Jr, D'Abreu A, Yasuda CL, et al. A combined voxel-based morphometry and 1H-MRS study in patients with Friedreich's ataxia. J Neurol 2009;256(7):1114–20.
15. Mantovan MC, Martinuzzi A, Squarzanti F, et al. Exploring mental status in Friedreich's ataxia: a combined neuropsychological, behavioral and neuroimaging study. Eur J Neurol 2006;13(8):827–35.
16. Koeppen AH, Ramirez RL, Becker AB, et al. The pathogenesis of cardiomyopathy in Friedreich ataxia. PLoS One 2015;10(3):e0116396.
17. Rajagopalan B, Francis JM, Cooke F, et al. Analysis of the factors influencing the cardiac phenotype in Friedreich's ataxia. Mov Disord 2010;25(7):846–52.
18. Harding AE. Friedreich's ataxia: a clinical and genetic study of 90 families with an analysis of early diagnostic criteria and intrafamilial clustering of clinical features. Brain 1981;104(3):589–620.
19. Geoffroy G, Barbeau A, Breton G, et al. Clinical description and roentgenologic evaluation of patients with Friedreich's ataxia. Can J Neurol Sci 1976;3(4):279–86.
20. Hoffman-Zacharska D, Mazurczak T, Zajkowski T, et al. Friedreich ataxia is not only a GAA repeats expansion disorder: implications for molecular

testing and counselling. J Appl Genet 2016;57(3):349–55.

21. de Silva R, Greenfield J, Cook A, et al. Guidelines on the diagnosis and management of the progressive ataxias. Orphanet J Rare Dis 2019;14(1):51.

22. Norrish G, Field E, Mcleod K, et al. Clinical presentation and survival of childhood hypertrophic cardiomyopathy: a retrospective study in United Kingdom. Eur Heart J 2019;40(12):986–93.

23. Colan SD, Lipshultz SE, Lowe AM, et al. Epidemiology and cause-specific outcome of hypertrophic cardiomyopathy in children: findings from the Pediatric Cardiomyopathy Registry. Circulation 2007;115(6):773–81.

24. Monda E, Rubino M, Lioncino M, et al. Hypertrophic cardiomyopathy in children: pathophysiology, diagnosis, and treatment of non-sarcomeric causes. Front Pediatr 2021;9:632293.

25. Limongelli G, Monda E, Tramonte S, et al. Prevalence and clinical significance of red flags in patients with hypertrophic cardiomyopathy. Int J Cardiol 2020;299:186–91.

26. Pousset F, Legrand L, Monin ML, et al. A 22-year follow-up study of long-term cardiac outcome and predictors of survival in Friedreich ataxia. JAMA Neurol 2015;72(11):1334–41.

27. Meyer C, Schmid G, Görlitz S, et al. Cardiomyopathy in Friedreich's ataxia-assessment by cardiac MRI. Mov Disord 2007;22(11):1615–22.

28. Kawai C, Kato S, Takashima M, et al. Heart disease in Friedreich's ataxia: observation of a case for half a century. JPN Circ J 2000;64(3):229–36.

29. Casazza F, Morpurgo M. The varying evolution of Friedreich's ataxia cardiomyopathy. Am J Cardiol 1996;77(10):895–8.

30. Weidemann F, Rummey C, Bijnens B, et al, Mitochondrial Protection with Idebenone in Cardiac or Neurological Outcome (MICONOS) study group. The heart in Friedreich ataxia: definition of cardiomyopathy, disease severity, and correlation with neurological symptoms. Circulation 2012;125(13):1626–34.

31. Vyas PM, Tomamichel WJ, Pride PM, et al. A TAT-Frataxin fusion protein increases lifespan and cardiac function in a conditional Friedreich's ataxia mouse model. Hum Mol Genet 2012;21(6):1230–47.

32. Michael S, Petrocine SV, Qian J, et al. Iron and iron-responsive proteins in the cardiomyopathy of Friedreich's ataxia. Cerebellum 2006;5(4):257–67.

33. Bradley JL, Blake JC, Chamberlain S, et al. Clinical, biochemical and molecular genetic correlations in Friedreich's ataxia. Hum Mol Genet 2000;9(2):275–82.

34. Ramirez RL, Qian J, Santambrogio P, et al. Relation of cytosolic iron excess to cardiomyopathy of Friedreich's ataxia. Am J Cardiol 2012;110(12):1820–7.

35. Child JS, Perloff JK, Bach PM, et al. Cardiac involvement in Friedreich's ataxia: a clinical study of 75 patients. J Am Coll Cardiol 1986;7(6):1370–8.

36. Asaad N, El-Menyar A, Al Suwaidi J. Recurrent ventricular tachycardia in patient with Friedreich's ataxia in the absence of clinical myocardial disease. Pacing Clin Electrophysiol 2010;33(1):109–12.

37. Raman SV, Phatak K, Hoyle JC, et al. Impaired myocardial perfusion reserve and fibrosis in Friedreich ataxia: a mitochondrial cardiomyopathy with metabolic syndrome. Eur Heart J 2011;32(5):561–7.

38. Weidemann F, Liu D, Hu K, et al. The cardiomyopathy in Friedreich's ataxia - new biomarker for staging cardiac involvement. Int J Cardiol 2015;194:50–7.

39. Dutka DP, Donnelly JE, Nihoyannopoulos P, et al. Marked variation in the cardiomyopathy associated with Friedreich's ataxia. Heart 1999;81(2):141–7.

40. Mastroianno S, Germano M, Maggio A, et al. Electrocardiogram in Friedreich's ataxia: a short-term surrogate endpoint for treatment efficacy. Ann Noninvasive Electrocardiol 2020;5:e12813.

41. Regner SR, Lagedrost SJ, Plappert T, et al. Analysis of echocardiograms in a large heterogeneous cohort of patients with Friedreich ataxia. Am J Cardiol 2012;109(3):401–5.

42. St John Sutton M, Ky B, Regner SR, et al. Longitudinal strain in Friedreich ataxia: a potential marker for early left ventricular dysfunction. Echocardiography 2014;31(1):50–7.

43. Liu D, Hu K, Nordbeck P, et al. Longitudinal strain bull's eye plot patterns in patients with cardiomyopathy and concentric left ventricular hypertrophy. Eur J Med Res 2016;21(1):21.

44. Tops LF, Delgado V, Marsan NA, et al. Myocardial strain to detect subtle left ventricular systolic dysfunction. Eur J Heart Fail 2017;19(3):307–13.

45. Milano EG, Harries IB, Bucciarelli-Ducci C. Young adult with Friedreich ataxia. Heart 2019;105(10):797–806.

46. Elliott PM, Anastasakis A, Borger MA, et al. 2014 ESC guidelines on diagnosis and management of hypertrophic cardiomyopathy: the task force for the diagnosis and management of hypertrophic cardiomyopathy of the European Society of Cardiology (ESC). Eur Heart J 2014;35(39):2733–79.

47. Ommen SR, Mital S, Burke MA, et al. 2020 AHA/ACC guideline for the diagnosis and treatment of patients with hypertrophic cardiomyopathy: a report of the American College of Cardiology/American Heart Association Joint Committee on clinical practice guidelines [published correction appears in Circulation. 2020 Dec 22;142(25):e633]. Circulation 2020;142(25):e558–631.

48. Anderson HN, Burkhart HM, Johnson JN. Septal myectomy for hypertrophic obstructive cardiomyopathy in Friedreich's ataxia. Cardiol Young 2016;26(1):175–8.

49. Chen A, Stecker E, Warden A. Direct oral anticoagulant use: a practical guide to common clinical challenges. J Am Heart Assoc 2020;9(13):e017559.

50. Payne RM, Wagner GR. Cardiomyopathy in Friedreich ataxia: clinical findings and research. J Child Neurol 2012;27(9):1179–86.

51. Payne RM, Peverill RE. Cardiomyopathy of Friedreich's ataxia (FRDA). Ir J Med Sci 2012;181(4): 569–70.

52. Brignole M, Auricchio A, Baron-Esquivias G, et al. 2013 ESC guidelines on cardiac pacing and cardiac resynchronization therapy: the Task Force on Cardiac Pacing and Resynchronization Therapy of the European Society of Cardiology (ESC). Developed in collaboration with the European Heart Rhythm Association (EHRA). Eur Heart J 2013;34(29):2281–329.

53. Kusumoto FM, Schoenfeld MH, Barrett C, et al. 2018 ACC/AHA/HRS guideline on the evaluation and management of patients with bradycardia and cardiac conduction delay: executive summary: a report of the American College of Cardiology/American Heart Association Task Force on Clinical Practice Guidelines, and the Heart Rhythm Society [published correction appears in J Am Coll Cardiol. 2019 Aug 20;74(7):1014-1016]. J Am Coll Cardiol 2019;74(7):932–87.

54. Ponikowski P, Voors AA, Anker SD, et al. 2016 ESC guidelines for the diagnosis and treatment of acute and chronic heart failure: the Task Force for the Diagnosis and Treatment of Acute and Chronic Heart Failure of the European Society of Cardiology (ESC) Developed with the special contribution of the Heart Failure Association (HFA) of the ESC [published correction appears in Eur Heart J. 2016 Dec 30]. Eur Heart J 2016;37(27):2129–200.

55. Yancy CW, Jessup M, Bozkurt B, et al. 2013 ACCF/AHA guideline for the management of heart failure: a report of the American College of Cardiology Foundation/American Heart Association Task Force on Practice Guidelines. J Am Coll Cardiol 2013; 62(16):e147–239.

56. Corben LA, Lynch D, Pandolfo M, et al, Clinical Management Guidelines Writing Group. Consensus clinical management guidelines for Friedreich ataxia. Orphanet J Rare Dis 2014;9:184.

57. Lynch DR, Willi SM, Wilson RB, et al. A0001 in Friedreich ataxia: biochemical characterization and effects in a clinical trial. Mov Disord 2012;27(8):1026–33.

58. Qureshi MY, Patterson MC, Clark V, et al. Safety and efficacy of (+)-epicatechin in subjects with Friedreich's ataxia: a phase II, open-label, prospective study. J Inherit Metab Dis 2021;44(2):502–14.

59. Costantini A, Laureti T, Pala MI, et al. Long-term treatment with thiamine as possible medical therapy for Friedreich ataxia. J Neurol 2016;263(11):2170–8.

60. Lynch DR, Farmer J, Hauser L, et al. Safety, pharmacodynamics, and potential benefit of omaveloxolone in Friedreich ataxia. Ann Clin Transl Neurol 2018; 6(1):15–26.

61. Yiu EM, Tai G, Peverill RE, et al. An open-label trial in Friedreich ataxia suggests clinical benefit with high-dose resveratrol, without effect on frataxin levels. J Neurol 2015;262(5):1344–53.

62. Schöls L, Zange J, Abele M, et al. L-carnitine and creatine in Friedreich's ataxia. A randomized, placebo-controlled crossover trial. J Neural Transm (Vienna) 2005;112(6):789–96.

63. Pandolfo M, Arpa J, Delatycki MB, et al. Deferiprone in Friedreich ataxia: a 6-month randomized controlled trial. Ann Neurol 2014;76(4):509–21.

64. Velasco-Sánchez D, Aracil A, Montero R, et al. Combined therapy with idebenone and deferiprone in patients with Friedreich's ataxia. Cerebellum 2011; 10(1):1–8.

65. Arpa J, Sanz-Gallego I, Rodríguez-de-Rivera FJ, et al. Triple therapy with deferiprone, idebenone and riboflavin in Friedreich's ataxia - open-label trial. Acta Neurol Scand 2014;129(1):32–40.

66. Zesiewicz T, Salemi JL, Perlman S, et al. Double-blind, randomized and controlled trial of EPI-743 in Friedreich's ataxia. Neurodegener Dis Manag 2018;8(4):233–42.

67. Zesiewicz T, Heerinckx F, De Jager R, et al. Randomized, clinical trial of RT001: early signals of efficacy in Friedreich's ataxia. Mov Disord 2018;33(6): 1000–5.

68. Meier T, Buyse G. Idebenone: an emerging therapy for Friedreich ataxia. J Neurol 2009;256(Suppl 1): 25–30.

69. Rustin P, von Kleist-Retzow JC, Chantrel-Groussard K, et al. Effect of idebenone on cardiomyopathy in Friedreich's ataxia: a preliminary study. Lancet 1999;354(9177):477–9.

70. Di Prospero NA, Baker A, Jeffries N, et al. Neurological effects of high-dose idebenone in patients with Friedreich's ataxia: a randomised, placebo-controlled trial. Lancet Neurol 2007;6(10):878–86.

71. Lynch DR, Perlman SL, Meier T. A phase 3, double-blind, placebo-controlled trial of idebenone in Friedreich ataxia. Arch Neurol 2010;67(8):941–7.

72. Lagedrost SJ, Sutton MS, Cohen MS, et al. Idebenone in Friedreich ataxia cardiomyopathy-results from a 6-month phase III study (IONIA). Am Heart J 2011;161(3):639–45.e1.

73. Cook A, Boesch S, Heck S, et al. Patient-reported outcomes in Friedreich's ataxia after withdrawal from idebenone. Acta Neurol Scand 2019;139(6): 533–9.

74. Perdomini M, Belbellaa B, Monassier L, et al. Prevention and reversal of severe mitochondrial cardiomyopathy by gene therapy in a mouse model of Friedreich's ataxia. Nat Med 2014;20(5):542–7.

75. Shroff G. A novel approach of human embryonic stem cells therapy in treatment of Friedrich's Ataxia. Int J Case Rep Images 2015;6:261.

Diagnosis and Management of Cardiovascular Involvement in Fabry Disease

Marta Rubino, MD[a,1], Emanuele Monda, MD[a,1], Michele Lioncino, MD[a],
Martina Caiazza, MD[a], Giuseppe Palmiero, MD[a], Francesca Dongiglio, MD[a],
Adelaide Fusco, MD[a], Annapaola Cirillo, MD[a], Arturo Cesaro, MD[a],
Laura Capodicasa, MD[b], Marialuisa Mazzella, MD[a], Flavia Chiosi, MD[c],
Paolo Orabona, MD[c], Eduardo Bossone, MD, PhD[d], Paolo Calabrò, MD, PhD[a],
Antonio Pisani, MD, PhD[e], Dominique P. Germain, MD, PhD[f],
Elena Biagini, MD, PhD[g], Maurizio Pieroni, MD, PhD[h],
Giuseppe Limongelli, MD, PhD[a,i],*

KEYWORDS

• Fabry disease • Hypertrophic cardiomyopathy • Diagnosis • Therapy

KEY POINTS

• Fabry disease is a multisystemic disease that can affect several organs, resulting in cardiac, neurologic, ocular, cutaneous, and renal manifestations.
• Age at onset and clinical presentation of Fabry disease largely depend on the gender and the degree of α-galactosidase A deficiency.
• Cardiac involvement represents a significant component of Fabry disease and is responsible for premature death and impaired quality of life.
• Treatment of adult patients with Fabry disease should aim at preventing the disease progression to irreversible organ damage and organ failure.

INTRODUCTION, EPIDEMIOLOGY, PATHOPHYSIOLOGY, CLINICAL FEATURES

Fabry disease (FD) is an X-linked lysosomal storage disease caused by pathogenic variants in the *GLA* gene leading to a greatly reduced or absent activity of the enzyme α-galactosidase A (α-Gal A),

responsible for metabolizing glycosphingolipids.[1] This condition is associated with a progressive accumulation of globotriaosylceramide (Gb$_3$) and its deacylated form, globotriaosylsphingosine (lysoGb$_3$), potentially affecting any organ or tissue.[1]

Although initially considered an extremely rare disease, neonatal screening programs have shown

[a] Department of Translational Medical Sciences, University of Campania "Luigi Vanvitelli", Via L. Bianchi, Naples 80131, Italy; [b] Department of Nephrology, Monaldi Hospital, Via L. Bianchi, Naples 80131, Italy; [c] Department of Ophthalmology, Monaldi Hospital, Via L. Bianchi, Naples 80131, Italy; [d] Division of Cardiology, Antonio Cardarelli Hospital, Via A. Cardarelli, Naples 80131, Italy; [e] Department of Public Health, University Federico II of Naples, Via Pansini, Naples 80131, Italy; [f] French Referral Centre for Fabry Disease, Division of Medical Genetics, Hôpital Raymond-Poincare, AP-HP, Garches 92380, France; [g] Cardiology Unit, St. Orsola Hospital, IRCCS Azienda Ospedaliero-Universitaria di Bologna, 40138 Bologna, Italy; [h] Cardiovascular Department, San Donato Hospital, Arezzo, Italy; [i] Institute of Cardiovascular Sciences, University College of London and St. Bartholomew's Hospital, Grower Street, London WC1E 6DD, UK
[1] These authors equally contributed.
* Corresponding author.
E-mail address: limongelligiuseppe@libero.it

Heart Failure Clin 18 (2022) 39–49
https://doi.org/10.1016/j.hfc.2021.07.005
1551-7136/22/© 2021 Elsevier Inc. All rights reserved.

a high incidence of disease-causing mutations (1 in 1,250–7,800 newborns).[2–5] Prevalence data are mainly based on systematic screening of high-risk subjects with clinical features belonging to the phenotype of FD, such as late-onset hypertrophic cardiomyopathy (HCM), cryptogenic stroke, and end-stage renal disease.[6,7] Accordingly, different studies have evaluated the frequency of FD among patients with late-onset HCM and have shown a prevalence of 0.8% to 1.2%.[8–13]

The classic form of FD usually manifests during childhood or adolescence, and typical manifestations include neuropathic pain, gastrointestinal symptoms, angiokeratomas, hypohidrosis, and autonomic dysfunction.[1] In adulthood, the involvement of kidneys, heart, and central nervous system progressively occurs and is responsible of decreased quality of life and increased risk of morbidity and mortality.[1,14]

The age at onset and clinical presentation of FD depend on the degree of α-Gal A deficiency, which depends on the type of GLA gene variant and the patient's sex (Table 1). With an X-linked transmission, men are usually significantly affected, whereas women can have a variable presentation, ranging from an asymptomatic to a severe phenotype; this variability in part depends on the pathogenic variant and the X chromosome inactivation profile, which occur in all cells of a female organism.[15] Therefore, men with higher residual activity tend to have predominantly nonclassic or later-onset single organ forms of the disease,[8,9] whereas, as a whole, women tend to have a milder disease phenotype than men.[16,17]

Cardiac involvement is common in FD, occurring in 40% to 60% of patients, and is similar in both the classic and the later-onset FD, including HCM, conduction abnormalities, bradycardia, chronotropic incompetence, atrial fibrillation (AF), ventricular arrhythmias, myocardial fibrosis, valve disease, and microvascular dysfunction.[18–23]

Recently, it has emerged that Gb$_3$ storage does not explain alone the entire spectrum of pathophysiological changes in the heart.[24,25] The storage itself acts as a trigger for numerous other complex processes that lead to myocyte biochemical and functional alterations. Those proposed additional processes range from endocytosis and autophagy processes with interference on energy production by the mitochondria, to altered expression of ion channels and/or membrane cell traffic and alteration of the electrical properties of the cardiomyocytes, activation of trophic factors such as sphingosine-1-phosphate leading to the activation of cell hypertrophy pathways common to other CMPs, up to inflammatory processes that proceed parallel to the Gb$_3$ storage with consequent extracellular matrix production and chronic inflammatory-autoimmunity phenomena.[24,25]

DIAGNOSIS OF FABRY DISEASE

FD is a multisystemic disease that can affect several organs, resulting in cardiac, neurologic, ocular, cutaneous, and renal manifestations. Therefore, specialists should consider the possibility of FD, depending on the patient's clinical presentation.

The diagnosis of FD varies on patient gender and disease phenotype (Fig. 1). In male patients,

---

Table 1
Clinical manifestations of Fabry disease according to phenotype

Phenotype	Residual Enzyme Activity	Sex	Age at Onset	Typical Manifestation
Classic FD	Very low or absent residual enzyme activity	Male (or rarely female with skewed X chromosome inactivation)[a]	Childhood or adolescence	*Severe phenotype with multiorgan involvement.* In childhood: neuropathic pain, gastrointestinal disorders, angiokeratomas, hypohidrosis, autonomic dysfunction. In adulthood: TIA or stroke, HCM, proteinuria, chronic kidney disease.
Nonclassic or later-onset FD	Low residual enzyme activity	Male or female[a]	Adulthood	*Mild phenotype with single organ.* TIA or stroke, HCM, proteinuria, chronic kidney disease.

Abbreviation: TIA, transient ischemic attack.
[a] Female patients can have a variable presentation, which depends on the mutation and the X chromosome inactivation profile, which occur at random in all cells.

reduced or absent α-Gal A activity is diagnostic.[1,26] In these patients, genetic testing with the identification of the *GLA* pathogenic variant is required to confirm the diagnosis,[1,26] to rule out benign polymorphisms that may partially reduce levels of α-Gal A activity, to evaluate the presence of an amenable *GLA* mutation (ie, *GLA* variants that retain their catalytic activity despite abnormal protein folding)[25] and to perform a cascade genotype screening in family members.[26,27] In female patients, because the levels of α-Gal A activity are often normal, the demonstration of a *GLA* pathogenic variant is required for the diagnosis.[1,26,28–31]

In patients carrying a *GLA* variant of uncertain significance (VUS), clinical, biochemical, and/or histopathologic evidence of FD is mandatory for the interpretation of the pathogenic nature of the variant.[26,27] The assessment of plasma lyso-Gb$_3$ has been proposed to determine the pathogenicity of the VUS.[32] The interpretation of a VUS by a team of health care providers with expertise in genetics and rare diseases may be useful. When the interpretation of the *GLA* variant is challenging, the evidence of lysosomal Gb$_3$ accumulation in the affected organs may be required for the diagnosis.[1,26,27,33–36]

DIAGNOSIS OF CARDIOVASCULAR INVOLVEMENT IN FABRY DISEASE

Cardiac, and, to a lesser extent, respiratory[36] involvement represents significant components of FD accounting for impaired quality of life and premature death.[23] The typical cardiac involvement is a nonobstructive form of HCM, usually manifesting as concentric left ventricular hypertrophy (LVH); however, apical, asymmetrical, and/or obstructive LVH has also been reported.[9,37] In male patients with FD, LVH usually develops after the third or fourth decade of life, whereas in women the onset is delayed by 10 years.[38] In the first 2 decades of life, although patients do not present with overt cardiovascular symptoms, the cardiac damage progresses subclinically and patients may present with electrocardiographic and mild echocardiographic abnormalities.[39,40]

The assessment of cardiac involvement in FD includes a comprehensive clinical and instrumental evaluation, including medical history, physical examination, electrocardiography (ECG), ambulatory ECG monitoring, echocardiography, cardiac magnetic resonance (CMR), and laboratory testing. In absence of systemic manifestations, differential diagnosis from other forms of unexplained HCM may be challenging.[41–47] Indeed, several pathogenic variants in *GLA,* such as p.Asn215Ser (p.N215S),[48] are associated with significant residual α-Gal A activity, responsible for later-onset forms of FD with predominant cardiac involvement.[38,48–50] Thus, in patients with unexplained LVH, the diagnosis of FD should be considered.[48]

In patients with isolated cardiovascular involvement, several red flags, defined as clinical or instrumental features that help for the diagnosis of a specific disorder, have been proposed to suspect FD[13,51,52] (**Table 2**).

Electrocardiography

In the first 2 decades of life, typical electrocardiographic abnormalities include a short PR interval without evidence of an accessory pathway, due to shortening of P-wave duration, which represents one of the first signs of cardiac involvement.[40,50,52] Signs of LVH, altered strain pattern, and negative T-wave in precordial leads usually manifest in patients with FD cardiomyopathy.[53] Other electrocardiographic manifestations are represented by sinus bradycardia and

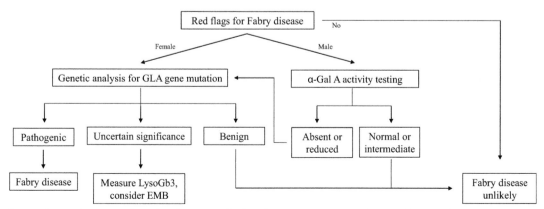

Fig. 1. Diagnostic approach to the diagnosis of Fabry disease in patients with unexplained left ventricular hypertrophy. α-Gal A, α-galactosidase A; EMB, endomyocardial biopsy; LysoGb3, globotriaosylsphingosine; LVH, left ventricular hypertrophy.

Table 2
Fabry disease–related red flags to consider in patients with unexplained left ventricular hypertrophy

Family history	Family history of left ventricular hypertrophy Family history of chronic kidney disease
Signs and symptoms	Gastrointestinal symptoms Angiokeratomas Cornea verticillata Hyperhidrosis Cryptogenic TIA or stroke Neurosensorial deafness Lymphedema
Laboratory abnormalities	Proteinuria Renal failure
Electrocardiographic abnormalities	Short PR interval or preexcitation (usually in first 2 decades) Bradycardia Chronotropic incompetence Atrioventricular block (usually from the third decades)
Echo abnormalities	Left ventricular hypertrophy Disproportionate hypertrophy of papillary muscles Presence of the "binary sign" Reduced GLS (in particular in the posterolateral basal segment)
CMR abnormalities	Midmyocardial distribution of LGE (in particular in the posterolateral basal segment) Low-native T1

Abbreviations: GLS, global longitudinal strain; GRS, global radial strain; TIA, transient ischemic stroke.

atrioventricular block[54]; the atrioventricular conduction delay is a common finding in the natural history of FD and likely reflects the progressive disease burden and the degenerative aging process.[55] Left bundle brunch block is quite rare, whereas right bundle brunch block is often present in the overt form of the disease with fragmented aspects of QRS.[55]

Ambulatory Electrocardiogram Monitoring

Patients with FD have an increased risk of developing symptomatic bradycardia, atrioventricular block, paroxysmal supraventricular tachycardia, AF, or ventricular arrhythmia. Thus, 24- to 48-hour ECG Holter monitoring or, when appropriate, an implantable loop recorder is recommended in patients with cardiac involvement.[54,56]

Echocardiography

Echocardiography is recommended for the diagnosis and monitoring of patients with FD and cardiovascular involvement. Typically, it manifests as concentric LVH without LV outflow tract obstruction (**Fig. 2**); however, various patterns have been described.[37] Other main findings are represented by disproportionate hypertrophy of papillary muscles[57] and normokinetic right ventricular hypertrophy.[58] Diastolic dysfunction is common and worsens with disease progression; however, a restrictive filling pattern is rarely present even in advanced cardiomyopathy.[58] The "binary sign" is frequently observed but shows low sensitivity and specificity.[59] Myocardial strain and strain rate are usually abnormal in patients with FD cardiomyopathy, with the greatest reduction occurring in the posterolateral basal LV segment,[60,61] and correlate with LV mass index, storage, and ECG abnormalities.[62]

Cardiac Magnetic Resonance

CMR represents the gold standard for measuring ventricular dimensions, wall thicknesses, LV mass, and systolic function. Moreover, it offers the possibility for tissue characterization. CMR in FD accurately detects LV apical hypertrophy and papillary muscle hypertrophy.[63,64] With the use of gadolinium contrast agents, it can, although late enhancement, visualize the myocardial fibrosis,

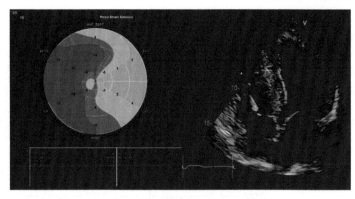

Fig. 2. Severe concentric left ventricular hypertrophy with reduced global longitudinal strain in a patient with Fabry disease.

typically localized, when present, in the midmyocardial of the posterolateral basal LV segment.[65] It also has a role as a prognostic tool, because the presence of extensive fibrosis is associated with increased risk of ventricular arrhythmias and sudden cardiac death (SCD)[50,66] and with reduced response to enzyme replacement therapy (ERT). Replacement fibrosis can be present also in the pre-clinical phase, before the development of LVH, thus favoring the early detection of the cardiac involvement in asymptomatic patients.[67]

Low-native T1 mapping is observed in patients with FD with and without LVH[68–71]; in the latter case, low-native T1 is observed in more than half of subjects and correlates with early electrocardiographic and echocardiographic abnormalities and predict future disease progression.[68] However, in more advanced cases, T1 values may become "pseudonormal" due to coexistence of Gb_3-laden hypertrophied myocytes and interstitial and replacement fibrosis.[69] Furthermore, T2 mapping sequences can be used to evaluate myocardial inflammation, which has been showed to be an early manifestation of FD, in particular in the basal inferolateral region.[72] Recently, it was evidenced that patients with FD has reduced stress myocardial blood flow even before LVH development, suggesting that microvascular dysfunction is an early disease marker and could contribute to the progression from storage to fibrosis.[73]

Endomyocardial Biopsy

Endomyocardial biopsy with a comprehensive evaluation including photonic and electron microscopy, should be considered in patients with *GLA* VUS, high residual enzyme activity and/or low lyso-Gb_3 levels, to confirm FD as the cause of LVH.[1,26,33–35]

Laboratory Tests

Elevated high-sensitivity troponin levels are observed in patients with FD with advanced cardiomyopathy and have been associated with adverse prognosis.[74] Plasma *N*-terminal pro-B-type natriuretic peptide (NT-proBNP) is also elevated in patients with cardiac involvement and correlates with symptoms severity with the highest values presenting in patients with advanced disease.[75,76] Plasma lyso-Gb_3 may be considered for biochemical characterization of clinical phenotype and treatment monitoring,[77] but this warrants further studies.

MANAGEMENT OF CARDIAC INVOLVEMENT IN FABRY DISEASE

Treatment of adult patients with FD should aim at preventing disease progression to irreversible organ damage and organ failure. Care should include both general cardiovascular management and specific therapy.

General Cardiovascular Management

Cardiovascular risk factors

Patients with FD may have one or more general risk factors for cardiovascular disease (eg, diabetes, hypertension, smoking, hypercholesterolemia), and those resulting from FD (eg, chronic kidney disease) and its treatment (eg, antiepileptic agents). A recent study has shown that the modification of cardiovascular risk factors can reduce the risk of adverse events related to the disease.[78] Thus, in patients with FD the modification of the cardiovascular risk factor is adviced, as described in the current guidelines.[79–82]

In particular, elevated systemic blood pressure has been shown to negatively impact on the progression of FD cardiomyopathy and also minor increases in systolic blood pressure were strongly associated with an advanced course of FD cardiomyopathy in a recent study.[83] This association seems to be related to the increased wall stress induced by the elevated blood pressure in the already damages and thus vulnerable heart segments, accelerating fibrosis progression. These findings suggest that systemic blood pressure should be adequately controlled, independent of the stage of the disease.

Conduction abnormalities

In case of symptomatic bradyarrhythmias, such as sinus node disease, including inappropriate sinus bradycardia and/or chronotropic incompetence, or high-degree atrioventricular block, permanent cardiac pacing should be considered, as described in the current guidelines.[84,85]

Supraventricular arrhythmias

In a prospective study of 207 patients with FD followed for 7 years, 6% of patients developed AF.[21] The occurrence of AF in patients with FD may have a significant impact on the natural history of the disease.[21] The choice of antiarrhythmic drugs in these patients is limited. In particular, the use of beta-blockers should be monitored carefully because of the risk of exacerbating bradycardia and chronotropic incompetence, while the use of amiodarone should be carefully weighted in patients receiving ERT due to its potential inhibitory effect on α-Gal A activity.[1,26,37]

Isolated reports data suggest that catheter ablation according to general guidelines can be considered.[86] Moreover, patients with FD who develop paroxysmal, persistent, or permanent AF or flutter should receive early oral anticoagulation therapy, irrespectively of age or gender, because the current scoring systems (ie, CHA_2DS_2VASc) may underestimate the risk of systemic embolization in young patients.[52] If not contraindicated for renal impairment, new oral anticoagulants should be preferred for the lower risks of cerebral microbleedings and lower renal toxicity compared with warfarin.

Ventricular arrhythmias and prevention of sudden cardiac death

Clinical experience in the FD population indicates that SCD is an uncommon event.[22] Unfortunately, there are no sufficient data to establish a clear model for SCD risk prediction in FD or to formulate specific recommendations in SCD prevention. To date, severe LVH, extensive fibrosis, and unexplained syncope have been considered predictors of SCD, and in their presence, the implantation of an ICD in primary prevention should be considered.[66,87]

Heart failure

Heart failure (HF) is related to age and disease progression. According to data from Fabry Registry, HF was a common cardiovascular event and occurred in 3.5% of men and 2.3% of women with FD.[21] HF should be treated according to the current guidelines, to improve exercise tolerance and normal daily activities, as well as to improve or prevent progression of New York Heart Association class, although there is no evidence for a prognostic benefit from standard management of HF in patients with FD.[81] As mentioned earlier, beta-blockers should be used with caution due to the risk of exacerbating bradycardia and chronotropic incompetence.[1,26,37]

Disease-specific therapy

The current therapeutic options for FD included ERT and chaperone therapy. ERT is available to treat patients with FD through intravenous infusions of agalsidase alfa or agalsidase beta at the dosage of 0.2 mg/kg and 1.0 mg/kg of body weight every other week, respectively. Long-term clinical studies showed a significant effect of ERT on renal and cardiovascular complication rate[88,89]; these clinical benefits were principally observed in patients who started therapy at an early stage of FD, before the occurrence of irreversible organ damage.[14,87,90,91] ERT can improve mild-to-moderate LVH and stabilize severe LVH; however, patients with cardiac fibrosis showed a minor reduction in LVH and no myocardial function improvement.[78,92–96] Therefore, ERT does not prevent the development of fibrosis in patients with severe cardiomyopathy.[92] Moreover, ERT is limited by several factors, including high costs, a frequent incident of infusion-related reactions, and a lifelong burden of intravenous infusion.[97]

More recently, new treatment options for FD have been developed to overcome some limitations of ERT. Among these, pharmacologic chaperone therapy, using migalastat, a small molecule agent that partially restores the deficient endogenous enzyme activity,[98,99] has been recently approved in patients with FD with amenable GLA pathogenic variants. Migalastat treatment is associated with increased and sustained endogenous α-Gal A activity levels, stability of renal function, and cardiac mass reduction.[100,101] Several factors make migalastat an attractive alternative option to ERT for treating FD: firstly, the oral administration, thus eliminating the requirement for lifelong intravenous infusions and related complications.[97] Secondly, migalastat has a high tissue distribution and has the potential to cross the blood-brain barrier.[102,103] Finally, in one clinical trial it showed improved efficacy compared with ERT in reducing cardiac mass.[100] In contrast, recent real-world data raised caution about the possible differences between in vitro and in vivo amenability for some genetic variants, likely responsible for worsening of renal function and increase of lysoGb$_3$ levels in some patients.[104] Plasma lysoGb$_3$ correlated with LVH and fibrosis in recent studies.[105,106]

However, its use for treatment monitoring has not been validated, and it seems that neither the absolute decrease of lysoGb$_3$ nor its relative decrease predict the risk of clinical events in patients receiving ERT[105] or migalastat.[106]

CLINICS CARE POINTS

- The diagnosis of FD varies depending on the patient gender and disease phenotype. In male patients, dramatically reduced or absent α-Gal A activity is diagnostic, whereas in female patients, the demonstration of a *GLA* pathogenic variant is required for the diagnosis.

- In patients with later-onset isolated cardiovascular involvement, several red flags, defined as clinical or instrumental features that help for the diagnosis of a specific disorder, have been proposed to suspect FD.

- Among patients with late-onset HCM, FD shows a prevalence of 0.8% to 1.1%. Thus, in patients with unexplained LVH, diagnosis of FD should be considered.

ACKNOWLEDGMENTS

The authors would like to acknowledge Michela Piscopo, Daniela Lafera, and Ciro De Prisco who made possible our research and clinical activity.

DISCLOSURE

The authors have nothing to disclose. D.P. Germain is a consultant for Sanofi Genzyme and Takeda.

REFERENCES

1. Germain DP. Fabry disease. Orphanet J Rare Dis 2010;5:30.
2. Lin HY, Chong KW, Hsu JH, et al. High incidence of the cardiac variant of fabry disease revealed by newborn screening in the Taiwan Chinese population. Circ Cardiovasc Genet 2009;2(5):450–6.
3. Spada M, Pagliardini S, Yasuda M, et al. High incidence of later-onset fabry disease revealed by newborn screening. Am J Hum Genet 2006;79(1):31–40.
4. Gelb MH, Turecek F, Scott CR, et al. Direct multiplex assay of enzymes in dried blood spots by tandem mass spectrometry for the newborn screening of lysosomal storage disorders. J Inherit Metab Dis 2006;29(2–3):397–404.
5. Scott CR, Elliott S, Buroker N, et al. Identification of infants at risk for developing Fabry, Pompe, or mucopolysaccharidosis-I from newborn blood spots by tandem mass spectrometry. J Pediatr 2013;163(2):498–503.
6. Reuser AJ, Verheijen FW, Bali D, et al. The use of dried blood spot samples in the diagnosis of lysosomal storage disorders–current status and perspectives. Mol Genet Metab 2011;104(1–2):144–8.
7. Linthorst GE, Bouwman MG, Wijburg FA, et al. Screening for Fabry disease in high-risk populations: a systematic review. J Med Genet 2010; 47(4):217–22.
8. Chimenti C, Pieroni M, Morgante E, et al. Prevalence of Fabry disease in female patients with late-onset hypertrophic cardiomyopathy. Circulation 2004;110(9):1047–53.
9. Sachdev B, Takenaka T, Teraguchi H, et al. Prevalence of Anderson-Fabry disease in male patients with late onset hypertrophic cardiomyopathy. Circulation 2002;105(12):1407–11.
10. Palecek T, Honzikova J, Poupetova H, et al. Prevalence of Fabry disease in male patients with unexplained left ventricular hypertrophy in primary cardiology practice: prospective Fabry cardiomyopathy screening study (FACSS). J Inherit Metab Dis 2014;37(3):455–60.
11. Elliott P, Baker R, Pasquale F, et al. Prevalence of Anderson-Fabry disease in patients with hypertrophic cardiomyopathy: the European Anderson-Fabry Disease survey. Heart 2011;97(23):1957–60.
12. Doheny D, Srinivasan R, Pagant S, et al. Fabry disease: prevalence of affected males and heterozygotes with pathogenic GLA mutations identified by screening renal, cardiac and stroke clinics, 1995-2017. J Med Genet 2018;55(4):261–8.
13. Limongelli G, Monda E, Tramonte S, et al. Prevalence and clinical significance of red flags in patients with hypertrophic cardiomyopathy. Int J Cardiol 2020;299:186–91.
14. Germain DP, Charrow J, Desnick RJ, et al. Ten-year outcome of enzyme replacement therapy with agalsidase beta in patients with Fabry disease. J Med Genet 2015;52(5):353–8.
15. Echevarria L, Benistan K, Toussaint A, et al. X-chromosome inactivation in female patients with Fabry disease. Clin Genet 2016;89(1):44–54.
16. Wilcox WR, Oliveira JP, Hopkin RJ, et al. Females with Fabry disease frequently have major organ involvement: lessons from the Fabry Registry. Mol Genet Metab 2008;93(2):112–28.
17. Arends M, Wanner C, Hughes D, et al. Characterization of classical and nonclassical fabry disease: a multicenter study. J Am Soc Nephrol 2017;28(5):1631–41.
18. Kampmann C, Baehner F, Whybra C, et al. Cardiac manifestations of Anderson-Fabry disease in

heterozygous females. J Am Coll Cardiol 2002; 40(9):1668–74.

19. Krämer J, Niemann M, Störk S, et al. Relation of burden of myocardial fibrosis to malignant ventricular arrhythmias and outcomes in Fabry disease. Am J Cardiol 2014;114(6):895–900.

20. Pieroni M, Moon JC, Arbustini E, et al. Cardiac involvement in fabry disease: JACC review topic of the week. J Am Coll Cardiol 2021;77:922–36.

21. Patel MR, Cecchi F, Cizmarik M, et al. Cardiovascular events in patients with fabry disease natural history data from the fabry registry. J Am Coll Cardiol 2011;57(9):1093–9.

22. Patel V, O'Mahony C, Hughes D, et al. Clinical and genetic predictors of major cardiac events in patients with Anderson-Fabry Disease. Heart 2015; 101(12):961–6.

23. Mehta A, Clarke JT, Giugliani R, et al. Natural course of Fabry disease: changing pattern of causes of death in FOS - Fabry Outcome Survey. J Med Genet 2009;46(8):548–52.

24. Platt FM, d'Azzo A, Davidson BL, et al. Lysosomal storage diseases [published correction appears in Nat Rev Dis Primers. 2018 Oct 18;4(1):36] [published correction appears in Nat Rev Dis Primers. 2019 May 17;5(1):34]. Nat Rev Dis Primers 2018; 4(1):27.

25. Ivanova M. Altered sphingolipids metabolism damaged mitochondrial functions: lessons learned from gaucher and fabry diseases. J Clin Med 2020; 9(4):1116.

26. Ortiz A, Germain DP, Desnick RJ, et al. Fabry disease revisited: management and treatment recommendations for adult patients. Mol Genet Metab 2018;123(4):416–27.

27. Miller EM, Wang Y, Ware SM. Uptake of cardiac screening and genetic testing among hypertrophic and dilated cardiomyopathy families. J Genet Couns 2013;22(2):258–67.

28. Benjamin ER, Della Valle MC, Wu X, et al. The validation of pharmacogenetics for the identification of Fabry patients to be treated with migalastat. Genet Med 2017;19(4):430–8.

29. Wang RY, Lelis A, Mirocha J, et al. Heterozygous Fabry women are not just carriers, but have a significant burden of disease and impaired quality of life. Genet Med 2007;9(1):34–45.

30. Weidemann F, Niemann M, Sommer C, et al. Interdisciplinary approach towards female patients with Fabry disease. Eur J Clin Invest 2012;42(4):455–62.

31. Pasqualim G, Simon L, Sperb-Ludwig F, et al. Fabry disease: a new approach for the screening of females in high-risk groups. Clin Biochem 2014;47(7–8):657–62.

32. Nair V, Belanger EC, Veinot JP. Lysosomal storage disorders affecting the heart: a review. Cardiovasc Pathol 2019;39:12–24.

33. Smid BE, van der Tol L, Cecchi F, et al. Uncertain diagnosis of Fabry disease: consensus recommendation on diagnosis in adults with left ventricular hypertrophy and genetic variants of unknown significance. Int J Cardiol 2014;177(2):400–8.

34. Tschöpe C, Dominguez F, Canaan-Kühl S, et al. Endomyocardial biopsy in Anderson-Fabry disease: the key in uncertain cases. Int J Cardiol 2015; 190:284–6.

35. Cooper LT, Baughman KL, Feldman AM, et al. The role of endomyocardial biopsy in the management of cardiovascular disease: a scientific statement from the American Heart Association, the American College of Cardiology, and the European Society of Cardiology. Endorsed by the Heart Failure Society of America and the Heart Failure Association of the European Society of Cardiology. J Am Coll Cardiol 2007;50(19):1914–31.

36. Girolami F, Frisso G, Benelli M, et al. Contemporary genetic testing in inherited cardiac disease: tools, ethical issues, and clinical applications. J Cardiovasc Med (Hagerstown) 2018;19(1):1–11.

37. Linhart A, Elliott PM. The heart in Anderson-Fabry disease and other lysosomal storage disorders. Heart 2007;93:528–35.

38. Kampmann C, Linhart A, Baehner F, et al. Onset and progression of the Anderson-Fabry disease related cardiomyopathy. Int J Cardiol 2008;130(3):367–73.

39. Havranek S, Linhart A, Urbanova Z, et al. Early cardiac changes in children with Anderson-Fabry disease. JIMD Rep 2013;11:53–64.

40. Wijburg FA, Bénichou B, Bichet DG, et al. Characterization of early disease status in treatment-naive male paediatric patients with Fabry disease enrolled in a randomized clinical trial. PLoS One 2015;10(5):e0124987.

41. Monda E, Rubino M, Lioncino M, et al. Hypertrophic cardiomyopathy in children: pathophysiology, diagnosis, and treatment of non-sarcomeric causes. Front Pediatr 2021;9:632293.

42. Limongelli G, Monda E, D'Aponte A, et al. Combined effect of mediterranean diet and aerobic exercise on weight loss and clinical status in obese symptomatic patients with hypertrophic cardiomyopathy. Heart Fail Clin 2021;17(2):303–13.

43. Caiazza M, Rubino M, Monda E, et al. Combined PTPN11 and MYBPC3 Gene mutations in an adult patient with noonan syndrome and hypertrophic cardiomyopathy. Genes (Basel) 2020;11(8):947.

44. Esposito A, Monda E, Gragnano F, et al. Prevalence and clinical implications of hyperhomocysteinaemia in patients with hypertrophic cardiomyopathy and MTHFR C6777T polymorphism. Eur J Prev Cardiol 2020;27(17):1906–8.

45. Limongelli G, Nunziato M, D'Argenio V, et al. Yield and clinical significance of genetic screening in

elite and amateur athletes. Eur J Prev Cardiol. 2020 Jul 2:2047487320934265. https://doi.org/10.1177/2047487320934265.

46. Monda E, Sarubbi B, Russo MG, et al. Unexplained sudden cardiac arrest in children: clinical and genetic characteristics of survivors. Eur J Prev Cardiol. 2020 Jul 26:2047487320940863. https://doi.org/10.1177/2047487320940863.

47. Monda E, Palmiero G, Rubino M, et al. Molecular Basis of Inflammation in the Pathogenesis of Cardiomyopathies. Int J Mol Sci 2020;21(18):6462.

48. Linhart A, Germain DP, Olivotto I, et al. An expert consensus document on the management of cardiovascular manifestations of Fabry disease. Eur J Heart Fail 2020;22(7):1076–96.

49. Wu JC, Ho CY, Skali H, et al. Cardiovascular manifestations of Fabry disease: relationships between left ventricular hypertrophy, disease severity, and alpha-galactosidase A activity. Eur Heart J 2010; 31(9):1088–97.

50. Hsu TR, Hung SC, Chang FP, et al. Later onset fabry disease, cardiac damage progress in silence: experience with a highly prevalent mutation. J Am Coll Cardiol 2016;68(23):2554–63.

51. Rapezzi C, Arbustini E, Caforio AL, et al. Diagnostic work-up in cardiomyopathies: bridging the gap between clinical phenotypes and final diagnosis. A position statement from the ESC Working Group on Myocardial and Pericardial Diseases. Eur Heart J 2013;34(19):1448–58.

52. Authors/Task Force Members, Elliott PM, Anastasakis A, et al. 2014 ESC Guidelines on diagnosis and management of hypertrophic cardiomyopathy: the task force for the diagnosis and management of hypertrophic cardiomyopathy of the European Society of Cardiology (ESC). Eur Heart J 2014;35(39):2733–79.

53. Namdar M, Steffel J, Vidovic M, et al. Electrocardiographic changes in early recognition of Fabry disease. Heart 2011;97(6):485–90.

54. O'Mahony C, Coats C, Cardona M, et al. Incidence and predictors of anti-bradycardia pacing in patients with Anderson-Fabry disease. Europace 2011;13(12):1781–8.

55. Namdar M. Electrocardiographic changes and arrhythmia in fabry disease. Front Cardiovasc Med 2016;3:7.

56. Sené T, Lidove O, Sebbah J, et al. Cardiac device implantation in Fabry disease: a retrospective monocentric study. Medicine (Baltimore) 2016; 95(40):e4996.

57. Niemann M, Liu D, Hu K, et al. Prominent papillary muscles in Fabry disease: a diagnostic marker? Ultrasound Med Biol 2011;37(1):37–43.

58. Graziani F, Laurito M, Pieroni M, et al. Right ventricular hypertrophy, systolic function, and disease severity in anderson-fabry disease: an echocardiographic study. J Am Soc Echocardiogr 2017;30(3):282–91.

59. Mundigler G, Gaggl M, Heinze G, et al. The endocardial binary appearance ('binary sign') is an unreliable marker for echocardiographic detection of Fabry disease in patients with left ventricular hypertrophy. Eur J Echocardiogr 2011;12(10): 744–9.

60. Esposito R, Galderisi M, Santoro C, et al. Prominent longitudinal strain reduction of left ventricular basal segments in treatment-naïve Anderson-Fabry disease patients. Eur Heart J Cardiovasc Imaging 2019;20(4):438–45.

61. Shanks M, Thompson RB, Paterson ID, et al. Systolic and diastolic function assessment in fabry disease patients using speckle-tracking imaging and comparison with conventional echocardiographic measurements. J Am Soc Echocardiogr 2013; 26(12):1407–14.

62. Vijapurapu R, Nordin S, Baig S, et al. Global longitudinal strain, myocardial storage and hypertrophy in Fabry disease. Heart 2019;105(6):470–6.

63. Ommen SR, Nishimura RA, Edwards WD. Fabry disease: a mimic for obstructive hypertrophic cardiomyopathy? Heart 2003;89:929–30.

64. Nakao S, Takenaka T, Maeda M, et al. An atypical variant of Fabry's disease in men with left ventricular hypertrophy. N Engl J Med 1995;333(5):288–93.

65. Militaru S, Ginghina C, Popescu BA, et al. Multimodality imaging in Fabry cardiomyopathy: from early diagnosis to therapeutic targets. Eur Heart J Cardiovasc Imaging 2018;19(12):1313–22.

66. Baig S, Edward NC, Kotecha D, et al. Ventricular arrhythmia and sudden cardiac death in Fabry disease: a systematic review of risk factors in clinical practice. Europace 2018;20(Fl2):f153–61.

67. Kozor R, Grieve SM, Tchan MC, et al. Cardiac involvement in genotype-positive Fabry disease patients assessed by cardiovascular MR. Heart 2016;102(4):298–302.

68. Camporeale A, Pieroni M, Pieruzzi F, et al. Predictors of clinical evolution in prehypertrophic fabry disease. Circ Cardiovasc Imaging 2019;12(4):e008424.

69. Haaf P, Garg P, Messroghli DR, et al. Cardiac T1 Mapping and Extracellular Volume (ECV) in clinical practice: a comprehensive review. J Cardiovasc Magn Reson 2016;18(1):89.

70. Pica S, Sado DM, Maestrini V, et al. Reproducibility of native myocardial T1 mapping in the assessment of Fabry disease and its role in early detection of cardiac involvement by cardiovascular magnetic resonance. J Cardiovasc Magn Reson 2014;16(1):99.

71. Thompson RB, Chow K, Khan A, et al. T_1 mapping with cardiovascular MRI is highly sensitive for Fabry disease independent of hypertrophy and sex. Circ Cardiovasc Imaging 2013;6(5):637–45.

72. Nordin S, Kozor R, Bulluck H, et al. Cardiac Fabry disease with late gadolinium enhancement is a chronic inflammatory cardiomyopathy. J Am Coll Cardiol 2016;68:1707–8.

73. Knott KD, Augusto JB, Nordin S, et al. Quantitative myocardial perfusion in fabry disease. Circ Cardiovasc Imaging 2019;12(7):e008872.

74. Seydelmann N, Liu D, Krämer J, et al. High-sensitivity troponin: a clinical blood biomarker for staging cardiomyopathy in fabry disease [published correction appears in. J Am Heart Assoc 2016; 5(9):e002839.

75. Coats CJ, Parisi V, Ramos M, et al. Role of serum N-terminal pro-brain natriuretic peptide measurement in diagnosis of cardiac involvement in patients with anderson-fabry disease. Am J Cardiol 2013;111(1):111–7.

76. Nordin S, Kozor R, Medina-Menacho K, et al. Proposed stages of myocardial phenotype development in fabry disease. JACC Cardiovasc Imaging 2019;12(8 Pt 2):1673–83.

77. Kramer J, Weidemann F. Biomarkers for Diagnosing and Staging of Fabry Disease. Curr Med Chem 2018;25:1530–7.

78. Sirrs SM, Bichet DG, Casey R, et al. Outcomes of patients treated through the Canadian Fabry disease initiative. Mol Genet Metab 2014;111(4): 499–506.

79. Cosentino F, Grant PJ, Aboyans V, et al. 2019 ESC guidelines on diabetes, pre-diabetes, and cardiovascular diseases developed in collaboration with the EASD [published correction appears in Eur Heart J. 2020 Dec 1;41(45):4317]. Eur Heart J 2020;41(2):255–323.

80. Mach F, Baigent C, Catapano AL, et al. 2019 ESC/ EAS guidelines for the management of dyslipidaemias: lipid modification to reduce cardiovascular risk [published correction appears in Eur Heart J. 2020 Nov 21;41(44):4255]. Eur Heart J 2020; 41(1):111–88.

81. Williams B, Mancia G, Spiering W, et al. 2018 ESC/ ESH guidelines for the management of arterial hypertension [published correction appears in Eur Heart J. 2019 Feb 1;40(5):475]. Eur Heart J 2018; 39(33):3021–104.

82. Piepoli MF, Hoes AW, Agewall S, et al. 2016 European guidelines on cardiovascular disease prevention in clinical practice: the sixth joint task force of the European Society of Cardiology and Other Societies on Cardiovascular Disease Prevention in Clinical Practice (constituted by representatives of 10 societies and by invited experts)Developed with the special contribution of the European Association for Cardiovascular Prevention & Rehabilitation (EACPR). Eur Heart J 2016;37(29):2315–81.

83. Krämer J, Bijnens B, Störk S, et al. Left ventricular geometry and blood pressure as predictors of adverse progression of fabry cardiomyopathy. PLoS One 2015;10(11):e0140627.

84. Acharya D, Doppalapudi H, Tallaj JA. Arrhythmias in Fabry cardiomyopathy. Card Electrophysiol Clin 2015;7:283–91.

85. Brignole M, Auricchio A, Baron-Esquivias G, et al. 2013 ESC guidelines on cardiac pacing and cardiac resynchronization therapy: the task force on cardiac pacing and resynchronization therapy of the European Society of Cardiology (ESC). Developed in collaboration with the European Heart Rhythm Association (EHRA). Eur Heart J 2013; 34(29):2281–329.

86. Qian P, Ross D, Tchan M, et al. A patient with recurrent disabling atrial fibrillation and Fabry cardiomyopathy successfully treated with single ring pulmonary vein isolation. Int J Cardiol 2015;182:375–6.

87. Weidemann F, Niemann M, Störk S, et al. Long-term outcome of enzyme-replacement therapy in advanced Fabry disease: evidence for disease progression towards serious complications. J Intern Med 2013;274(4):331–41.

88. Arends M, Biegstraaten M, Wanner C, et al. Agalsidase alfa versus agalsidase beta for the treatment of Fabry disease: an international cohort study. J Med Genet 2018;55(5):351–8.

89. El Dib R, Gomaa H, Ortiz A, et al. Enzyme replacement therapy for Anderson-Fabry disease: a complementary overview of a cochrane publication through a linear regression and a pooled analysis of proportions from cohort studies. PLoS One 2017;12(3):e0173358.

90. Tøndel C, Bostad L, Larsen KK, et al. Agalsidase benefits renal histology in young patients with Fabry disease. J Am Soc Nephrol 2013;24(1): 137–48.

91. Arends M, Wijburg FA, Wanner C, et al. Favourable effect of early versus late start of enzyme replacement therapy on plasma globotriaosylsphingosine levels in men with classical Fabry disease. Mol Genet Metab 2017;121(2):157–61.

92. Germain DP, Weidemann F, Abiose A, et al. Analysis of left ventricular mass in untreated men and in men treated with agalsidase-β: data from the Fabry Registry. Genet Med 2013;15(12):958–65.

93. Eng CM, Guffon N, Wilcox WR, et al. Safety and efficacy of recombinant human alpha-galactosidase A replacement therapy in Fabry's disease. N Engl J Med 2001;345(1):9–16.

94. Thurberg BL, Fallon JT, Mitchell R, et al. Cardiac microvascular pathology in Fabry disease: evaluation of endomyocardial biopsies before and after enzyme replacement therapy. Circulation 2009; 119(19):2561–7.

95. Hughes DA, Elliott PM, Shah J, et al. Effects of enzyme replacement therapy on the cardiomyopathy of Anderson-Fabry disease: a randomised,

double-blind, placebo-controlled clinical trial of agalsidase alfa. Heart 2008;94(2):153–8.

96. Beer M, Weidemann F, Breunig F, et al. Impact of enzyme replacement therapy on cardiac morphology and function and late enhancement in Fabry's cardiomyopathy. Am J Cardiol 2006; 97(10):1515–8.

97. Lidove O, West ML, Pintos-Morell G, et al. Effects of enzyme replacement therapy in Fabry disease–a comprehensive review of the medical literature. Genet Med 2010;12(11):668–79.

98. Parenti G, Andria G, Valenzano KJ. Pharmacological chaperone therapy: preclinical development, clinical translation, and prospects for the treatment of lysosomal storage disorders. Mol Ther 2015; 23(7):1138–48.

99. Benjamin ER, Flanagan JJ, Schilling A, et al. The pharmacological chaperone 1-deoxygalactonojiri-mycin increases alpha-galactosidase A levels in Fabry patient cell lines. J Inherit Metab Dis 2009; 32(3):424–40.

100. Hughes DA, Nicholls K, Shankar SP, et al. Oral pharmacological chaperone migalastat compared with enzyme replacement therapy in Fabry disease: 18-month results from the randomised phase III ATTRACT study [published correction appears in J Med Genet. 2018 Apr 16;:]. J Med Genet 2017; 54(4):288–96.

101. Germain DP, Hughes DA, Nicholls K, et al. Treatment of fabry's disease with the pharmacologic chaperone migalastat. N Engl J Med 2016;375(6): 545–55.

102. Parenti G. Treating lysosomal storage diseases with pharmacological chaperones: from concept to clinics. EMBO Mol Med 2009;1(5):268–79.

103. Mohamed FE, Al-Gazali L, Al-Jasmi F, et al. Pharmaceutical chaperones and proteostasis regulators in the therapy of lysosomal storage disorders: current perspective and future promises. Front Pharmacol 2017;8:448.

104. Lenders M, Nordbeck P, Kurschat C, et al. Treatment of fabry disease with migalastat-outcome from a prospective 24 months observational multicenter study (FAMOUS). Eur Heart J Cardiovasc Pharmacother. 2021 Mar 16:pvab025. https://doi.org/10.1093/ehjcvp/pvab025.

105. Arends M, Biegstraaten M, Hughes DA, et al. Retrospective study of longterm outcomes of enzyme replacement therapy in Fabry disease: analysis of prognostic factors. PLoS ONE 2017;12:e0182379.

106. Franzen D, Haile SR, Kasper DC, et al. Pulmonary involvement in Fabry disease: effect of plasma globotriaosylsphingosine and time to initiation of enzyme replacement therapy. BMJ Open Respir Res 2018;5:e000277.

Cardiovascular Involvement in mtDNA Disease
Diagnosis, Management, and Therapeutic Options

Michele Lioncino, MD[a], Emanuele Monda, MD[a], Martina Caiazza, MD[a],
Adelaide Fusco, MD[a], Annapaola Cirillo, MD, PhD[a],
Francesca Dongiglio, MD[a], Vicenzo Simonelli, MD[b], Simone Sampaolo, MD[c],
Lucia Ruggiero, MD[d], Gioacchino Scarano, MD[a], Vicenzo Pota, MD, PhD[e],
Giulia Frisso, MD[f,g,h], Cristina Mazzaccara, MD[f,g,h], Giulia D'Amati, MD, PhD[i],
Gerardo Nigro, MD, PhD[j], Maria Giovanna Russo, MD, PhD[k],
Karim Wahbi, MD, PhD[l], Giuseppe Limongelli, MD, PhD[a],*

KEYWORDS

- Mitochondrial diseases • MELAS syndrome • mtDNA • Hypertrophic cardiomyopathy

KEY POINTS

- Mitochondrial diseases include an heterogenous group of systemic disorders caused by sporadic or inherited mutations in nuclear or mitochondrial DNA (mtDNA), causing impairment of oxidative phosphorylation system.
- Hypertrophic cardiomyopathy is the dominant pattern of cardiomyopathy in all forms of mtDNA diseases (mtDNA-D), being observed in almost 40% of the patients.
- The diagnosis of mtDNA-D is challenging because of wide clinical and genetic heterogeneity and requires a multisystemic approach.

INTRODUCTION

Mitochondrial diseases (MD) include an heterogenous group of systemic disorders caused by sporadic or inherited mutations in nuclear (nDNA) or mitochondrial DNA (mtDNA), causing impairment of oxidative phosphorylation system (OXPHOS) and subsequent reduction in adenosine triphosphate production, leading to different phenotypes, depending on the tissue involved, type of

[a] Inherited and Rare Cardiovascular Disease Unit, Department of Translational Medical Sciences, University of Campania "Luigi Vanvitelli", Naples; [b] Division of Neurology, AORN Dei Colli, Monaldi Hospital, Naples; [c] Second Division of Neurology, Department of Advanced Medical and Surgical Sciences, University of Campania Luigi Vanvitelli, Naples, Italy; [d] Department of Neurosciences, Reproductive Sciences and Odontostomatology, University of Naples Federico II, Naples, Italy; [e] Department of Women, Child and General and Specialized Surgery, University of Campania "Luigi Vanvitelli", Piazza L. Miraglia 2, 80138 Naples, Italy; [f] Dipartimento di Medicina Molecolare e Biotecnologie Mediche, Università di Napoli Federico II, Naples, Italy; [g] CEINGE Biotecnologie Avanzate, Scarl, Naples, Italy; [h] CEINGE Advanced Biotechnologies, 80145 Naples, Italy; [i] Department of Radiological, Oncological and Pathological Sciences, Sapienza University of Rome, Rome, Italy; [j] Department of Medical Translational Sciences, Division of Cardiology, Monaldi Hospital, University of Campania "Luigi Vanvitelli", Naples, Italy; [k] Pediatric Cardiology Unit, Monaldi Hospital, University "Luigi Vanvitelli", Naples, Italy; [l] APHP, Cochin Hospital, Cardiology Department, FILNEMUS, Paris-Descartes, Sorbonne Paris Cité University, Paris, France
* Corresponding author.
E-mail address: limongelligiuseppe@libero.it

Heart Failure Clin 18 (2022) 51–60
https://doi.org/10.1016/j.hfc.2021.07.003
1551-7136/22/© 2021 Elsevier Inc. All rights reserved.

pathogenic mutations, and heteroplasmy level.[1–3] MD affect preferentially tissue with high energy demands and show multiorgan involvement, resulting in complex multisystemic diseases mainly characterized by neurologic, ophthalmologic, audiological, endocrine, and cardiovascular disease.[4,5] In particular, myocardial involvement is present in up to 60% of patients with MD and represents an independent predictor of morbidity and early mortality.[6,7] Although the exact prevalence of MD is unknown, population-based studies report a prevalence of 9.2/100000 among adults younger than 65 years; such data are not completely accurate because of the lack of standardized criteria for diagnosis and may reflect an underestimation of the true prevalence of MD.[8,9] Currently, more than 250 nuclear genes over 37 mitochondrial genes are associated with OXPHOS defects.

Before the advent of next-generation sequencing (NGS) technology, few of the genes and mutations were known to be pathogenic or likely pathogenic for MD. In particular, the m.3243A>G mutation has been detected in up to 1/300 of the general population, and although many individuals are asymptomatic carriers of low levels of mutation, its clinical prevalence is estimated to be of 1/5000 in the general population.[9]

In this article, the authors discuss the current clinical knowledge on MD, focusing on diagnosis and management of MD caused by mtDNA mutations (mtDNA-D).

CLINICAL PRESENTATION AND RED FLAGS

The clinical spectrum of mtDNA disease (mtDNA-D) is heterogeneous and can range from oligo-symptomatic patients to severe multisystemic involvement.[10] Organs with high aerobic metabolic demands as brain tissue, heart, or skeletal muscle are more severely affected in patients with mtDNA-D.[11] Lactic acidosis may be present, but its absence should not be used to rule out mtDNA-D.[12]

Patients with neuromuscular mtDNA-D often present with increased creatine kinase levels and symptoms of skeletal myopathy; rarely nervous conduction tests show axonal sensorimotor neuropathy.[3,13–15] Almost 10% of the patients have abnormal liver function tests; gastrointestinal symptoms such as constipation, dysphagia, and chronic intestinal pseudoobstruction are common.[16,17] Renal involvement is characterized by proximal tubulopathy, Fanconi syndrome, and tubulointerstitial nephritis, causing a progressive reduction in glomerular filtration rate.[14,18] Endocrine disorders may include diabetes mellitus, hypothyroidism, hypoparathyroidism, diabetes

insipidus, and hypogonadism.[16] Short stature has been reported in up to 20% of the cases.[13] Ophthalmologic manifestations include retinitis pigmentosa, palpebral ptosis, external ophthalmoplegia, cataract, and optic atrophy.[3,11,13]

Central nervous system involvement is a major determinant of adverse events in patients with mtDNA-D and common clinical features such as encephalopathy, strokelike episodes, cognitive dysfunction, ataxia, seizures, migraine, or depression should raise the suspicion of an underlying mtDNA disorder.[7,11] Bilateral sensorineural deafness occurs in 7% to 26% of the patients, and its prevalence increases with age.[13,19]

Although there are no consensus statements evaluating the performance of clinical "red flags" for the diagnosis of mitochondrial cardiomyopathies, the presence of a maternal inheritance pattern or the identification of extra cardiac features of mtDNA-D should guide further investigations in order to exclude an underlying mitochondrial disorder.[20] Clinical clues for the diagnosis of mtDNA-D are listed in **Table 1**.

CARDIOVASCULAR INVOLVEMENT IN MITOCHONDRIAL DISEASE

Cardiovascular involvement in MD is progressive, and it is an independent predictor of morbidity and mortality,[6,21] both in pediatric and adult patients. In a cohort study including 113 children with mtDNA-D, survival rate to age 16 years was 18% in patients with cardiovascular involvement compared with 92% in patients without evidence of heart disease.[21]

In a large, retrospective study enrolling 260 adult patients, most of them with mtDNA-D, cardiovascular involvement was present in almost 31% of the patients at baseline. Over a 7-year follow-up, hypertrophic cardiomyopathy (HCM) was observed in 18% of the patients, mostly carriers of the m.3243A>G mutation.[7] Major adverse clinical events, including sudden death, death or hospitalization due to heart failure, resuscitated cardiac arrest, high-grade atrioventricular block, or cardiac transplantation, were observed in 10% of the patients; multivariate analysis showed hypertrophic phenotype to be an independent predictor of MACE (hazard ratio 2.5; 95% confidence interval: 1.1–5.8).[7]

HCM is the dominant pattern of cardiomyopathy in all forms of mtDNA-D, being observed in almost 40% of the patients.[6,22–24] Although different mtDNA mutations may have heterogeneous phenotypical expression, cross-sectional studies seem to show recurrent patterns of genotype-phenotype correlation.[24,25] Cardiomyopathies

Table 1
Clinical red flags for the suspicion of mitochondrial disorders

Organ System	
Neurologic	Hypotonia + metabolic acidosis Encephalopathy Myoclonus Ataxia Axonal neuropathy Skeletal myopathy
Ophthalmologic	Retinitis pigmentosa Palpebral ptosis External ophthalmoplegia Cataract Optic atrophy
ENT	Bilateral sensorineural deafness
Endocrine	Diabetes mellitus Hypothyroidism Diabetes insipidus Hypogonadism
Renal	Fanconi syndrome Proximal tubulopathy
Cardiovascular	HCM Ventricular preexcitation Left ventricular noncompaction Conduction system disease
Biomarkers	Increased CK enzyme Lactic acidosis Lactate/pyruvate ratio>20 Leukocytopenia (Barth syndrome)
Brain magnetic resonance	Diffuse, fluctuating strokelike lesion in nonvascular distribution pattern, with elevated T2 and ECV signal and normal DWI Symmetric abnormalities of deep gray matter, with high T2 and FLAIR and low T1 signal Delayed myelination pattern

Abbreviations: CK, creatine kinase; DWI, diffusion-weighted imaging; ECV, extracellular volume.

with hypertrophic remodeling seem to be associated to mt-tRNA mutations, whereas single, large-scale deletions are more often associated to conduction disturbances, such as atrioventricular (AV) block in Kearns-Sayre syndrome (KSS).[6,26,27] According to recent studies, the echocardiographic prevalence of left ventricular hypertrophy (LVH) ranges from 38% to 56% in carriers of m3243A>G mutation; noteworthy mutation load seemed to predict the severity of hypertrophy[23,24] and heart failure. Of note, LVH is less common in association with mt-rRNA gene and protein-coding-genes mutations.[28–31]

The natural history of mitochondrial cardiomyopathies shows many important differences with sarcomeric HCM: left ventricular outflow tract obstruction is less common in mtDNA-D, and the risk of progression to end-stage clinical variants, characterized by LV chamber dilatation and systolic dysfunction, is higher than in sarcomeric forms.[10,23] In patients with mtDNA-D, dilated cardiomyopathy often results from the end-stage progression of HCM rather than being the initial pattern of clinical presentation and has been reported in carriers of m.8344A>G, m.3243A>G, m4317A>G, and m.4269A>G gene mutations.[2,25,26,29,32]

Recently, left ventricular noncompaction has been described in mtDNA-D, especially in pediatric patients with multisystemic involvement.[21,33] Restrictive cardiomyopathy is rare in mtDNA-D, but it has been associated to diabetes and inherited bilateral deafness in patients with m3243A>G mutation and in otherwise healthy carriers of the m1555A>G gene mutation.[34,35]

Conduction system disease commonly occurs in patients with mtDNA-D. Conduction disturbances represent a major diagnostic criterion in patients with KSS, among which high-grade AV block has a reported prevalence of 84%.[36] Bradyarrhythmias can present as syncope, Adam-Stokes syndrome, or sudden death; noteworthy, their onset usually occurs after the development of ophthalmoplegia and retinopathy.[11,36–38] Therefore, close clinical monitoring with 24-ECG Holter or internal loop recorder is recommended in patients with KSS after the development of ophthalmic involvement. Albeit less commonly, AV conduction disturbances have been reported in other mtDNA-D, with a prevalence that ranges up to 10%, in association with m.3243A>G and m.8344A>G mutations.[7,24] The risk of progression of conduction disease to high-grade AV block is often unpredictable in patients with mtDNA-D, particularly among patients with large-scale deletions who carry a significantly higher risk of SCD and sudden AV block; therefore, prophylactic pacing should be considered only in this subgroup of patients.[39]

Ventricular preexcitation and Wolff Parkinson White syndrome were first described in association with Leber hereditary optic neuropathy, with a prevalence of 10% and 8% among affected individuals and their maternal relatives, respectively, compared with 1.6% among paternal relatives.[40]

Case series and cohort studies have reported a prevalence of manifest preexcitation pattern ranging from 3% to 27% among carriers of m.3243A>G and m.8433A>G gene mutations; interestingly, Wolff-Parkinson-White preceded the manifestations of mitochondrial encephalomyopathy with lactic acidosis and strokelike episodes (MELAS) syndrome in a subgroup of patients.[7,22,24,26,41]

DIAGNOSIS OF mtDNA DISEASE

The diagnosis of mtDNA-D is challenging because of wide clinical and genetic heterogeneity and requires a multisystemic approach including extensive medical, laboratory, and neuroimaging investigations. Cardiologists should be aware of the complexity of diagnosis and management in MD; an integrated approach constituting of assessment by a multidisciplinary specialist team is recommended.

Two clinical scenarios are possible: (1) patients with confirmed mtDNA-D being periodically evaluated for cardiovascular involvement and (2) patients with cardiovascular disease and red flags for the suspicion of mtDNA-D. The diagnostic algorithm in patients with cardiovascular involvement and suspected mtDNA-D is shown in **Fig. 1**.

Patients with Suspected mtDNA Disease

A comprehensive evaluation by a specialized team with expertise in mtDNA-D, including cardiologists, neurologists, and pathologists, is advised.

Patients with suspected mtDNA-D should undergo a complete diagnostic workup: a pedigree up to third-generation relatives should be collected to identify the inheritance pattern (matrilinear vs recessive).[42] Clinicians should evaluate the extent of organ involvement and detect specific clues for differential diagnosis at physical

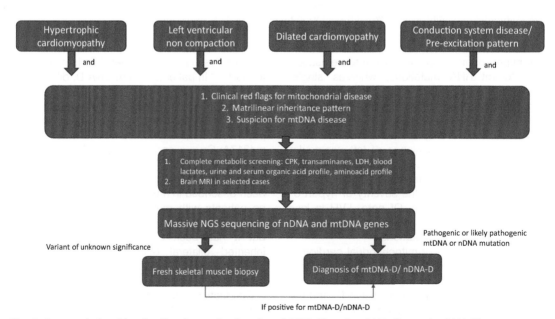

Fig. 1. Proposed algorithm for the diagnosis of nuclear (nDNA-D) and mtDNA disease (mtDNA-D).

examination.[43] Although most of the brain lesions in mtDNA-D are not specific, their pattern of distribution can be suggestive. A global delay in cortical myelination is common; strokelike lesions in a nonvascular distribution, symmetric signal abnormalities of deep gray matter presenting with hyperintensity on T2 and FLAIR images, and hypointensity on T1 images are common findings in mtDNA-D.[44,45] Diffusion-weighted sequences can be useful to differentiate strokelike lesions in MELAS syndrome from acute ischemic foci: noteworthy strokelike foci are fluctuating and they lack the reduction in diffusion coefficient usually found in vascular lesions.[44]

Laboratory investigations of suspected mtDNA-D are complex, and recently, the Mitochondrial Medicine Society has provided consensus recommendations on the diagnosis and management of mtDNA-D.[46]

The baseline evaluation should include complete blood count and determination of glycated hemoglobin, iron status, creatine kinase, plasma proteins and transaminases, serum, and urine amino acids; the presence of lactic acidosis should be systematically assessed.[42] An increased postprandial lactate to pyruvate molar ratio (>20), although not specific of MD, could help in the differential diagnosis of congenital lactic acidosis.[47]

A urine organic acid panel is recommended in patients with suspected mtDNA-D and could be diagnostic in case of propionic and methylmalonic aciduria or show a 3-methylglutaconic aciduria. Although acylcarnitine profile may be normal in absence of metabolic stress, plasma and urine carnitine and acylcarnitine levels should be dosed in patients with suspected mtDNA-D to detect fatty acid beta oxidation or carnitine uptake defects.[43,48]

When the metabolic screening or the clinical evaluation can suggest a specific diagnosis, molecular testing with mtDNA or nDNA sequencing of target genes should be considered.[10,43]

Growing evidence support screening in lymphocytes or urine samples for mtDNA mutations in specific clinical scenarios.[10,39] Among patients with unexplained LVH and suspected mtDNA-D if biochemical panel is inconclusive, a first-level molecular screening for the most common mtDNA mutations (such as m.3243A>G or m.4300A>G) is recommended to rule out an OXPHOS deficiency.[10,43,49–51]

Fresh skeletal muscle biopsy is considered the gold standard for the diagnosis of mtDNA-D.[52,53] Under light microscopy, affected muscles contain peripheral and interfibrillar accumulation of abnormal mitochondria, nonetheless the hallmark of mtDNA-D is represented by red ragged fibers that can be demonstrated using modified trichrome Gomori stains.[5,54] Tissue samples should undergo biochemical and spectrophotometrical analysis to measure enzymatic activity of each OXPHOS complex.[55,56] Blue native polyacrylamide gel electrophoresis allows assessment of proper assembly of the 5 OXPHOS complexes, whereas spectrophotometric assays may be used to assess the enzymatic activity of each complex, to quantify ATP production and proper oxidation of substrate. Recently, new high-resolution respirometry techniques have been proposed to assess oxidative chain function in frozen samples.[57]

Skeletal muscle biopsy is a low-risk procedure, and it is recommended as first-line approach in patients requiring definitive diagnosis. However, in patients with isolated heart involvement or in case of mutations with tissue specificity, endomyocardial biopsy may represent another diagnostic option.[58,59] In consideration of the relatively low rate of serious complications, opportunistic assessment of cardiac tissue obtained during other cardiac procedures should be considered.[60] Molecular diagnostic testing performed by Sanger or next-generation sequencing is recommended to assess the presence of single missense or nonsense point mutations and large rearrangements, both in nuclear genes and mtDNA to confirm diagnosis.[61–63]

Molecular Diagnosis of mtDNA Disease

The use of molecular analysis in the evaluation and prevention of cardiovascular risk, with particular emphasis on sudden cardiac death risk stratification, in patients, healthy subjects, and athletes is an important issue in clinical practice.[64]

Traditionally, the genetic diagnosis of mitochondrial cardiomyopathies provides analysis of "candidate genes." This approach is achieved by Sanger sequencing of known genes in order to assess the presence of single missense or nonsense point mutations.[61–63] In fact, the mitochondrial genome is often initially sequenced in patients with a clinical diagnosis and a strongly suggestive family history of MD, to exclude a primary defect of mtDNA.[65] However, due to the complexity of genetic testing, many patients still lack a molecular diagnosis.

To date, the widespread application of NGS technology has allowed to investigate, at the same time, both the entire mitochondrial genome and different nuclear genes.

In this scenario, the distinction between rare or novel pathogenetic variants from nonpathogenic polymorphisms in known/unknown genes represents the main difficulty.[66] Although the correct classification of these variants needs functional studies, requiring specific laboratory competences, in silico evaluations using several bioinformatics tools are, currently, used to predict the likelihood of pathogenicity of missense and splicing variants. Furthermore, Guidelines from the American College of Medical Genetics allows to classify variants by using different criteria, also including in silico analysis.[67]

Cardiac Investigations in Patients with Confirmed mtDNA Disease

Cardiac involvement in mtDNA-D may remain silent until an advanced state, because of the limitation in the exercise capacity in this subset of patients.[10]

A complete cardiovascular assessment, comprehensive of patient's history, 12-lead ECG, and transthoracic echocardiogram should be performed in patients with mtDNA-D and in carriers of a mitochondrial mutation at initial evaluation and should be repeated at annual interval and with the development of new symptoms, if cardiovascular disease is present. In patients without cardiovascular involvement, repeated assessment at 3-year intervals should be considered, with the exclusion of patients with KSS, proximal myopathy, or large-scale deletions, for whom an annual ECG could be useful.[68–71]

Electrocardiogram and 24-hour holter monitoring

A 12-lead ECG can show prolongation of the PR interval and signs of AV block, a Wolff-Parkinson-White pattern, or repolarization abnormalities such as inverted T waves and prolonged corrected QT interval (>440 msec); an abnormal ECG represents the most common cardiovascular manifestation in mtDNA disease.[6,68,72]

Cardiac conduction abnormalities with an unpredictable course are frequent in mtDNA-D, with a higher prevalence in Kearns-Sayre syndrome and in carriers of m.3243A>G mutations.[7] Patients with large mtDNA deletions or carriers of m.3243A<G mutation, diabetes, intraventricular conduction blocks, LVH, or evidence of premature ventricular complexes seem to carry the highest risk for sudden AV block.[7] A 24-hour ECG Holter monitoring should be performed in patients with mtDNA-D and asymptomatic carriers of mtDNA mutations at initial evaluation and repeated at 1-year intervals.[69] In selected patients with risk factors for sudden AV block, Holter monitoring should be performed more frequently.[7,25,69]

Echocardiography

Transthoracic echocardiography is recommended in patients with mtDNA-D to assess cardiovascular involvement and should be performed at initial diagnosis and with the development of new symptoms and repeated on annual basis.

Of note, hypertrophic cardiomyopathy and LVH seem to be more prevalent in patients with point missense or nonsense mutation (such as m.3243A>G "MELAS" mutation or in myoclonic epilepsy with ragged red fibers syndrome), whereas patients with KSS or mitochondrial myopathy display a bradyarrhythmic phenotype, with lower prevalence of LVH.[7,10,25,42,68]

Cardiac magnetic resonance

Cardiac magnetic resonance has unique tissue-characterizing features and should be considered in patients with suspected mtDNA disease when transthoracic echocardiography is inconclusive, for the quantification of chamber volumes and left ventricular mass, and to exclude other differential diagnoses.[73,74] Specific patterns of late gadolinium enhancement have been described: compared with controls, patients with Kearns Sayre Syndrome and Chronic Progressive External Ophthalmoplegia show a higher prevalence of late gadolinium enhancement (LGE) confined to an intramural pattern in the inferolateral wall; a predominantly focal, patchy LGE with homogeneous distribution among left ventricular segments and severe concentric LVH is common in MELAS-like patients.[75–77]

Extracellular volume imaging and quantitative T2 mapping can be useful in patients without LGE, showing an expanded extracellular volume and diffuse increase in T2 signal.[78]

Cardiopulmonary exercise test

Cardiopulmonary exercise test in mtDNA-D often shows a reduced peak V_{O_2} and early lactic acidosis during exercise, because of increased reliance on anaerobic metabolism. Respiratory exchange ratio is increased in MD (often >1.5), reflecting a high rate of bicarbonate buffer. Other specific findings of mtDNA-D include a large increment in VE/VCO2 between the nadir and peak exercise and reduced mean arteriovenous oxygen difference.[79,80]

MANAGEMENT OF mtDNA DISORDERS
General Measures

To date, there is no drug treatment that has shown clinical benefit in mtDNA-D.[81] When possible, patients with mtDNA-D should avoid medications that could interfere with respiratory chain and precipitate acute metabolic crisis, such as metformin;

statins; valproic acid; high-dose acetaminophen; and antibiotics, including aminoglycosides, linezolid, tetracycline, and macrolides.[46] Patients affected by mtDNA-D should prevent entering catabolism and avoid prolonged fasting.[82] Intravenous dextrose-containing solutions may be considered for caloric supplementation in patients undergoing surgery or medical procedures, or in acute clinical settings, unless contraindicated. Patients with pyruvate metabolism disorders, ketogenic diet, or glucose intolerance should undergo careful nutritional supplementation during acute illness.[46]

There is growing evidence demonstrating the benefits of endurance exercise in patients with mtDNA-D.[83–88] Individuals with mtDNA-D undergoing exercise training showed improved exercise tolerance and reduced postexercise blood lactates,[86] recruitment of satellite cells in muscle fibers, and increased peripheral muscle strength.

Bradyarrhythmias

According to current 2018 AHA/ACC/HRS Guidelines,[89] permanent pacemaker implantation is recommended in patients with neuromuscular disease, including mtDNA-D, with evidence of second-degree AV block, third-degree AV block, or an HV interval of 70 ms or greater, regardless of symptoms. Pacemaker implantation has been proposed at earlier stage in patients with mtDNA-D than general population, as this subgroup of patients show an unpredictable rate of progression to high-grade AV block, mainly in carriers of single large-scale deletions. Thus, according to current guidelines[89] permanent pacemaker implantation may be considered in patients with MD with a PR interval greater than 240 ms, a QRS duration greater than 120 ms, or any grade of fascicular block.

Supraventricular Tachyarrhythmias

Current treatment options for the management of supraventricular tachyarrhythmias can be used in patients with mtDNA-D. In case of symptomatic ventricular preexcitation with recurrent episodes of AVNRT, accessory pathway ablation has been successfully performed in patients with mtDNA-D.[40,41,90,91] In asymptomatic patients with intermittent ventricular preexcitation, the role of electrophysiological study (EPS) and catheter accessory pathway ablation is more controversial. Although data are lacking, there is general consensus that catheter ablation of accessory pathway should be performed in asymptomatic patients in whom invasive EPS risk stratification

identifies high-risk properties, according to current guidelines.[92]

CLINICS CARE POINTS

- The clinical spectrum of mtDNA-D is heterogeneous and can range from oligosymptomatic patients to severe multisystemic involvement.
- The presence of a maternal inheritance pattern or the identification of extra cardiac features of mtDNA-D should guide further investigations in order to exclude an underlying mitochondrial disorder.
- Patients with neuromuscular mtDNA-D often present with increased creatine kinase levels and symptoms of skeletal myopathy.
- In the suspicion of mtDNA-D, the baseline evaluation should include complete blood count and determination of glycated hemoglobin, iron status, creatine kinase, plasma proteins, transaminases, serum and urine aminoacids, and blood lactates.
- When the metabolic screening or the clinical evaluation can suggest a specific diagnosis, molecular testing with mtDNA or nDNA sequencing of target genes should be considered.
- Skeletal muscle biopsy is considered the gold standard for the diagnosis of mtDNA-D.

DISCLOSURE

The authors declare that they have no conflict of interest.

REFERENCES

1. Hanna MG, Nelson IP. Genetics and molecular pathogenesis of mitochondrial respiratory chain diseases. Cell Mol Life Sci 1999;55(5):691–706.
2. Ino H, Tanaka M, Ohno K, et al. Mitochondrial leucine tRNA mutation in a mitochondrial encephalomyopathy. Lancet 1991;337(8735):234–5.
3. DiMauro S, Schon EA. Mitochondrial respiratory-chain diseases. N Engl J Med 2003;348(26):2656–68.
4. Mazzaccara C, Iafusco D, Liguori R, et al. Mitochondrial diabetes in children: Seek and you will find it. PLoS One 2012;7(4):e34956.
5. El-Hattab AW, Scaglia F. Mitochondrial cardiomyopathies. Front Cardiovasc Med 2016;3:25.

6. Limongelli G, Tome-Esteban M, Dejthevaporn C, et al. Prevalence and natural history of heart disease in adults with primary mitochondrial respiratory chain disease. Eur J Heart Fail 2010;12(2):114–21.

7. Wahbi K, Bougouin W, Béhin A, et al. Long-term cardiac prognosis and risk stratification in 260 adults presenting with mitochondrial diseases. Eur Heart J 2015;36(42):2886–93.

8. Schaefer AM, McFarland R, Blakely EL, et al. Prevalence of mitochondrial DNA disease in adults. Ann Neurol 2008;63(1):35–9.

9. Elliott HR, Samuels DC, Eden JA, et al. Pathogenic mitochondrial DNA mutations are common in the general population. Am J Hum Genet 2008;83(2):254–60.

10. Bates MGD, Bourke JP, Giordano C, et al. Cardiac involvement in mitochondrial DNA disease: clinical spectrum, diagnosis, and management. Eur Heart J 2012;33(24):3023–33.

11. Meyers DE, Basha HI, Koenig MK. Mitochondrial cardiomyopathy: pathophysiology, diagnosis, and management. Tex Hear Inst J 2013;40(4):385–94.

12. Saudubray JM, Desguerre I, Sedel F, et al. A clinical approach to inherited metabolic diseases. In: Inborn metabolic diseases: diagnosis and treatment. Springer Berlin Heidelberg; 2006. p. 3–48. https://doi.org/10.1007/978-3-540-28785-8_1.

13. Petty RKH, Harding AE, Morgan-hughes JA. The clinical features of mitochondrial myopathy. Brain 1986;109(5):915–38.

14. Munnich A, Rötig A, Chretien D, et al. Clinical presentation of mitochondrial disorders in childhood. J Inherit Metab Dis 1996;19:521–7.

15. Jackson MJ, Schaefer JA, Johnson MA, et al. Presentation and clinical investigation of mitochondrial respiratory chain disease. A study of 51 patients. Brain 1995;118(2):339–57.

16. Koenig MK. Presentation and diagnosis of mitochondrial disorders in children. Pediatr Neurol 2008;38(5):305–13.

17. Gillis LA, Sokol RJ. Gastrointestinal manifestations of mitochondrial disease. Gastroenterol Clin North Am 2003;32(3):789–817.

18. Niaudet P, Rötig A. Renal involvement in mitochondrial cytopathies. Pediatr Nephrol 1996;10:368–73.

19. Hsu CH, Kwon H, Perng CL, et al. Hearing loss in mitochondrial disorders. Ann N Y Acad Sci 2005;1042:36–47.

20. Rapezzi C, Arbustini E, Caforio ALP, et al. Diagnostic work-up in cardiomyopathies: bridging the gap between clinical phenotypes and final diagnosis. A position statement from the ESC Working Group on Myocardial and Pericardial Diseases. Eur Heart J 2013;34(19):1448–58.

21. Scaglia F, Towbin JA, Craigen WJ, et al. Clinical spectrum, morbidity, and mortality in 113 pediatric patients with mitochondrial disease. Pediatrics 2004;114(4):925–31.

22. Sorajja P, Sweeney MG, Chalmers R, et al. Cardiac abnormalities in patients with Leber's hereditary optic neuropathy. Heart 2003;89(7):791–2.

23. Vydt TCG, de Coo RFM, Soliman OII, et al. Cardiac involvement in adults with m.3243A>G MELAS gene mutation. Am J Cardiol 2007;99(2):264–9.

24. Majamaa-Voltti K, Peuhkurinen K, Kortelainen ML, et al. Cardiac abnormalities in patients with mitochondrial DNA mutation 3243A>G. BMC Cardiovasc Disord 2002;2:12.

25. Wahbi K, Larue S, Jardel C, et al. Cardiac involvement is frequent in patients with the m.8344A>G mutation of mitochondrial DNA. Neurology 2010;74(8):674–7.

26. Anan R, Nakagawa M, Miyata M, et al. Cardiac involvement in mitochondrial diseases: a study on 17 patients with documented mitochondrial DNA defects. Circulation 1995;91(4):955–61.

27. Merante F, Tein I, Benson L, et al. Maternally inherited hypertrophic cardiomyopathy due to a novel T-to-C transition at nucleotide 9997 in the mitochondrial tRNA(glycine) gene. Am J Hum Genet 1994;55(3):437–46.

28. Pastores GM, Santorelli FM, Shanske S, et al. Leigh syndrome and hypertrophic cardiomyopathy in an infant with a mitochondrial DNA point mutation (T8993G). Am J Med Genet 1994;50(3):265–71.

29. Taniike M, Fukushima H, Yanagihara I, et al. Mitochondrial tRNAIle mutation in fatal cardiomyopathy. Biochem Biophys Res Commun 1992;186(1):47–53.

30. Tanaka M, Ino H, Ohno K, et al. Mitochondrial mutation in fatal infantile cardiomyopathy. Lancet 1990;336(8728):1452.

31. Ware SM, El-Hassan N, Kahler SG, et al. Infantile cardiomyopathy caused by a mutation in the overlapping region of mitochondrial ATPase 6 and 8 genes. J Med Genet 2009;46(5):308–14.

32. Stalder N, Yarol N, Tozzi P, et al. Mitochondrial A3243G mutation with manifestation of acute dilated cardiomyopathy. Circ Hear Fail 2012;5(1):e1–3.

33. Finsterer J, Stöllberger C, Maeztu C. Sudden cardiac death in neuromuscular disorders. Int J Cardiol 2016;203:508–15.

34. Thebault C, Ollivier R, Leurent G, et al. Mitochondriopathy: a rare aetiology of restrictive cardiomyopathy. Eur J Echocardiogr 2008;9(6):840–5.

35. Santorelli FM, Tanji K, Manta P, et al. Maternally inherited cardiomyopathy: an atypical presentation of the mtDNA 12S rRNA gene A1555G mutation [3]. Am J Hum Genet 1999;64(1):295–300.

36. Tsang SH, Aycinena ARP, Sharma T. Mitochondrial disorder: Kearns-Sayre syndrome. Adv Exp Med Biol 2018;1085:161–2.

37. Tueskov C, Angelo-Nielsen K. Kearns-sayre syndrome and dilated cardiomyopathy. Neurology 1990;40(3):553–4.

38. Smits BW, Fermont J, Delnooz CCS, et al. Disease impact in chronic progressive external ophthalmoplegia: more than meets the eye. Neuromuscul Disord 2011;21(4):272–8.

39. Ommen SR, Mital S, Burke MA, et al. 2020 AHA/ACC guideline for the diagnosis and treatment of patients with hypertrophic cardiomyopathy. Circulation 2020. https://doi.org/10.1161/cir.0000000000000937.

40. Nikoskelainen EK, Savontaus ML, Huoponen K, et al. Pre-excitation syndrome in Leber's hereditary optic neuropathy. Lancet 1994;344(8926):857–8.

41. Sproule DM, Kaufmann P, Engelstad K, et al. Wolff-Parkinson-White syndrome in patients with MELAS. Arch Neurol 2007;64(11):1625–7.

42. Limongelli G, Masarone D, Pacileo G. Mitochondrial disease and the heart. Heart 2017;103(5):390–8.

43. Brunel-Guitton C, Levtova A, Sasarman F. Mitochondrial diseases and cardiomyopathies. Can J Cardiol 2015;31(11):1360–76.

44. Alves CAPF, Gonçalves FG, Grieb D, et al. Neuroimaging of mitochondrial cytopathies. Top Magn Reson Imaging 2018;27(4):219–40.

45. Saneto RP, Friedman SD, Shaw DWW. Neuroimaging of mitochondrial disease. Mitochondrion 2008; 8(5–6):396–413.

46. Parikh S, Goldstein A, Koenig MK, et al. Diagnosis and management of mitochondrial disease: a consensus statement from the Mitochondrial Medicine Society. Genet Med 2015;17(9):689–701.

47. Debray FG, Mitchell GA, Allard P, et al. Diagnostic accuracy of blood lactate-to-pyruvate molar ratio in the differential diagnosis of congenital lactic acidosis. Clin Chem 2007;53(5):916–21.

48. Vishwanath VA. Fatty acid beta-oxidation disorders: a brief review. Ann Neurosci 2016;23(1):51–5.

49. Marin-Garcia J, Goldenthal MJ. Mitochondrial DNA defects in cardiomyopathy. Cardiovasc Pathol 1998;7(4):205–13.

50. Zaragoza MV, Brandon MC, Diegoli M, et al. Mitochondrial cardiomyopathies: how to identify candidate pathogenic mutations by mitochondrial DNA sequencing, MITOMASTER and phylogeny. Eur J Hum Genet 2011;19(2):200–7.

51. Lieber DS, Calvo SE, Shanahan K, et al. Targeted exome sequencing of suspected mitochondrial disorders. Neurology 2013;80(19):1762–70.

52. Bernier FP, Boneh A, Dennett X, et al. Diagnostic criteria for respiratory chain disorders in adults and children. Neurology 2002;59(9):1406–11.

53. Wolf NI, Smeitink JAM. Mitochondrial disorders: a proposal for consensus diagnostic criteria in infants and children. Neurology 2002;59(9):1402–5.

54. Bourgeois JM, Tarnopolsky MA. Pathology of skeletal muscle in mitochondrial disorders. Mitochondrion 2004;4(5–6 SPEC. ISS):441–52.

55. Jha P, Wang X, Auwerx J. Analysis of mitochondrial respiratory chain supercomplexes using blue native polyacrylamide gel electrophoresis (BN-PAGE). Curr Protoc Mouse Biol 2016;6(1):1–14.

56. Birch-Machin MA, Turnbull DM. Assaying mitochondrial respiratory complex activity in mitochondria isolated from human cells and tissues. Methods Cell Biol 2001;65(65):97–117.

57. Acin-Perez R, Benador IY, Petcherski A, et al. A novel approach to measure mitochondrial respiration in frozen biological samples. EMBO J 2020; 39(13):e104073.

58. Leone O, Veinot JP, Angelini A, et al. 2011 Consensus statement on endomyocardial biopsy from the Association for European Cardiovascular Pathology and the Society for Cardiovascular Pathology. Cardiovasc Pathol 2012;21(4):245–74.

59. Cooper LT, Baughman KL, Feldman AM, et al. The role of endomyocardial biopsy in the management of cardiovascular disease. A scientific statement from the American Heart Association, the American College of Cardiology, and the European Society of Cardiology Endorsed by the Heart Failure Society of America and the Heart Failure Association of the European Society of Cardiology. J Am Coll Cardiol 2007;50(19):1914–31.

60. Stone JR, Basso C, Baandrup UT, et al. Recommendations for processing cardiovascular surgical pathology specimens: a consensus statement from the Standards and Definitions Committee of the Society for Cardiovascular Pathology and the Association for European Cardiovascular Pathology. Cardiovasc Pathol 2012;21(1):2–16.

61. Carroll CJ, Brilhante V, Suomalainen A. Next-generation sequencing for mitochondrial disorders. Br J Pharmacol 2014;171(8):1837–53.

62. Neveling K, Feenstra I, Gilissen C, et al. A post-hoc comparison of the utility of sanger sequencing and exome sequencing for the diagnosis of heterogeneous diseases. Hum Mutat 2013;34(12):1721–6.

63. Taylor RW, Pyle A, Griffin H, et al. Use of whole-exome sequencing to determine the genetic basis of multiple mitochondrial respiratory chain complex deficiencies. JAMA 2014;312(1):68–77.

64. Limongelli G, Nunziato M, D'Argenio V, et al. Yield and clinical significance of genetic screening in elite and amateur athletes. Eur J Prev Cardiol 2020. https://doi.org/10.1177/2047487320934265.

65. Ng YS, Turnbull DM. Mitochondrial disease: genetics and management. J Neurol 2016;263(1):179–91.

66. Frisso G, Detta N, Coppola P, et al. Functional studies and in silico analyses to evaluate non-coding variants in inherited cardiomyopathies. Int J Mol Sci 2016;17(11):1883.

67. Richards S, Aziz N, Bale S, et al. Standards and guidelines for the interpretation of sequence variants: a joint consensus recommendation of the American College of Medical Genetics and

Genomics and the Association for Molecular Pathology. Genet Med 2015;17(5):405–24.

68. Anan R, Nakagawa M, Miyata M, et al. Cardiac involvement in mitochondrial diseases. Circulation 1995;91(4):955–61.

69. Parikh S, Goldstein A, Karaa A, et al. Patient care standards for primary mitochondrial disease: a consensus statement from the mitochondrial medicine society. Genet Med 2017;19(12):1–18.

70. Holmgren D. Cardiomyopathy in children with mitochondrial disease clinical course and cardiological findings. Eur Heart J 2003;24(3):280–8.

71. Quadir A, Pontifex CS, Robertson HL, et al. Systematic review and meta-analysis of cardiac involvement in mitochondrial myopathy. Neurol Genet 2019;5(4):e339.

72. Baik R, Chae JH, Lee YM, et al. Electrocardiography as an early cardiac screening test in children with mitochondrial disease. Korean J Pediatr 2010; 53(5):644–7.

73. Nakanishi M, Harada M, Tadamura E, et al. Mitochondrial cardiomyopathy evaluated with cardiac magnetic resonance. Circulation 2007;116(2):e25–6.

74. Partington SL, Givertz MM, Gupta S, et al. Cardiac magnetic resonance aids in the diagnosis of mitochondrial cardiomyopathy. Circulation 2011;123(6):227–9.

75. Jose T, Gdynia H-J, Mahrholdt H, et al. CMR gives clue to "ragged red fibers" in the heart in a patient with mitochondrial myopathy. Int J Cardiol 2011; 149(1):e24–7.

76. Florian A, Ludwig A, Stubbe-Dräger B, et al. Characteristic cardiac phenotypes are detected by cardiovascular magnetic resonance in patients with different clinical phenotypes and genotypes of mitochondrial myopathy. J Cardiovasc Magn Reson 2015;17(1):40.

77. Yilmaz A, Gdynia HJ, Ponfick M, et al. Cardiovascular magnetic resonance imaging (CMR) reveals characteristic pattern of myocardial damage in patients with mitochondrial myopathy. Clin Res Cardiol 2012;101(4):255–61.

78. Lee KH, Park HS, Park CH, et al. Extracellular volume imaging and quantitative T2 mapping for the diagnosis of mitochondrial cardiomyopathy. Circulation 2014;130(20):1832–4.

79. Riley MS, Nicholls DP, Cooper CB. Cardiopulmonary exercise testing and metabolic myopathies. Ann Am Thorac Soc 2017;14:S129–39.

80. Taivassalo T, Jensen TD, Kennaway N, et al. The spectrum of exercise tolerance in mitochondrial myopathies: a study of 40 patients. Brain 2003;126(2): 413–23.

81. Pfeffer G, Majamaa K, Turnbull DM, et al. Treatment for mitochondrial disorders. The Cochrane database of systematic reviews, 2012. https://doi.org/10.1002/14651858.CD004426.pub3.

82. Rinninella E, Pizzoferrato M, Cintoni M, et al. Nutritional support in mitochondrial diseases: the state of the art. Eur Rev Med Pharmacol Sci 2018; 22(13):4288–98.

83. Taivassalo T, Gardner JL, Taylor RW, et al. Endurance training and detraining in mitochondrial myopathies due to single large-scale mtDNA deletions. Brain 2006;129(12):3391–401.

84. Jeppesen TD, Schwartz M, Olsen DB, et al. Aerobic training is safe and improves exercise capacity in patients with mitochondrial myopathy. Brain 2006; 129(12):3402–12.

85. Voet NBM, van der Kooi EL, van Engelen BGM, et al. Strength training and aerobic exercise training for muscle disease. Cochrane Database Syst Rev. 9(7); 2013. https://doi.org/10.1002/14651858.CD003907.pub4.

86. Taivassalo T, De Stefano N, Argov Z, et al. Effects of aerobic training in patients with mitochondrial myopathies. Neurology 1998;50(4):1055–60.

87. Jeppesen TD. Aerobic exercise training in patients with mtdna-related mitochondrial myopathy. Front Physiol 2020;11:349.

88. Fernández-de la Torre M, Fiuza-Luces C, Valenzuela PL, et al. Exercise training and neurodegeneration in mitochondrial disorders: insights from the harlequin mouse. Front Physiol 2020;11:594223.

89. Kusumoto FM, Schoenfeld MH, Barrett C, et al. 2018 ACC/AHA/HRS guideline on the evaluation and management of patients with bradycardia and cardiac conduction delay: a report of the American College of Cardiology/American Heart Association Task Force on Clinical Practice Guidelines and the Heart Rhythm Society. J Am Coll Cardiol 2019;74(7): e51–156.

90. Finsterer J, Stöllberger C, Kopsa W, et al. Wolff-Parkinson-White syndrome and isolated left ventricular abnormal trabeculation as a manifestation of Leber's hereditary optic neuropathy. Can J Cardiol 2001; 17(4):464–6.

91. Finsterer J, Stollberger C, Gatterer E. Wolff-Parkinson-White syndrome and noncompaction in Leber's hereditary optic neuropathy due to the variant m.3460G>A. J Int Med Res 2018;46(5):2054–60.

92. Brugada J, Katritsis DG, Arbelo E, et al. 2019 ESC Guidelines for the management of patients with supraventricular tachycardia. Eur Heart J 2020;41(5): 655–720.

The Role of New Imaging Technologies in the Diagnosis of Cardiac Amyloidosis

Giuseppe Palmiero, MD[a,b,*], Erica Vetrano, MD[b], Marta Rubino, MD[b],
Emanuele Monda, MD[b], Francesca Dongiglio, MD[b], Michele Lioncino, MD[b],
Francesco Di Fraia, MD[b], Martina Caiazza, MD[b], Federica Verrillo, MD[b],
Laura Capodicasa, MD[b], Giuseppe Cerciello, MD[c],
Fiore Manganelli, MD, PhD[d], Mara Catalano, MD[e], Davide D'Arienzo, MD[f],
Maria Luisa De Rimini, MD[f], Raffaele Ascione, MD[g], Paolo Golino, MD, PhD[h],
Pio Caso, MD[a], Luigi Ascione, MD[a], Giuseppe Limongelli, MD, PhD[b,i]

KEYWORDS

- Cardiac amyloidosis • Multimodality imaging • Echocardiography • Cardiac magnetic resonance
- Nuclear imaging

KEY POINTS

- Multimodality imaging has revolutionized the diagnostic process in cardiac amyloidosis by enabling noninvasive diagnosis in most forms of ATTR.
- In this era of specific treatment, cardiac amyloidosis early diagnosis is able to significantly modify the prognosis.
- Echocardiography and cardiac magnetic resonance are pivotal for cardiac morphologic and functional characterization and crucial for diagnosis, prognosis, disease progression, and response to therapy.
- Radionuclide imaging provides additional and critical information on amyloid type and burden that completes the findings provided by echocardiography and cardiac magnetic resonance.
- Understanding the properties and the limits of each technique and selecting the optimal imaging modality to achieve each goal is the cornerstone of the multimodality application.

[a] Department of Cardiology, AORN Ospedale dei Colli – Monaldi Hospital, via Leonardo Bianchi SNC, 80131 Naples, Italy; [b] Inherited and Rare Cardiovascular Diseases Unit, AORN Ospedale dei Colli – Monaldi Hospital, via Leonardo Bianchi SNC, 80131 Naples, Italy; [c] Haematology Unit (Building n. 2), Department of Clinical Medicine and Surgery, AOU Policlinico "Federico II", via Sergio Pansini 5, 80131 Naples, Italy; [d] Neurology Unit (Building n. 17), Department of Neurosciences, Reproductive Medicine and Odontostomatology, AOU Policlinico "Federico II", via Sergio Pansini 5, 80131 Naples, Italy; [e] Department of Nuclear Imaging, AORN Cardarelli Hospital, via Antonio Cardarelli 9, 80131 Naples, Italy; [f] Department of Nuclear Medicine, AORN Ospedale dei Colli – Monaldi Hospital, via Leonardo Bianchi SNC, 80131 Naples, Italy; [g] Department of Advanced Biomedical Sciences, University of Naples Federico II, Naples, Italy; [h] Department of Cardiology, University of Campania "Luigi Vanvitelli", Naples, Italy; [i] Institute of Cardiovascular Sciences, University College of London and St. Bartholomew's Hospital, London, UK
* Corresponding author. Inherited and Rare Cardiovascular Diseases Unit, Department of Translational Medical Sciences, University of Campania "Luigi Vanvitelli", AORN Ospedale dei Colli – Monaldi Hospital, 80131 Naples, Italy.
E-mail address: g.palmiero@hotmail.it

Heart Failure Clin 18 (2022) 61–72
https://doi.org/10.1016/j.hfc.2021.07.014
1551-7136/22/© 2021 Elsevier Inc. All rights reserved.

INTRODUCTION

Amyloidosis includes a group of diseases characterized by the accumulation of amyloid fibrils derived from the aggregation of misfolded proteins in the extracellular spaces of different organs, whose function is consequently progressively compromised. The most common proteins that form amyloid fibrils with common cardiac involvement are immunoglobulin light chains (AL) and transthyretin (TTR).[1] Those forms of cardiac amyloidosis (CA) have similar phenotypic expressions, but are markedly different for prognosis and therapy.

AL amyloidosis results from an uncontrolled proliferation of a single clone of plasma cells (plasma cells dyscrasia), resulting in an overproduction of immunoglobulin AL that deposits as amyloid in many tissues.[2,3] Thus, AL is a systemic disease characterized by a rapidly progressive clinical course with a prognosis that largely depends on toxic–infiltrative cardiomyopathy, consisting of a median survival of less than 6 months if left untreated.[4]

In ATTR amyloidosis, the misfolded TTR is the protein primarily produced in the liver. The transformation of this 127 amino acid protein into amyloid is stimulated by unknown mechanisms related to aging in wild-type ATTR or by at least 120 known point mutations in its gene, resulting in single amino acid substitutions in the ATTR hereditary or variant.[5] In contrast with AL amyloidosis, the cardiac consequences of ATTR primarily result from myocardial infiltration, with less evidence of direct toxic effects. The wild-type ATTR amyloidosis is characterized by an age-dependent penetrance and a better prognosis than AL-CA. Hereditary TTR-mediated amyloidosis is a progressively disabling inherited disease with a varied clinical course, depending on the mutations in the TTR gene and the consequent phenotype.

The diagnosis of amyloidosis is complex and usually delayed, because the symptoms may mimic those caused by other common disorders.[6] Diagnostic delays may bring detrimental consequences for patient outcomes.[7,8] Until recently, CA was considered a rare entity. However, advances in cardiac imaging and the availability of specific therapies for AL and ATTR amyloidosis only in recent years have led to an increased awareness of this entity as an underestimated cause of heart failure.[9]

An early diagnosis of CA is crucial owing to its worse prognosis when it affects the heart, and treatments can modify the patient's clinical outcome.[10–13] Furthermore, several noninvasive imaging tests exploring different features are available for CA diagnosis, reducing the need for an invasive procedure (with endomyocardial biopsy above all others) to obtain a definitive diagnosis, especially in the ATTR setting.

This review aims to describe the different imaging tools, from the traditional to the more novel ones, useful for CA diagnosis and highlight the prognostic value of the different approaches.

ROLE OF MULTIMODALITY IMAGING IN CARDIAC AMYLOIDOSIS

In multimodality imaging, the combination of morphofunctional information obtained by diverse image techniques in the field of diagnostic imaging, are interpreted together to better characterize different aspects of a specific disease with different objectives: (i) raising the diagnostic suspicion; (ii) allowing an early diagnosis; (iii) making a definitive diagnosis; (iv) evaluating the disease pathophysiology; (v) assessing the prognosis; and (vi) monitoring the disease progression and the response to therapy. All imaging methods have the same goal: identifying the cardiac infiltration and its consequence on cardiac morphology and function. Understanding the properties and the limits of each technique and selecting the optimal imaging modality to achieve each goal is the cornerstone of the multimodality application.

ECHOCARDIOGRAPHY

Transthoracic echocardiography is the first-line examination in patient with suspected or confirmed CA. Left ventricular thickening is due to amyloid deposition within the extracellular space and determines a characteristic pattern of concentric pseudohypertrophy. However, a typical asymmetric hypertrophy pattern in common in CA, predominantly characterized by septal involvement.[14] In the early stages of the disease, left ventricular wall thickening may be overlooked or attributed to more common conditions (eg, arterial hypertension or aortic stenosis).

The suspicion of an underlying CA should be raised by the finding of an interventricular septum wall thickness of 12 mm or greater, measured in the parasternal long axis view, in the absence of alternative causes of left ventricular hypertrophy.[15] Many 2-dimensional echocardiographic findings have been reported: a granular sparkling appearance has been long attributed to myocardial infiltration; however, it shows low specificity for the diagnosis of CA. Other findings suggestive of CA include valvular or interatrial septal thickening and mild pericardial effusion. Atrioventricular (mitral and tricuspid) and aortic involvement (in

50% and 25% of patients, respectively) has been associated with a more advanced Ney York Heart Association functional class, lower left ventricular ejection fraction (LVEF), and lower 5-year survival rates.[16] Most patients with CA exhibit diastolic dysfunction, with progression from an impaired relaxation to a restrictive pattern.[17] Signs of impaired diastolic function may anticipate biventricular thickening via atrial dilatation, increased E/e ratio[18] owing to increased filling pressures and dilatation of the vena cava owing to the restrictive diastolic pattern. In addition, left atrial function may be decreased based on the assessment of atrial deformation.[19] Transmitral E-wave deceleration time, transmitral flow E/A ratio, and pulmonary venous flow D/S ratio are independent predictors of mortality,[20] while the ejection fraction is typically preserved until late stages of the disease.[21–23] However, in recent studies, a prevalence of a LVEF of less than 50% in up to 50% of patients with wild-type ATTR-CA was observed.[24] In AL-CA, patients with a normal LVEF and elevated cardiac biomarker values, a stroke volume of less than 33 mL/min, a myocardial contraction fraction (calculated as the ratio of the left ventricular stroke volume to the left ventricular myocardial volume) of less than 34%, and a cardiac index of less than 2.4 $L/min/m^2$ result in higher mortality, and these measurements are modified before the LVEF changes. Hence, they represent an early index of left ventricular dysfunction with low infiltration.[25]

Global longitudinal strain (GLS) has been considered a useful clinical marker of CA, which may help to distinguish CA from other causes of unexplained left ventricular hypertrophy. GLS is decreased in the early stages of the disease.[26,27] A typical pattern in patients with CA consists of a preserved apical strain and a decreased strain at the base of the heart and in intermediate segments of the myocardium.[28] This phenomenon creates a characteristic bullseye pattern when segmental deformation is traced, which is rarely seen in other cardiomyopathies (**Fig. 1**). The pathophysiological mechanism underlying this phenomenon remains unclear. Several mechanisms have been proposed, including the presence of less amyloid deposition at the apex than at the base, differences in the orientation of myocardial fibers at the apex, and a greater tendency to apoptosis and remodeling of basal segments related to increased parietal stress and turbulent flow.[29] Phelan and colleagues[26] have observed that the relative apical longitudinal strain (medium apical longitudinal strain/[medium basal + medium longitudinal strain]) of greater than 1 could differentiate CA from hypertrophic cardiomyopathy and aortic

stenosis with high diagnostic accuracy (sensitivity 93%, specificity 82%). Moreover, Pagourelias and colleagues[30] have proposed the LVEF/GLS ratio as a helpful parameter in the differential diagnostic process, describing the unique behavior of CA (preserved LVEF in presence of early reduction of GLS) among other potential causes of left ventricular hypertrophy. In patients with AL amyloidosis, low baseline GLS levels before the initiation of immunotherapy are predictive of survival.[31] Of note, longitudinal strain is related to the extent of amyloid deposit, quantified by histopathology. Therefore, longitudinal strain and 2-dimensional global longitudinal strain could improve diagnostic accuracy of widely accepted parameters, such as N-terminal pro B-type natriuretic peptide, troponin, and clinical evaluation.[32]

A recent study has evaluated the right ventricle in patients with infiltrative diseases to discriminate AL amyloidosis from other causes of unexplained left ventricular hypertrophy and to assess whether right ventricular dysfunction predicts overall mortality in AL amyloidosis. A decreased longitudinal right ventricular free wall strain (with a cutoff of approximately −21.2%) discriminates AL amyloidosis from patients with other infiltrative diseases. In AL amyloidosis, the longitudinal right ventricular free wall strain is associated significantly with mortality and is the only independent echocardiographic predictor of overall mortality, even when adjusted for Mayo staging and global left ventricular longitudinal strain.[33]

Right ventricular wall thickening and impaired right ventricular function are common findings in patients with CA. Patients with AL-CA with a normal LVEF show impaired tricuspid annular plane systolic excursion and right ventricular longitudinal deformation (right ventricular longitudinal strain) in basal lateral segments of control patients, thus suggesting an early right ventricular systolic dysfunction.[34] Reduced tricuspid annular plane systolic excursion, low longitudinal strain, and impaired right ventricular function are also predictive of severe cardiovascular events.[35–37]

There are many structural and functional differences between AL-CA and ATTR-CA. AL-CA is associated with only slightly increased wall thickness, but has a more significant hemodynamic imbalance than ATTR-CA.[38] In contrast, ATTR-CA is predominantly characterized by increased left ventricular and right ventricular mass and more systolic dysfunction. The discrepancy between the 2 types of amyloid cardiomyopathy on imaging and the clinical course reinforces the concept that AL-CA is not a simple infiltrative disorder and should be more accurately characterized as toxic and infiltrative cardiomyopathy.[39]

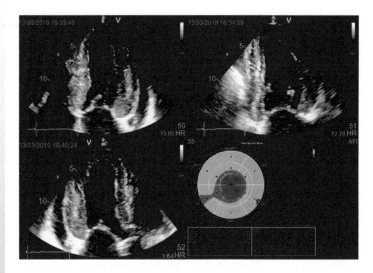

Fig. 1. Apical sparing pattern on strain imaging bullseye. Note the impaired longitudinal strain values in medium and basal segments in contrast with the spared apical segments.

Recently, left ventricular myocardial work indices derived from pressure–strain loop analysis, have been implied in left ventricular function evaluation in patients with CA. Left ventricular myocardial work indices are more impaired in CA compared with healthy subjects with a prevalent basal and medium segment impairment compared with the relatively spared apical ones, following the typical pattern on strain imaging (**Fig. 2**). Clemmensen and colleagues[40] have shown a significant correlation between the abnormal myocardial oxidative metabolism, evaluated with ^{11}C-acetate PET and the decreased myocardial work efficiency calculated by echocardiography-derived work, both in AL and ATTR-CA. Recent evidence seems to suggest that the magnitude of left ventricular myocardial work indices reduction is increased with exercise, despite being present at rest.[41] Of note, the left ventricular myocardial work index seems also able to predict prognosis in this setting.[42,43]

Given the several echocardiographic features common to the 2 different forms of CA and other cardiomyopathies, echocardiography alone cannot be used to differentiate the many different pathologies associated with an increased wall thickness but should require a low threshold for further multimodality assessment.

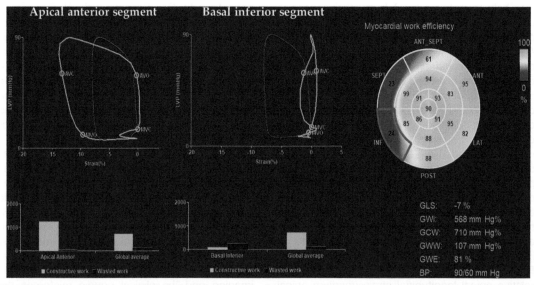

Fig. 2. Pressure–strain loop (PSL)-derived left ventricular myocardial work indices (LVMWI) in CA. Note the impaired constructive work (CW) in the basal inferior segment compared with the preserved CW in the apical anterior segment with a consequent decrease in the Global Word Index (GWI) Efficiency (GWE 81% vs 95% as referral value). BP, blood pressure; GCW, global constructive work.

CARDIAC MAGNETIC RESONANCE

Cardiac magnetic resonance (CMR) allows to obtain a broad range of information on cardiac morphology and function and, after the administration of contrast medium, on tissue characterization, distinguishing fibrotic from healthy myocardial tissue and, thus, playing a central role in the diagnosis of CA.[44–47] In amyloidosis, intrinsic myocardial signaling can be measured using T1/T2-weighted imaging sequences, T1 mapping (pre- and post-contrast), late gadolinium enhancement (LGE), and extracellular volume (ECV) imaging.[48] Although pathognomonic in patients with biopsy-confirmed amyloidosis, these markers are nonspecific and may also be found in other forms of cardiovascular disease, including reactive or replacement fibrosis and inflammation. As a result, we have different patterns, named hyperenhancement, that differ about the underlying pathology.

CA shows a unique gadolinium-kinetics and the pattern of myocardial nulling in the inversion scout sequence (time of inversion scout) is an accurate tool to detect CA. In CA, the myocardium nulls before or coincident with the blood pool at 10 minutes after gadolinium injection as opposed to the normal pattern observed in patients with other disease or without cardiac involvement. The nulling pattern in the time of inversion scout sequence in CA seems to be time dependent and is likely related to the load of amyloid deposition. Indeed, the earlier onset of reverse nulling pattern shows a trend toward a greater left ventricular mass and, consequently, more amyloid infiltration.[49]

LGE technique has evolved over the years by using the phase-sensitive image reconstruction, a more reliable and less operator-dependent technique. With the phase-sensitive image reconstruction LGE approach, several patterns of LGE have been recognized, with the subendocardial enhancement being the most common[50,51] and the transmural showing the best correlation with the degree of myocardial infiltration.[52] Unfortunately, gadolinium-based contrast agents have been associated with nephrogenic systemic fibrosis, a severe and potentially fatal condition.[53,54] These limitations could be overcome by using T1 mapping, which directly measures an intrinsic signal from the myocardium. Native myocardial T1 (precontrast) reflects cardiac amyloid infiltration, systolic and diastolic dysfunction markers, and disease severity.[55] T1 can be used to measure the progression of infiltration from early stages without LGE, up to diffuse transmural involvement.[56]

The essential advantages of native myocardial T1 are its diagnostic accuracy in detecting both AL and ATTR-CA, and its early sensitivity, because an increased native T1 has been reported before the onset of left ventricular hypertrophy or LGE.[57] Native T1 and ECV are elevated in both forms of CA, and both have been validated as indicators of cardiac infiltration, especially when compared with infiltration obtained using other techniques such as 99mTc-3,3- diphosphono-1,2-propanodicarboxylic acid (99mTc-DPD) scintigraphy.[58] Baggiano and colleagues[59] developed an algorithm using native myocardial T1 to enable the diagnosis of amyloidosis in many patients with suspected systemic amyloidosis. In particular, a native T1 value of less than 1.036 ms seems to exclude a cardiac involvement (negative predictive value, 98% insert CI: 0.91-0.95), whereas a native T1 value of greater than 1.164 ms to confirm the presence of CA (positive predictive value, 98% insert CI: 0.91-0.95), without the need for gadolinium-based contrast agents, with obvious advantages in patients with chronic kidney disease. Although at first T1 and ECV had been supposed to play a similar role in identifying the 2 types of amyloidosis, later native T1 has been found as more reliable in identifying AL-CA, with ECV more in those with ATTR-CA.[60] This factor more likely derives from the intrinsic characteristics of the 2 methods. T1 is strongly affected by the water content, resulting in more cases of myocardial edema, although it could be decreased in cases of hypertrophy (especially in ATTR-CA). Conversely, the ECV is less affected by the intrinsic pathophysiological mechanisms of amyloidosis and can accurately measure the degree of infiltration of the extracellular space, resulting in an accurate marker of infiltration[60] and early illness.[61] The ECV correlates with markers of disease severity such as cardiac function, blood biomarkers, and functional status. Native T1 and ECV are predictors of prognosis in the 2 types of CA. However, ECV is an independent predictor of prognosis in patients with ATTR-CA and the first cardiac amyloid regression marker after successful therapy in patients with AL-CA.[58,62,63]

T2-weighted imaging is of pivotal importance in CA. The T2 relaxation time is a time constant representing the decay of transverse magnetization.[64] T2 levels were shown to be higher in a cohort of patients with untreated AL-CA than treated AL and ATTR-CA, thus showing that edema has important pathophysiologic and prognostic roles.[65] Although native T1 and T2 values tend to be higher in patients with AL-CA (especially in untreated patients), and the ECV is higher in patients with ATTR-CA, none of these CMR techniques can be used to differentiate between the 2 types of CA in a single patient definitively.

CMR diffusion tensor imaging (DTI) has emerged as a promising method for determining myocardial fiber orientation[66,67] and tissue characterization without the need for a gadolinium contrast agent. CMR DTI allows the investigation of water diffusion within the tissue and derivation of additional scalar metrics, such as mean diffusivity and fractional anisotropy for the quantification of structural integrity. Gotschy and colleagues[72] have applied CMR DTI in CA to assess microstructural alterations and their consequences on myocardial function compared with healthy controls. CMR DTI analysis showed a strong correlation between the (more) circumferential myofibers orientation and GLS observed in CA, indicating in the microstructural a potential determinant of loss of longitudinal function in this setting[68–72].

Finally, CMR also allows the study of myocardial perfusion.[73] Intramyocardial vessels are frequently infiltrated by amyloid, resulting in reduced vasodilation, which can cause global myocardial ischemia. In addition, levels of cardiac biomarkers, such as troponin T and N-terminal pro B-type natriuretic peptide, are usually consistently elevated in patients with CA.[74] Myocardial perfusion in these patients seems reduced even at rest.[75] A recent study assessed the diagnostic value of the new cardiovascular magnetic resonance parameter called the myocardial transit time in distinguishing CA from other hypertrophic cardiomyopathies. The myocardial transit time was defined as the circulation time of blood from the orifice of coronary arteries to stagnation in the coronary sinus, reflecting the transit time of gadolinium in the myocardial microvasculature.[76] The present study results show that mapping-based ECV is superior to myocardial transit time to diagnose an infiltrative and predominantly extracellular disease such as CA. However, myocardial transit time is a new, highly sensitive parameter allowing both the detection and characterization of cardiac diseases such as conventional hypertrophic cardiomyopathy that are characterized by less pronounced extracellular remodeling, but they are instead dominated by intracellular and subsequent intravascular changes. Coronary myocardial dysfunction severity has been reported to correlate with longitudinal deformation in both hypertrophic cardiomyopathy and CA.[76,77] Decreased longitudinal strain and coronary myocardial dysfunction are frequently observed in patients with CA, because the decreased longitudinal strain is partially owing to disturbed microvascular function. Most longitudinal fibers are located in the subendocardium, which in turn is more susceptible to (microvascular) ischemia.[78] The correlation between the myocardial transit time and longitudinal deformation is of great interest: because an association between an abnormal myocardial deformation and a higher rate of adverse cardiac events in patients with hypertrophic cardiomyopathy has been reported[79] and worse survival in patients with CA,[80] the new CMR parameter myocardial transit time may have a novel prognostic value. However, future studies are needed to confirm this hypothesis.

RADIONUCLIDE IMAGING

Radionuclide imaging offers an additional noninvasive imaging modality that provides additional and critical information on amyloid type and burden that completes the morphologic and functional characterization provided by echocardiography and CMR. Indeed, recent but large pieces of evidence suggests a higher potential for earlier CA diagnosis than echocardiography and CMR,[81] a better diagnostic accuracy than CMR,[82] a capability to quantify the amyloid burden,[83] distinguish between types of CA,[84] and provide prognostic data.[85–89]

Radionuclide bone scintigraphy with technetium-labelled bisphosphonates is the gold standard for noninvasive diagnosis of ATTR-CA[18,90–93] and is highly sensitive and specific for detecting ATTR-CA, even in patients in the early stages of the disease[94] (**Fig. 3**). However, as mentioned elsewhere in this article, cardiac localization of a radiotracer is also possible in patients with AL-CA. Thus, nuclear scintigraphy alone is not appropriated for the diagnosis of ATTR-CA.[89] Therefore, a definitive noninvasive ATTR-CA diagnosis requires always excluding a plasma cell dyscrasia to rule out AL-CA (sensitivity or >99%).[95] Bone scans can be evaluated with semiquantitative or quantitative methods. In quantitative analysis, a region of interest is placed over the heart, and the mean counts are compared with a similar-sized region placed over the contralateral chest. Semiquantitative techniques are based on the comparison between bone and rib uptake, and patients are classified as grade 2 or 3 if cardiac uptake is equal or greater than bone uptake. Thus, radionuclide scintigraphy is diagnostic of ATTR-CA if there is a grade 2 or 3 cardiac uptake or in the presence of a heart/contralateral chest ratio of greater than 1.58.[33,93] Moreover, a heart/contralateral chest ratio of greater than 1.58 is associated with poor survival.[33]

However, up to 5% of the patients aged greater than 65 have a monoclonal gammopathy of uncertain significance, and this condition could lead to an incorrect diagnosis of AL-CA in patients with

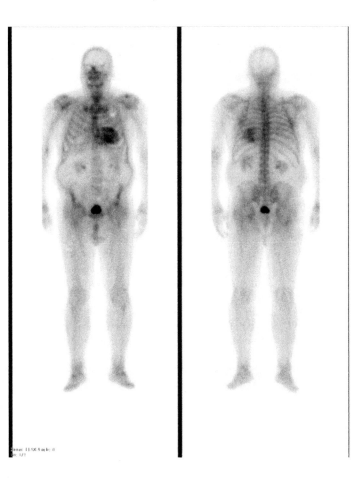

Fig. 3. Bone tracers cardiac uptake score 3 according to the Perugini Scoring System.

coexistence of monoclonal gammopathy of uncertain significance and ATTR-CA.[96] Based on these findings, the endomyocardial biopsy is recommended in patients with a positive screening for a monoclonal AL to exclude a superimposed AL-CA.[97] Hence, advances in nuclear imaging have changed the diagnostic pathway for patients with CA, and only a minority of patients with ATTR-CA requires an endomyocardial biopsy.

Intense bone tracer uptake in ATTR-CA seems to suggest also a greater burden of amyloid infiltration and has prognostic relevance. Bokhari and colleagues[89] reported a significantly greater uptake of 99m Tc-PYP in patients with ATTR-CA than in patients with AL-CA, and increased cardiac uptake has been associated with increased all-cause mortality. Sperry and colleagues described a pattern of apical sparing and increased mortality dependent on the regional distribution of 99m Tc-PYP uptake.[90,98] Patients showing diffuse infiltration had a more apical uptake and consequently a worse survival.

Interestingly, Ser77Tyr-associated ATTR-CA may present on bone scintigraphy only with grade 1 uptake, despite clinical, morphologic, and functional features on echocardiography and CMR (typical LGE imaging and elevated ECV) is expected to increase in cardiac biomarker levels. This observation suggests that patients with ATTR-CA associated with the Ser77Tyr variant, given the amyloid burden, have less bone tracer uptake than expected. In addition, ATTR-CA could be associated with rare mutations in which amyloid deposits primarily consisting of full-length TTR that either do not show or show minimal cardiac uptake of bone tracer research.[45]

The potential assessment of extracardiac amyloid involvement by bone tracers is still under investigation. A typical muscle pattern and soft-tissue uptake of 99mTc-DPD has been reported previously, and amyloid tissue infiltration has been subsequently demonstrated by soft tissue biopsy in a larger series of patients.[99] Pulmonary uptake can be found at 99mTc-HMDP scintigraphy and is highly selective in the case of ATTR-CA.[100] More likely, extracardiac uptake depends on the tracer used. This limitation can be overcome by other techniques such as a PET scan. PET imaging offers high spatial resolution and can facilitate the quantification of amyloid at cardiac and extracardiac levels.[83] Amyloid-binding PET radiotracers investigated in patients with AL and ATTR-CA include 11C-Pittsburgh compound B,[82] 18F-florbetapir,[84] and 18F-vlorbetaben.[101] These tracers more likely bind to the β-folded structure of amyloid fibrils, thus facilitating the identification of amyloid deposits, and have also been found helpful for the early diagnosis and follow-up of patients with Alzheimer's disease.[102] In a study by Lee and colleagues, 11C-PIB was significantly decreased in the 5 patients with AL-CA who had previously received chemotherapy, suggesting the possibility of using this tracer to assess disease burden/activity by quantifying the maximum standard uptake value of the myocardium relative to the blood cavity. Recent studies have also demonstrated increased uptake of 18F-florbetapir in patients with AL-CA compared with those with ATTR-CA, which further supports the concept that 18F-florbetapir may preferentially bind to AL fibrils and that its uptake measurements may be able to differentiate between subgroups.[103] A recent systematic review including 6 studies (n = 98) on the application of PET imaging with 11C-PIB, 18F-florbetapir, and 18F-florbetaben reported a sensitivity of 92% and specificity of 83% for the detection of AL and ATTR-CA.[104]

In CA, autonomic dysfunction is caused by amyloid infiltration of myocardial conduction pathways and is common in ATTR-CA, especially in the hereditary form that has been studied extensively; it is present only in approximately 9% of cases of wild-type ATTR.[105] The use of iodine 123-labelled metaiodobenzylguanidine (^{123}I-MIBG), a modified chemical analogue of norepinephrine, is well-established in patients with heart failure and also plays an essential role in the assessment of sympathetic innervation in CA.[106] In patients with amyloidosis, myocardial sympathetic denervation often precedes neurologic and cardiac manifestations, especially in carriers of pathogenic genetic variants. A semiquantitative analysis of ^{123}I-MIBG cardiac uptake compared with background (heart-to-mediastinal ratio) provides indirect information of amyloid infiltration in the sympathetic nervous system. Increased ventricular arrhythmias and the 5-year mortality rate is observed in ATTR-CA with decreased heart-to-mediastinal ^{123}I-MIBG uptake (heart-to-mediastinum ratio od <1.6) at 4 hours after tracer administration and reflects the cardiovascular dysautonomia caused by myocardial infiltration.[107] Cardiac sympathetic denervation documented by decreased MIGB uptake has also been detected before amyloid burden by 99mTc-DPD scintigraphy in patients with hereditary ATTR, thus highlighting the importance of this tool

for early diagnosis in this subgroup of patients.[108] PET imaging benefits from a superior spatial resolution as compared with single-photon emission computed tomography scans. In addition, it provides a quantitative analysis of tracer uptake and has the potential to quantify amyloid burden accurately, facilitate prognosis, and assess disease progression and response to therapy. These questions are of particular interest for future research and may improve our understanding of the underlying molecular mechanism of amyloidosis.

SUMMARY

Multimodality imaging has been proposed for many cardiovascular disorders, including cardiomyopathy, to ameliorate the diagnostic performance and management of patients affected. CA represent the paradigm of multimodality application in the recent era. Multimodality imaging has revolutionized CA diagnosis and management in the last few years. Its application in daily practice has permitted the noninvasive diagnosis of ATTR-CA, diagnosis in the earlier stages of the disease the AL and ATTR-CA, stratification by the patient risk, and monitoring the performance of therapy in this setting.

CLINICS CARE POINTS

- In the presence of cardiomyopathies with a hypertrophic phenotype, a decreased GLS, especially in the basal and intermediate segments, the presence of a preserved LVEF is useful in the diagnosis of suspected pseudo-hypertrophy owing to amyloid infiltration.

- ECV imaging by CMR can measure the degree of infiltration of the extracellular space accurately, resulting in an accurate marker of infiltration and helping in the differential diagnosis, prognostic stratification, and monitoring disease progression and response to therapy.

- Radionuclide bone scintigraphy with technetium-labelled bisphosphonates is the gold standard for noninvasive diagnosis of ATTR-CA, but requires always excluding a plasma cell dyscrasia to rule out AL-CA.

DISCLOSURE

The author(s) received no financial support for the research, authorship, and/or publication of this article.

REFERENCES

1. Benson MD, Buxbaum JN, Eisenberg DS, et al. Amyloid nomenclature 2018: recommendations by the International Society of Amyloidosis (ISA) nomenclature committee. Amyloid 2018;25(4): 215–9.
2. Merlini G, Bellotti V. Molecular mechanisms of amyloidosis. N Engl J Med 2003;349:583–96.
3. Muchtar E, Gertz MA, Kyle RA, et al. A modern primer on light chain amyloidosis in 592 patients with mass spectrometry-verified typing. Mayo Clin Proc 2019;94(3):472–83.
4. Shi J, Guan J, Jiang B, et al. Amyloidogenic light chains induce cardiomyocyte contractile dysfunction and apoptosis via a non-canonical p38a MAPK pathway. Proc Natl Acad Sci U S A 2010; 107:4188–93.
5. Ruberg FL, Grogan M, Hanna M, et al. Transthyretin amyloid cardiomyopathy: JACC state-of-the-art review. J Am Coll Cardiol 2019;73:2872–91.
6. Maurer MS, Elliott P, Comenzo R, et al. Addressing common questions encountered in the diagnosis and management of cardiac amyloidosis. Circulation 2017;135(14):1357–77.
7. Lousada I, Comenzo RL, Landau H, et al. Light chain amyloidosis: patient experience survey from the Amyloidosis Research Consortium. Adv Ther 2015;32:920–8.
8. Lane T, Fontana M, Martinez-Naharro A, et al. Natural history, quality of life, and outcome in cardiac transthyretin amyloidosis. Circulation 2019;140:16–26.
9. Wechalekar AD, Gillmore JD, Hawkins PN. Systemic amyloidosis. Lancet 2016;387(10038): 2641–54.
10. Grogan M, Dispenzieri A, Gertz MA. Light-chain cardiac amyloidosis: strategies to promote early diagnosis and cardiac response. Heart 2017; 103(14):1065–72.
11. Pereira NL, Grogan M, Dec GW. Spectrum of restrictive and infiltrative cardiomyopathies: part 2 of a 2-part series. J Am Coll Cardiol 2018;71(10): 1149–66.
12. Maurer MS, Schwartz JH, Gundapaneni B, et al. Tafamidis treatment for patients with transthyretin amyloid cardiomyopathy. N Engl J Med 2018;379(11): 1007–16.
13. Siddiqi OK, Ruberg FL. Cardiac amyloidosis: an update on pathophysiology, diagnosis, and treatment. Trends Cardiovasc Med 2018;28:10–21.
14. González-López E, Gagliardi C, Dominguez F, et al. Clinical characteristics of wild-type transthyretin cardiac amyloidosis: disproving myths. Eur Heart J 2017;38(24):1895–904.
15. Barros-Gomes S, Williams B, Nhola LF, et al. Prognosis of light chain amyloidosis with preserved LVEF: added value of 2D speckle-tracking echocardiography to the current prognostic staging system. JACC Cardiovasc Imaging 2017;10(4): 398–407.
16. Mohty D, Pradel S, Magne J, et al. Prevalence and prognostic impact of left-sided valve thickening in systemic light-chain amyloidosis. Clin Res Cardiol 2017;106(5):331–40.
17. Klein AL, Hatle LK, Burstow DJ, et al. Doppler characterization of left ventricular diastolic function in cardiac amyloidosis. J Am Coll Cardiol 1989; 13(5):1017–26.
18. Modesto KM, Dispenzieri A, Cauduro SA, et al. Left atrial myopathy in cardiac amyloidosis: implications of novel echocardiographic techniques. Eur Heart J 2005;26(2):173–9.
19. Nochioka K, Quarta CC, Claggett B, et al. Left atrial structure and function in cardiac amyloidosis. Eur Heart J Cardiovasc Imaging 2017;18(10):1128–37.
20. Koyama J, Ray-Sequin PA, Falk RH. Prognostic significance of ultrasound myocardial tissue characterization in patients with cardiac amyloidosis. Circulation 2002;106:556–61.
21. Austin BA, Duffy B, Tan C, et al. Comparison of functional status, electrocardiographic, and echocardiographic parameters to mortality in endomyocardial-biopsy proven cardiac amyloidosis. Am J Cardiol 2009;103(10):1429–33.
22. Knight DS, Zumbo G, Barcella W, et al. Cardiac structural and functional consequences of amyloid deposition by cardiac magnetic resonance and echocardiography and their prognostic roles. JACC Cardiovasc Imaging 2019;12(5):823–33.
23. Tsang W, Lang RM. Echocardiographic evaluation of cardiac amyloid. Curr Cardiol Rep 2010 May; 12(3):272–6.
24. Grogan M, Scott CG, Kyle RA, et al. Natural history of wild-type transthyretin cardiac amyloidosis and risk stratification using a novel staging system. J Am Coll Cardiol 2016;68(10):1014–20.
25. Milani P, Dispenzieri A, Scott CG, et al. Independent prognostic value of stroke volume index in patients with immunoglobulin light chain amyloidosis. Circ Cardiovasc Imaging 2018;11(5):e006588.
26. Phelan D, Collier P, Thavendiranathan P, et al. Relative apical sparing of longitudinal strain using two-dimensional speckle-tracking echocardiography is both sensitive and specific for the diagnosis of cardiac amyloidosis. Heart 2012;98(19):1442–8.
27. Salinaro F, Meier-Ewert HK, Miller EJ, et al. Longitudinal systolic strain, cardiac function improvement, and survival following treatment of light-chain (AL) cardiac amyloidosis. Eur Heart J Cardiovasc Imaging 2017;18(9):1057–64.
28. Belkin RN, Kupersmith AC, Khalique O, et al. A novel two-dimensional echocardiographic finding in cardiac amyloidosis. Echocardiography 2010;27(10):1171–6.

29. Rapezzi C, Fontana M. Relative left ventricular apical sparing of longitudinal strain in cardiac amyloidosis: is it just amyloid infiltration? JACC Cardiovasc Imaging 2019;12:1174–6.

30. Pagourelias ED, Mirea O, Duchenne J, et al. Echo parameters for differential diagnosis in cardiac amyloidosis: a head-to-head comparison of deformation and nondeformation parameters. Circ Cardiovasc Imaging 2017;10(3):e005588.

31. Buss SJ, Emami M, Mereles D, et al. Longitudinal left ventricular function for prediction of survival in systemic light-chain amyloidosis: incremental value compared with clinical and biochemical markers. J Am Coll Cardiol 2012;60:1067–76.

32. Ternacle J, Bodez D, Guellich A, et al. Causes and consequences of longitudinal LV dysfunction assessed by 2D strain echocardiography in cardiac amyloidosis. JACC Cardiovasc Imaging 2016;9:126–38.

33. Uzan C, Lairez O, Raud-Raynier P, et al. Right ventricular longitudinal strain: a tool for diagnosis and prognosis in light-chain amyloidosis. Amyloid 2018;25(1):18–25.

34. Bellavia D, Pellikka PA, Dispenzieri A, et al. Comparison of right ventricular longitudinal strain imaging, tricuspid annular plane systolic excursion, and cardiac biomarkers for early diagnosis of cardiac involvement and risk stratification in primary systematic (AL) amyloidosis: a 5-year cohort study. Eur Heart J Cardiovasc Imaging 2012;13(8):680–9.

35. Binder C, Duca F, Stelzer PD, et al. Mechanisms of heart failure in transthyretin vs light chain amyloidosis. Eur Heart J Cardiovasc Imaging 2019;20(5):512–24.

36. Cappelli F, Porciani MC, Bergesio F, et al. Right ventricular function in AL amyloidosis: characteristics and prognostic implication. Eur Heart J Cardiovasc Imaging 2012;13(5):416–22.

37. Bodez D, Ternacle J, Guellich A, et al. Prognostic value of the right ventricular systolic function in cardiac amyloidosis. Amyloid 2016;23(3):158–67.

38. Rapezzi C, Merlini G, Quarta CC, et al. Systemic cardiac amyloidosis: disease profiles and clinical courses of the 3 main types. Circulation 2009; 120(13):1203–12.

39. Falk RH, Alexander KM, Liao R, et al. (Light-chain) cardiac amyloidosis: a review of diagnosis and therapy. J Am Coll Cardiol 2016;68(12):1323–41.

40. Clemmensen TS, Soerensen J, Hansson NH, et al. Myocardial oxygen consumption and efficiency in patients with cardiac amyloidosis. J Am Heart Assoc 2018;7(21):e009974.

41. Clemmensen TS, Eiskjær H, Mikkelsen F, et al. Left ventricular pressure-strain-derived myocardial work at rest and during exercise in patients with cardiac amyloidosis. J Am Soc Echocardiogr 2020;33(5):573–82.

42. Clemmensen TS, Eiskjær H, Ladefoged B, et al. Prognostic implications of left ventricular myocardial work indices in cardiac amyloidosis. Eur Heart J Cardiovasc Imaging 2021;22(6): 695–704.

43. Roger-Rollé A, Cariou E, Rguez K, et al. Amyloidosis Research Network collaborators. Can myocardial work indices contribute to the exploration of patients with cardiac amyloidosis? Open Heart 2020;7(2):e001346.

44. Pennell DJ. Cardiovascular magnetic resonance: twenty-first-century solutions in cardiology. Clin Med 2003;3:273–8.

45. Martinez-Naharro A, Treibel TA, Abdel-Gadir A, et al. Magnetic resonance in transthyretin cardiac amyloidosis. J Am Coll Cardiol 2017;70(4):466–77.

46. van Geuns RJ, Wielopolski PA, de Bruin HG, al at. Basic principles of magnetic resonance imaging. Prog Cardiovasc Dis 1999;42(2):149–56.

47. Maceira AM, Joshi J, Prasad SK, et al. Cardiovascular magnetic resonance in cardiac amyloidosis. Circulation 2005;111(2):186–93.

48. White JA, Kim HW, Shah D, et al. CMR imaging with rapid visual T1 assessment predicts mortality in patients suspected of cardiac amyloidosis. J Am Coll Cardiol Img 2014;7:143–56.

49. Mahalingam H, Chacko BR, Irodi A, et al. Myocardial nulling pattern in cardiac amyloidosis on time of inversion scout magnetic resonance imaging sequence - a new observation of temporal variability. Indian J Radiol Imaging 2018;28(4):427–32.

50. Fontana M, Pica S, Reant P, et al. Prognostic value of late gadolinium enhancement cardiovascular magnetic resonance in cardiac amyloidosis. Circulation 2015;132:1570–9.

51. Vogelsberg H, Mahrholdt H, Deluigi CC, et al. Cardiovascular magnetic resonance in clinically suspected cardiac amyloidosis: noninvasive imaging compared to endomyocardial biopsy. J Am Coll Cardiol 2008;51:1022–30.

52. Selvanayagam JB, Hawkins PN, Paul B, et al. Evaluation and management of the cardiac amyloidosis. J Am Coll Cardiol 2007;50:2101–10.

53. Kanda T, Fukusato T, Matsuda M, et al. Gadolinium-based contrast agent accumulates in the brain even in subjects without severe renal dysfunction: evaluation of autopsy brain specimens with inductively coupled plasma mass spectroscopy. Radiology 2015;276:228–32.

54. Murata N, Gonzalez-Cuyar LF, Murata K, et al. Macrocyclic and other non-group 1 gadolinium contrast agents deposit low levels of gadolinium in brain and bone tissue: preliminary results from 9 patients with normal renal function. Investig Radiol 2016;51:447–53.

55. Karamitsos TD, Piechnik SK, Banypersad SM, et al. Noncontrast T1 mapping for the diagnosis of cardiac amyloidosis. JACC Cardiovasc Imaging 2013;6(4):488–97.

56. Martinez-Naharro A, Kotecha T, Norrington K, et al. Native T1 and extracellular volume in transthyretin amyloidosis. JACC Cardiovasc Imaging 2019; 12(5):810–9.

57. Fontana M, Banypersad SM, Treibel TA, et al. Native T1 mapping in transthyretin amyloidosis. JACC Cardiovasc Imaging 2014;7:157–65.

58. Banypersad SM, Fontana M, Maestrini V, et al. T1 mapping and survival in systemic light-chain amyloidosis. Eur Heart J 2015;36(4):244–51.

59. Baggiano A, Boldrini M, Martinez-Naharro A, et al. Noncontrast magnetic resonance for the diagnosis of cardiac amyloidosis. JACC Cardiovasc Imaging 2020;13(1 Pt 1):69–80.

60. Fontana M, Banypersad SM, Treibel TA, et al. Differential myocyte responses in patients with cardiac transthyretin amyloidosis and light-chain amyloidosis: a cardiac MR imaging study. Radiology 2015;277(2):388–97.

61. Banypersad SM, Sado DM, Flett AS, et al. Quantification of myocardial extracellular volume fraction in systemic AL amyloidosis: an equilibrium contrast cardiovascular magnetic resonance study. Circ Cardiovasc Imaging 2013;6(1):34–9.

62. Martinez-Naharro A, Abdel-Gadir A, Treibel TA, et al. CMR-verified regression of cardiac AL amyloid after chemotherapy. JACC Cardiovasc Imaging 2018;11(1):152–4.

63. Lin L, Li X, Feng J, et al. The prognostic value of T1 mapping and late gadolinium enhancement cardiovascular magnetic resonance imaging in patients with light chain amyloidosis. J Cardiovasc Magn Reson 2018;20(1):2.

64. Ferreira VM, Piechnik SK, Robson MD, et al. Myocardial tissue characterization by magnetic resonance imaging: novel applications of T1 and T2 mapping. J Thorac Imaging 2014;29:147–54.

65. Kotecha T, Martinez-Naharro A, Treibel TA, et al. Myocardial edema and prognosis in amyloidosis. J Am Coll Cardiol 2018;71:2919–31.

66. Hales PW, Schneider JE, Burton RA, et al. Histo-anatomical structure of the living isolated rat heart in two contraction states assessed by diffusion tensor MRI. Prog Biophys Mol Biol 2012;110(2–3): 319–30.

67. Nielles-Vallespin S, Mekkaoui C, Gatehouse P, et al. In vivo diffusion tensor MRI of the human heart: reproducibility of breath-hold and navigator-based approaches. Magn Reson Med 2013;70(2): 454–65.

68. McGill LA, Scott AD, Ferreira PF, et al. Heterogeneity of fractional anisotropy and mean diffusivity measurements by in vivo diffusion tensor imaging in normal human hearts. PLoS One 2015;10(7): e0132360.

69. Wu MT, Tseng WY, Su MY, et al. Diffusion tensor magnetic resonance imaging mapping the fibre architecture remodelling in human myocardium after infarction: correlation with viability and wall motion. Circulation 2006;114(10):1036–45.

70. Mekkaoui C, Jackowski MP, Kostis WJ, et al. Myocardial scar delineation using diffusion tensor magnetic resonance tractography. J Am Heart Assoc 2018;7(3):e007834.

71. Nielles-Vallespin S, Khalique Z, Ferreira PF, et al. Assessment of myocardial microstructural dynamics by in vivo diffusion tensor cardiac magnetic resonance. J Am Coll Cardiol 2017;69(6):661–76.

72. Gotschy A, von Deuster C, van Gorkum RJH, et al. Characterizing cardiac involvement in amyloidosis using cardiovascular magnetic resonance diffusion tensor imaging. J Cardiovasc Magn Reson 2019; 21(1):56.

73. Kellman P, Hansen MS, Nielles-Vallespin S, et al. Myocardial perfusion cardiovascular magnetic resonance: optimized dual sequence and reconstruction for quantification. J Cardiovasc Magn Reson 2017;19(1):43.

74. Nordlinger M, Magnani B, Skinner M, et al. Is elevated plasma B-natriuretic peptide in amyloidosis simply a function of the presence of heart failure? Am J Cardiol 2005;96(7):982–4.

75. Martinez-Naharro A, Knight DS, Kotecha T, et al. Routine identification of hypoperfusion in cardiac amyloidosis by myocardial blood flow mapping [abstract 028]. Heart 2017;103(Suppl. 1):A24.

76. Chatzantonis G, Bietenbeck M, Florian A, et al. Diagnostic value of the novel CMR parameter "myocardial transit-time" (MyoTT) for the assessment of microvascular changes in cardiac amyloidosis and hypertrophic cardiomyopathy. Clin Res Cardiol 2021;110(1):136–45.

77. Betocchi S, Hess OM, Losi MA, et al. Regional left ventricular mechanics in hypertrophic cardiomyopathy. Circulation 1993;88(5 Pt 1):2206–14.

78. Dorbala S, Vangala D, Bruyere J Jr, et al. Coronary microvascular dysfunction is related to abnormalities in myocardial structure and function in cardiac amyloidosis. JACC Heart Fail 2014 Aug;2(4): 358–67.

79. Tower-Rader A, Mohananey D, To A, et al. Prognostic value of global longitudinal strain in hypertrophic cardiomyopathy: a systematic review of existing literature. JACC Cardiovasc Imaging 2019;12(10):1930–42.

80. Koyama J, Falk RH. Prognostic significance of strain Doppler imaging in light-chain amyloidosis. JACC Cardiovasc Imaging 2010;3(4):333–42.

81. Singh V, Falk R, Di Carli MF, et al. State-of-the-art radionuclide imaging in cardiac transthyretin amyloidosis. J Nucl Cardiol 2019;26(1):158–73.

82. Lee SP, Lee ES, Choi H, et al. 11C-Pittsburgh B PET imaging in cardiac amyloidosis. JACC Cardiovasc Imaging 2015;8:50–9.

83. Dorbala S, Vangala D, Semer J, et al. Imaging cardiac amyloidosis: a pilot study using 18F-florbetapir positron emission tomography. Eur J Nucl Med Mol Imaging 2014;41:1652–62.

84. Osborne DR, Acuff SN, Stuckey A, et al. A routine PET/CT protocol with streamlined calculations for assessing cardiac amyloidosis using (18)F-florbetapir. Front Cardiovasc Med 2015;2:23.

85. Castano A, Haq M, Narotsky DL, et al. Multicenter study of planar technetium 99m pyrophosphate cardiac imaging: predicting survival for patients with ATTR cardiac amyloidosis. JAMA Cardiol 2016;1:880–9.

86. Galat A, Rosso J, Guellich A, et al. Usefulness of (99m)Tc-HMDP scintigraphy for the etiologic diagnosis and prognosis of cardiac amyloidosis. Amyloid 2015;22:210–20.

87. Stats MA, Stone JR. Varying levels of small microcalcifications and macrophages in ATTR and AL cardiac amyloidosis: implications for utilizing nuclear medicine studies to subtype amyloidosis. Cardiovasc Pathol 2016;25:413–7.

88. Pepys MB, Dyck RF, de Beer FC, et al. Binding of serum amyloid P-component (SAP) by amyloid fibrils. Clin Exp Immunol 1979;38:284–93.

89. Bokhari S, Castano A, Pozniakoff T, et al. (99 m) Tc-pyrophosphate scintigraphy for differentiating light-chain cardiac amyloidosis from the transthyretin-related familial and senile cardiac amyloidoses. Circ Cardiovasc Imaging 2013;6:195–201.

90. Wizenberg TA, Muz J, Sohn YH, et al. Value of positive myocardial technetium-99m-pyrophosphate scintigraphy in the non-invasive diagnosis of cardiac amyloidosis. Am Heart J 1982;103(4 PART 1):468–73.

91. Falk RH, Lee VW, Rubinow A, et al. Sensitivity of technetium-99m-pyrophosphate scintigraphy in diagnosing cardiac amyloidosis. Am J Cardiol 1983;51(5):826–30.

92. Rapezzi C, Quarta CC, Guidalotti PL, et al. Usefulness and limitations of 99mTc-3, 3-diphosphono-1, 2-propanodicarboxylic acid scintigraphy in the aetiological diagnosis of amyloidotic cardiomyopathy. Eur J Nucl Med Mol Imaging 2011;38(3):470–8.

93. Rapezzi C, Guidalotti P, Salvi F, et al. Usefulness of 99mTc-DPD scintigraphy in cardiac amyloidosis. J Am Coll Cardiol 2008;51(15):1509–10.

94. Glaudemans AWJM, Van Rheenen RWJ, Van Den Berg MP, et al. Bone scintigraphy with 99mtechnetium-hydroxymethylene diphosphonate allows early diagnosis of cardiac involvement in patients with transthyretin-derived systemic amyloidosis. Amyloid 2014;21(1):35–444.

95. Katzmann JA, Abraham RS, Dispenzieri A, et al. Diagnostic performance of quantitative κ and λ free light chain assays in clinical practice. Clin Chem 2005;51(5):878–81.

96. Dispenzieri A, Katzmann JA, Kyle RA, et al. Prevalence and risk of progression of light-chain monoclonal gammopathy of undetermined significance: a retrospective population-based cohort study. Lancet 2010;375(9727):1721–8.

97. Kittleson MM, Maurer MS, Ambardekar AV, et al. Cardiac amyloidosis: evolving diagnosis and management: a scientific statement from the American Heart Association. Circulation 2020;142(1):E7–22.

98. Sperry BW, Vranian MN, Tower-Rader A, et al. Regional variation in technetium pyrophosphate uptake in transthyretin cardiac amyloidosis and impact on mortality. JACC Cardiovasc Imaging 2018;11(2 Pt 1):234–42.

99. Hutt DF, Fontana M, Burniston M, et al. Prognostic utility of the Perugini grading of 99mTc-DPD scintigraphy in transthyretin (ATTR) amyloidosis and its relationship with skeletal muscle and soft tissue amyloid. Eur Heart J Cardiovasc Imaging 2017;18:1344–50.

100. Cappelli F, Gallini C, Costanzo EN, et al. Lung uptake during 99mTc-hydroxymethylene diphosphonate scintigraphy in patients with TTR cardiac amyloidosis: an underestimated phenomenon. Int J Cardiol 2018;254:346–50.

101. Law WP, Wang WY, Moore PT, et al. Cardiac amyloid imaging with 18F-florbetaben PET: a pilot study. J Nucl Med 2016;57:1733–9.

102. Bateman RJ, Xiong C, Benzinger TL, et al. Dominantly Inherited Alzheimer Network. Clinical and biomarker changes in dominantly inherited Alzheimer's disease. N Engl J Med 2012;367(9):795–804.

103. Park MA, Padera RF, Belanger A, et al. 18F-florbetapir binds specifically to myocardial light chain and transthyretin amyloid deposits: autoradiography study. Circ Cardiovasc Imaging 2015;8: e002954.

104. Kim YJ, Ha S, Kim YI. Cardiac amyloidosis imaging with amyloid positron emission tomography: a systematic review and meta-analysis. J Nucl Cardiol 2020;27(1):123–32.

105. Dorbala S, Ando Y, Bokhari S, et al. ASNC/AHA/ ASE/EANM/HFSA/ISA/SCMR/SNMMI expert consensus recommendations for multimodality imaging in cardiac amyloidosis: Part 1 of 2-evidence base and standardized methods of imaging. J Nucl Cardiol 2019;26:2065–123.

106. Slart RHJA, Glaudemans AWJM, Hazenberg BPC, et al. Imaging cardiac innervation in amyloidosis. J Nucl Cardiol 2019;26(1):174–87.

107. Coutinho MC, Cortez-Dias N, Cantinho G, et al. Reduced myocardial 123-iodine metaiodobenzylguanidine uptake: a prognostic marker in familial amyloid polyneuropathy. Circ Cardiovasc Imaging 2013;6(5):627–36.

108. Piekarski E, Chequer R, Algalarrondo V, et al. Cardiac denervation evidenced by MIBG occurs earlier than amyloid deposits detection by diphosphonate scintigraphy in TTR mutation carriers. Eur J Nucl Med Mol Imaging 2018;45:1108–18.

Cardiovascular Involvement in Transthyretin Cardiac Amyloidosis

Michele Lioncino, MD[a,1], Emanuele Monda, MD[a,1],
Giuseppe Palmiero, MD[a], Martina Caiazza, MD[a], Erica Vetrano, MD[a,b],
Marta Rubino, MD[a], Augusto Esposito, MD[a], Gemma Salerno, MD[c],
Francesca Dongiglio, MD[a], Barbara D'Onofrio, MD[a], Federica Verrillo, MD[a],
Giuseppe Cerciello, MD[d], Fiore Manganelli, MD, PhD[e],
Giuseppe Pacileo, MD[f], Eduardo Bossone, MD, PhD[g],
Paolo Golino, MD, PhD[c,h], Paolo Calabrò, MD, PhD[h,i],
Giuseppe Limongelli, MD, PhD[a,j,*]

KEYWORDS

- Transthyretin cardiac amyloidosis • Hypertrophic cardiomyopathy • Left ventricular hypertrophy
- Heart failure • Atrial fibrillation • Management

KEY POINTS

- Cardiac amyloidosis is a great pretender, and its diagnosis requires a high index of suspicion. There is a significant diagnostic delay in the diagnosis of CA.
- Although 12-lead ECG has low specificity for the diagnosis of ATTR-CA, an unremarkable 12-lead ECG is a rare finding.
- Diagnosis of TTR-CA is complex and requires integration of multimodality imaging techniques.
- Atrial fibrillation and atrioventricular conduction disturbances are of major concern and require specific management in patients affected by ATTR-CA.

[a] Inherited and Rare Cardiovascular Disease Unit, Department of Translational Medical Sciences, University of Campania "Luigi Vanvitelli", AORN dei Colli, Monaldi Hospital, Naples, Italy; [b] Internal Medicine Unit, Department of Translational Sciences, University of Campania "Luigi Vanvitelli", Naples, Italy; [c] Vanvitelli Cardiology Unit, Monaldi Hospital, Naples 80131, Italy; [d] Haematology Unit, Department of Clinical Medicine and Surgery, University of Naples Federico II, Naples, Italy; [e] Department of Neuroscience, Reproductive Sciences and Odontostomatology, University of Naples 'Federico II', Via Pansini, 5, Naples 81025, Italy; [f] Heart Failure and Cardiac Rehabilitation Unit, Department of Cardiology, AORN dei Colli, Monaldi Hospital, Naples, Italy; [g] Division of Cardiology, "Antonio Cardarelli" Hospital, Naples 80131, Italy; [h] Department of Translational Sciences, University of Campania "Luigi Vanvitelli", Naples, Italy; [i] Division of Cardiology, A.O.R.N. "Sant'Anna & San Sebastiano", Caserta I-81100, Italy; [j] Institute of Cardiovascular Sciences, University College of London and St. Bartholomew's Hospital, London WC1E 6DD, UK
[1] The authors equally contributed to the manuscript.
* Corresponding author. Institute of Cardiovascular Sciences, University College of London and St. Bartholomew's Hospital, London WC1E 6DD, UK.
E-mail address: limongelligiuseppe@libero.it

Heart Failure Clin 18 (2022) 73–87
https://doi.org/10.1016/j.hfc.2021.07.006

TRANSTHYRETIN CARDIAC AMYLOIDOSIS
Introduction, Epidemiology, and Pathophysiology

Transthyretin cardiac amyloidosis (ATTR-CA) is a systemic disorder resulting from the extracellular deposition of amyloid fibrils of misfolded transthyretin protein in the heart.[1,2] Transthyretin, also known as prealbumin, is a protein primarily synthetized in the liver, whose functions involve transport of thyroid hormones and retinol binding protein-vitamin A complex.[3-5] ATTR-CA is a life-threatening disease, which can be caused by progressive deposition of wild-type transthyretin (wtATTR), a condition formerly known as senile cardiac amyloidosis, or by aggregation of an inherited mutated variant of transthyretin (mATTR).[2,6]

ATTR-CA is often overlooked in many clinical scenarios; although its prevalence is uncertain, recent autopsy data reveal that among patients with heart failure with preserved ejection fraction, amyloid deposits can be found in almost 32% of patients older than 75 years, compared with 8% in patients younger than 75 years.[7] Observational studies[8-10] seem to suggest a prevalence of 13% among patients with heart failure with preserved ejection fraction,[11] 16% among patients with severe aortic stenosis requiring aortic valve replacement,[10,12] and 5% among patients with a diagnosis of hypertrophic cardiomyopathy.[13] Subclinical cardiac deposition of transthyretin, evaluated by myocardial uptake of bone tracers, has been described in up to 3% of elderly patients with no previous clinical suspicious of ATTR, suggesting that the prevalence of wtATTR is underestimated.[14,15]

mATTR Is a rare condition transmitted in an autosomal dominant manner with incomplete penetrance, causing heterogenous phenotypes which can range from predominant neuropathic involvement (transthyretin-related familiar amyloid polyneuropathy), predominant cardiomyopathy (ATTR-CA), or mixed.[16-19] This heterogeneity is linked to different factors, such as age, sex, fibril type, maternal inheritance, and country of origin.[20-22] Since its first description, the prevalence of the Val122Ile substitution has been reported between 3% and 4% among individuals of African-American descent,[23,24] and ATTR-CA secondary to this mutation has been considered the most common variant worldwide. Compared with age-adjusted healthy controls, asymptomatic carriers of Val122Ile mutation did not show a significant difference in mortality, nonetheless their lifetime risk of incident heart failure was significantly higher (stratified hazard ratio, 1.47; 95% confidence interval [CI], 1.03–2.10; $P = .04$).[23] In subjects with mATTR in Western Europe, Val30-Met seems the most common mutation, being endemic in Portugal, Brazil, and Japan.[18,21,25,26] In individuals affected by Val30Met substitution, two clinical forms can be detected: Patients with *early-onset mTTR* are younger, they often show a prevalent neurologic phenotype, and cardiac abnormalities are limited to atrioventricular conduction disturbances without evidence of cardiac hypertrophy; whereas *in late-onset mTTR*, the clinical presentation is common over the fifth decade of life, especially in older male-sex individuals with overt cardiac hypertrophy.[18,26,27] While the clinical presentation and natural history of ATTR associated with the Val30Met mutation have been widely studied,[18,25,26] at least four mutations are responsible for an exclusively or predominant cardiac phenotype: Val122Ile,[24] Ile68Leu,[28] Thre60Ala,[29] and Leu111Met.[30] The Thre60Ala mutation is the second most common variant in the United States, and it is endemic in Northern Ireland.[31] This variant causes both neurologic and cardiac phenotypes, with symptoms onset between the fifth and the sixth decade of life.[29] The Ile68Leu is endemic in northern Italy, and carriers of this variant show an exclusively cardiac phonotype, with late, age-dependent onset, incomplete prevalence, and male predominance.[18] Subjects with cardiac mutations are more likely: male, older, with a history of cardiac disease or receiving a treatment for a cardiac disease, lower estimated glomerular filtration rate (eGFR), and higher circulating levels of troponin, brain natriuretic peptide (BNP), and NT-pro-BNP.[32] Furthermore, carriers of a cardiac mutation were more likely to have an abnormal baseline ECG and an increased diastolic interventricular septum thickness, with the exception of the individuals with an *early onset* Val30Met mutation.[32] Clinically relevant TTR genotypes and their relative distribution are listed in **Table 1**.

Clinical Presentation and Red Flags of Transthyretin Cardiac Amyloidosis

Cardiac amyloidosis is a great pretender, and its diagnosis requires a high index of suspicion.[33] In a recent survey including 533 subjects with confirmed diagnosis of amyloidosis, the average time between diagnosis and the onset of symptoms was 2 years; cardiologists were the most consulted specialists for referral, nonetheless a correct diagnosis was performed at first evaluation only in 18.7% of the cases.[34] In a descriptive study, almost 35% of patients affected by cardiac amyloidosis had been previously misdiagnosed with other cardiovascular diseases, such as

Table 1
Genotypes in transthyretin cardiac amyloidosis

Gene Variant	Distribution and Prevalence	Clinical Features	Age of Presentation
mATTR-CA - Val122Ile	4% of African-Americans	LVH, mild reduction in LVEF, peripheral neuropathy, bilateral carpal tunnel	60–65 yo
mATTR-CA- Ile68Leu	Italy	LVH, AS, low QRS voltage	>55yo
mATTR-CA Val30Met	Brazil, Portugal, and Japan	Peripheral ascending polyneuropathy, cardiac involvement in late onset forms	Early onset: 30–40 y.o Late onset: >55 y.o
mATTR-CA Thre60Ala	Ireland	Peripheral neuropathy, LVH	>60 y.o
wtATTR-CA	Elderly male	Lumbar spinal stenosis, bilateral carpal tunnel, biceps tendon rupture, LVH, HFpEF	>55 y.o

hypertensive cardiomyopathy (53%), HCM (23.5%), HpEF (8.8%), or aortic stenosis (8.8%)[35]

Patients affected by CA often present with dyspnea, congestion, and other signs of heart failure, but these findings are not specific and can be misdiagnosed with HFpEF.[36] Increased wall thickness caused by amyloid fibrils deposition is a cardinal feature of ATTR-CA and can lead to severe diastolic dysfunction.[11,37] In a cohort study including 120 patients older than 60 years, among individuals admitted for HFpEF with left ventricular wall thickness greater than 12 mm, the prevalence of wtATTR was 13.3%.[11] A significant male predominance and a clear association between increasing age and frequency of cardiac involvement have been described in both mATTR and wtATTR.[32,38,39] Based on these findings, an international panel of 11 amyloidosis experts has proposed a disease identification framework. The panel recommends screening for the possibility of an underlying ATTR-CA in men older than 65 or women older than 70 years in the presence of symptoms of HF, increased LV thickness, and at least one clinical "red flag."[40]

The clinical clues or red flags that should alert the clinician about the possibility of ATTR-CA are listed in **Table 2**.

A clinical history of bilateral carpal tunnel syndrome,[41–43] lumbar spinal stenosis,[44,45] or spontaneous biceps tendon rupture[46] can represent an early indicator of ATTR-CA and often precedes cardiac involvement. The suspicion of ATTR-CA should be triggered by a clinical history of intolerance to angiotensin-converting enzyme inhibitors (ACEi), angiotensin receptor blockers (ARBs), or beta-blockers, in case of symptomatic hypotension or after the resolution of hypertension in

previously hypertensive patients.[47,48] Unexplained peripheral neuropathy or signs of autonomic dysfunction could represent other hints of ATTR amyloidosis.[6] ATTR-CA should be systematically excluded in patients with a clinical history of premature pacemaker implantation[38,39,49] or predominant right heart failure, especially if associated to an increased RV wall thickness.[50]

The coexistence of aortic stenosis and ATTR represents a challenging clinical scenario, and it is likely underestimated because of the absence of a systematic screening and the complexity of diagnosis confirmation.[51,52] Furthermore, almost 50% of patients affected by ATTR and AS have a paradoxic low-flow low-gradient AS; in this scenario, additional test are required to differentiate a true-severe versus a pseudo-severe AS.[12,51–53]

Electrocardiography

A 12-lead ECG is a cost-effective, broadly available screening test and should be obtained at the initial evaluation of a patient with suspected ATTR-CA and with the development of new symptoms, to exclude other cardiovascular comorbidities and, in selected cases (ie, sudden AV block), to direct treatment strategies.[33,35,36,40] Classically, ATTR-CA is characterized by low QRS voltages despite increased LV wall thickness, nonetheless recent series have shown that the prevalence of low QRS voltages (defined by QRS amplitude <0.5 mV in all limb leads or Sokolow index <1.5 mV) ranges from 20% to 25% among patients affected by ATTR-CA.[40,54–58] Thus, the absence of low-amplitude QRS complexes should not be considered an exclusion criteria for the diagnosis of ATTR-CA because of its low sensitivity.[2,35] However, the disproportion between

Table 2
Clinical red flags for the suspicion of ATTR-CA

Clinical Red Flags for the Diagnosis of ATTR-CA	
Physical examination:	Bilateral carpal tunnel syndrome Spontaneous rupture of biceps tendon Lumbar spinal stenosis Intolerance to ACEi, beta-blockers, or ARBs Unexplained peripheral neuropathy Autonomic dysfunction (orthostatic hypotension) Signs of right heart failure Disproportion between symptoms and severity of HF Low-flow low-gradient AS
Electrocardiogram	Disproportion between low QRS voltages and LVH Pseudoinfarct Q waves
Biomarkers	Mild increase in circulating troponin I without myocardial ischemia High levels of NT pro BNP despite mild HF
Echocardiography	Severe LVH with nondilated cavities AV valve thickening (>2 mm) Interatrial septum thickening RV wall thickening (>5 mm) Granular sparkling appearance Apex to base longitudinal strain ratio>2 Relative apical sparing + transmitralic DT < 200 msec Increased ejection fraction to strain ratio
Cardiac magnetic resonance	Diffuse subendocardial or transmural LGE in a noncoronary artery distribution Abnormal gadolinium kinetics Elevated T1 relaxation times Elevated extracellular volume (ECV)

QRS voltages and LV wall thickness, expressed as QRS voltage/LV mass ratio, has been reported both in AL-CA and ATTR-CA and represents a frequently overlooked clinical red flag.[55,59] Broad Q waves and pseudo-infarction pattern in the anteroseptal and inferior leads can be present in up to 70% of the cases and could lead to a misdiagnosis of coronary artery disease.[54,56] Atrial fibrillation, supraventricular arrhythmias, or conduction disturbances are present in a significant number of patients affected by ATTR-CA.[54–57]

The relation between ECG findings and prognosis is not well delineated. Low-voltage pattern, increased PQ interval, and prolonged QRS duration have been shown to be independently associated to decreased survival in a combined cohort of patients with AL and ATTR-CA.[56] In a longitudinal study including 200 consecutive patients with confirmed diagnosis of CA, none of the ECG variables predicted mortality; nonetheless, a Sokolow index less than 1.5 mV was independently

associated to the combined endpoint of hospitalization, liver transplant, or death at multivariate analysis.[54]

Twenty-four-hour Holter monitoring

Atrial arrhythmias appear to be more prevalent in ATTR than in the general population, and in particular, wtATTR seems to be associated to the highest risk of comorbid AF.[39,54,60–62] AF is present in up to 70% of the patients with ATTR-CA and is often poorly tolerated.[63] In a longitudinal study including 238 amyloid patients,[60] Sanchis and colleagues reported an overall AF prevalence of 44% compared with a prevalence of 1% in the age-adjusted general population. The prevalence was higher among patients with wtATTR (71%) than that among patients affected by mATTR (19%) or AL-CA (26%).

Furthermore, premature ventricular beats, nonsustained ventricular tachycardia, and sustained ventricular tachycardia are common in patients affected by CA and have been associated with an increased risk of arrhythmic sudden cardiac death.[64–66] In addition, conduction disease is highly prevalent in ATTR-CA,[67–69] and, when compared with age-matched controls, patients affected by ATTR-CA had a significant HV interval prolongation often without evidence of QRS prolongation.[68] Patients with wtATTR-CA seem to show the highest prevalence of atrioventricular conduction disease compared with AL-CA.[68]

Echocardiography
Echocardiography is a first-line screening tool in patients with clinically suspected ATTR-CA and can be useful in the differential diagnosis of hypertensive, hypertrophic, and restrictive cardiomyopathies.[33,47,55,70–74] In the presence of a definite diagnosis of CA, echocardiographic screening should be obtained every 6 to 12 months and with new symptoms, to provide prognostic stratification and to assess the response to treatment.[33] Classical findings in ATTR-CA include symmetric hypertrophy of LV with nondilated cavities,[33,36,59] thickening of the atrioventricular valves (>2 mm) and the interatrial septum,[33,36,55,74] biatrial enlargement, RV free wall thickening (>5 mm),[33,72] pericardial effusion, or intracardiac thrombi.[75] Diastolic dysfunction is present in the very early stages of disease, evolving from an abnormal relaxation pattern, characterized by a decreased early filling velocity-to-atrial filling velocity ratio (E/A ratio), to a restrictive physiology in advanced stages of disease.[73] Although left ventricular ejection fraction may be preserved until the end stages of disease,[39,70,71,76,77] speckle tracking techniques can show an impairment of peak systolic wall motion velocities even in patients with mild hypertrophy.[78,79] Strain parameters are altered to a much greater extent in CA than in other cardiomyopathies,[70,71,79] and relative apical sparing is a clinical hallmark of CA.[70] Relative apical strain, which is the ratio between average apical and the sum of basal and mid-LS strain, has been validated as an highly sensitive and specific tool for the differential diagnosis of CA from other causes of cardiac hypertrophy such as AS or HCM (sensitivity 93%, specificity 82%, area under the curve [AUC] 0.91, $P < .001$).[70] A combined cutoff of deceleration time of early filling (DT<200 msec) and septal apical to basal longitudinal strain ratio greater than 2.1 can improve diagnostic accuracy for CA (88% sensitivity, 100% specificity, 100% predictive positive value, and 96% predictive negative value).[76] In patients with mild hypertrophy (defined as LV wall thickness between 12 and 16 mm) and preserved ejection fraction, the ejection fraction to strain ratio improves the diagnostic accuracy for

CA (sensitivity 89.7%, specificity 91.7%, AUC 0.96) compared with relative apical strain and should be considered in the differential diagnosis with other causes of hypertrophy, such as HCM, AS, and Fabry disease.[80]

Cardiac magnetic resonance
Cardiac magnetic resonance (CMR) with late gadolinium enhancement (LGE) is the gold standard for volume and chamber quantification and can offer unique information on myocardial tissue characterization in patients with CA.[81–84] The typical CMR findings of cardiac amyloidosis include diffuse subendocardial or transmural LGE in a noncoronary artery territory of distribution and a characteristic abnormal myocardial and blood pool gadolinium kinetics.[2,83,85,86] Other patterns of distribution are possible: diffuse, transmural, or patchy LGE has been described in patients with ATTR-CA.[2,85,86] However, the assessment of LGE in CA was technically challenging because of high myocardial uptake and fast blood washout, the relative enhancement was lower than previously reported, and false negatives can be obtained when scans are nulled using abnormal myocardium.[83] Phase-sensitive inversion recovery sequences can reduce the need for an optimal null point and should be performed in patients with suspected ATTR.[87] However, LGE sequences may not be specific and require contrast, which could be contraindicated in patients affected by chronic kidney disease.

In contrast, native T1 mapping sequences can evaluate the degree of myocardial infiltration in CA and correlate with the extent of systolic and diastolic dysfunction.[82,88,89] Elevated T1 relaxation times likely represent a direct marker of cardiac amyloid load and are more sensitive than LGE in detecting the early stages of ATTR-CA.[88,89] Native myocardial T1 and pregadolinium and postgadolinium contrast T1 can be used to calculate myocardial extracellular volume (ECV). Both native T1 and ECV correlate with mortality, but ECV has a significantly better correlation with all markers of amyloid burden and a better prognostic power.[88] CMR should be considered in patients with suspected ATTR to rule out other infiltrative cardiomyopathies such as hemochromatosis, Fabry disease, sarcoidosis, myocarditis, or constrictive pericarditis; in patients with a definite diagnosis of ATTR-CA, it can be used to assess amyloid burden and response to therapy every 24 months.[90]

Biomarkers
No plasma or urinary biomarker can be used for the diagnosis of ATTR-CA. Plasma levels of NT-

pro-BNP are often elevated in ATTR-CA, even in patients with mild cardiac involvement or in asymptomatic carriers of a mutation of the TTR gene.[91] The disproportion between high levels of plasma NT-pro-BNP and the severity of HF can represent a clinical clue for the diagnosis of CA.[33]

As a result of myocardial injury, plasma levels of troponin I are often elevated in patients with ATTR-CA, and dosing should be performed for the purposes of prognostic stratification.[91,92]

In individuals of African-American descent, the combination of low levels of retinol-binding protein 4 and classical electrocardiographic and echocardiographic "red flags" may suggest the diagnosis of Val122Ile ATTR-CA.[93]

Radionuclide bone scintigraphy

Radionuclide bone scintigraphy with technetium-labeled bisphosphonates (^{99m}Tc-labeled 3,3-diphosphono-1,2-propanodicarboxylic acid, ^{99m}Tc-labeled pyrophosphate, and ^{99m}Tc-labeled hydroxymethylene diphosphonate) is the gold standard for noninvasive diagnosis of ATTR-CA[94–98] and is highly sensitive and specific for detecting ATTR amyloid, even in patients in early stages of disease.[99] However, cardiac localization of radiotracer is possible in patients with AL amyloidosis, thus nuclear scintigraphy alone is not appropriated for the diagnosis of ATTR-CA.[100] Serum immunofixation electrophoresis and serum-free light chains concentration are mandatory in patients with suspected ATTR-CA to rule out AL-CA (sensitivity>99%).[101] Bone scans can be evaluated with semiquantitative or quantitative methods. In quantitative analysis, a region of interest is placed over the heart, and the mean counts are compared with a similar sized region placed over the contralateral chest. Semiquantitative techniques are based on the comparison between bone and rib uptake, and patients are classified as grade 2 or 3 if cardiac uptake is respectively equal or greater than rib uptake. In patients with suspected ATTR and a negative screening for presence of a monoclonal light chain, radionuclide scintigraphy is diagnostic of ATTR-CA if there is a grade 2 or 3 cardiac uptake or if heart/contralateral chest ratio is greater than 1.5.[8,9,96]

It is important to note that up to 5% of the patients older than 65 years have a monoclonal gammopathy of uncertain significance (MGUS), and this could lead to an incorrect diagnosis of AL-CA in patients with coexistence of MGUS and ATTR-CA.[102] Therefore, endomyocardial biopsy is advised in patients with a positive screening for monoclonal light chain to exclude a superimposed AL-CA.[36]

Biopsy

Endomyocardial biopsy with Congo staining is the gold standard for the diagnosis of ATTR-CA (sensitivity 100%, specificity 100%)[8,40,47,103] and should be performed in

- Patients with suspected ATTR-CA and a monoclonal free light chain,[8]
- When radionuclide scintigraphy is unavailable,[33,36]
- When there is high clinical suspicion of ATTR-CA despite a negative scan.[36]

Biopsy of noninvolved organs (fat pad, bone marrow) should not be considered an option because of low sensitivity both in wtATTR and mATTR (sensitivity 45% and 15%, respectively).[104] Histologic samples must undergo either mass spectrometry or immunofluorescence to confirm the subtype of CA.

Genetic testing

Regardless of age and familiar history of CA, genetic testing is underscored in patients with confirmed ATTR-CA.[33,36] In the Beta-Blocker Evaluation of Survival Trial, a high prevalence of the Val122Ile mutation was reported among individuals of African-American descent.[105] Regular monitoring should be considered in carriers of a mutation of interest 10 years before the predicted age of onset of symptoms.[106]

Management of Cardiac Involvement in Transthyretin Amyloidosis

Management of heart failure

Patients with ATTR-CA often present with symptoms of HF either with reduced or preserved ejection fraction.[7,11] Because of the lack of evidence in patients affected by ATTR-CA, guideline-derived treatment algorithms may have partial benefits.[107] ACEi and ARBs may be detrimental in hypotensive patients, can cause a worsening of renal function, and reduce preload.[33,36,107] Beta-blockers are often poorly tolerated because patients with ATTR-CA often show evidence of conduction disturbances and, in patients with restrictive physiology, stroke volume becomes critically dependent on heart rate. Almost 30% of the patients included in the ATTR-ACT trial were treated with beta-blockers, ACEi, or ARBs,[108] but prognostic data about efficacy and tolerability of guideline-derived medical therapy are lacking. Beta-blockers, ACEi, and ARBs may be a therapeutic option in patients with ATTR-CA unless contraindicated.[36,109] Nondihydropyridine calcium channel blockers can exert a negative inotropic effect; thus, they should be avoided in ATTR-CA.[48]

Digoxin may be considered in patients with ATTR-CA, but a significant risk of enhanced drug toxicity has been reported.[110] Diuretics remain the cornerstone of medical therapy in patients with ATTR-CA and symptoms of volume overloading. Intravenous loop diuretics and mineral corticoid receptor antagonists can be used in "wet" patients with signs of acute heart failure, according to current guidelines.[107,111] Of note, the dose of diuretics and New York Heart Association functional class are strong predictors of all-cause mortality in patients with ATTR-CA, and their prognostic value remained significant after adjustment for age, base demographics, eGFR, and clinical status.[112]

Atrial fibrillation and risk of stroke/Tansient ischemic attack and systemic embolism

AF is present in up to 70% of the patients with ATTR-CA and is often poorly tolerated.[63] Compared with general population, patients with ATTR-CA and AF have a higher risk of intracavitary thrombosis, stroke, and systemic embolism.[60,61,75,113,114] It has been suggested that myocardial amyloid infiltration involves both left and right atria, and the loss of atrial contractility can cause blood stasis and a consequent state of hypercoagulability.[61,113] The presence of left atrial appendage thrombus at transesophageal echocardiogram was not adequately predicted by the CHA2-DS2-VASc score.[115]

Based on these findings, patients with AF and ATTR-CA should be anticoagulated with VKA or DOAC, in the absence of contraindications, irrespective of CHA2-DS2-VASc score.[36,115] In the absence of prospective studies comparing different anticoagulation strategies, the choice of anticoagulant should follow current guidelines.[116]

Direct electrical cardioversion (DCV) should be performed in hemodynamically unstable AF.[114,116] Compared with controls, no significant difference in success rate was found for DCV in ATTR patients.[114] Despite optimal anticoagulation, the presence of intracavitary thrombus is more common in ATTR-CA patients programmed for a planned DCE than among general population and remains high even in patients who had a therapeutic level of anticoagulation for more than 3 weeks before DCV.[60,114] In light of these pieces of evidence, transesophageal echocardiography should be offered before DCV in patients with AF and ATTR-CA, irrespective of anticoagulation status.

If a rhythm control strategy is preferred, amiodarone is well tolerated in ATTR-CA patients and may be the antiarrhythmic of choice in this clinical setting.[63] Because of restrictive physiology, there is expert consensus that ATTR-CA patients should be maintained in sinus rhythm; however, no mortality benefit was found from the rhythm control versus rate control.[63]

Symptomatic bradycardia/atrioventricular block

Permanent pacing is recommended in patients with ATTR-CA and significant conduction disease, according to current guidelines.[117] In a series of patients with mATTR, prophylactic pacemaker was implanted in patients with (1) his-ventricle (HV) interval greater than 70 msec; (2) HV interval greater than 50 msec and fascicular block; (3) I grade atrioventricular block; (4) Wenckebach point less than 100 b.p.m. Over a follow-up period of 45 months, almost 25% of the patients developed high-grade AV block.[118] Although there are insufficient data to recommend routine electrophysiological testing in patients affected by ATTR-CA, close monitoring may be considered in patients with abnormal ECG at baseline.

In patients with ATTR-CA and an indication for permanent pacing, the use of CRT may be associated to better outcomes than RV pacing and is associated to improved left ventricular ejection fraction, reduced mitral regurgitation severity, and improved functional capacity[119]; nonetheless, there are insufficient data to recommend the use of CRT in this clinical subset.

Aortic stenosis

In patients with CA, the assessment of aortic stenosis severity should be performed according to current guidelines.[120] Patients with coexisting ATTR-CA and AS are more likely to have low-flow, low-gradient AS or paradoxic low-flow low-gradient AS.[51–53] The assessment of AS severity can be challenging in CA patients, and additional imaging tests are needed to discriminate a true severe versus moderate AS.[120] Dobutamine stress echocardiography often fails to increase stroke volume in CA patients, and it cannot be used to confirm AS severity. The use of noncontrast-CT to assess aortic calcium score should be considered if echocardiographic quantification of AS is inconclusive.

There are few studies reporting the outcomes of AVR in patients with severe AS and CA, but a high risk of mortality and nonimprovement in functional status and a high risk of periprocedural complications have been described.[52,121–124] Depressed LVEF, severely reduced global longitudinal strain (<10%), restrictive physiology, and moderate-to-severe low-flow state (defined as a stroke volume index <30 mL/m2) have been associated to a poor prognosis with futility of AVR in patients with CA and AS.[52,121] The choice and type of intervention must be based on careful evaluation of clinical status by local heart team, weighing the benefits and risk of each procedure. Although there are insufficient data to make recommendations, small studies suggest that TAVR should be preferred over SAVR in CA patients.[52]

Disease-modifying therapies

Disease-modifying therapies for ATTR-CA are listed in **Table 3**.

Tafamidis Tafamidis is a small molecule which binds to the thyroxine-binding sites of TTR and inhibits the dissociation of TTR tetramers into monomers.[125,126] In a multicentric phase 3 study,[108] 441 consecutive patients with a diagnosis of ATTR-CA were randomized to receive in 2:1:2 ratio tafamidis 80 mg versus tafamidis 20 mg versus placebo for 30 months. Tafamidis was associated to a lower all-cause mortality compared with placebo (hazard ratio 0.70, 95% CI 0.51 to 0.96) and to a lower rate of cardiovascular hospitalizations (relative risk 0.68, 95% CI 0.56–0.81).[108] Kaplan-Meier curve diverged substantially after 18 months of treatment. Furthermore, treatment with tafamidis was able to relieve symptoms as it lowered decline in sex-minute walking test and improved quality of life (measured through the Kansas City Cardiomyopathy Questionnaire Overall Summary).[108] Subgroup analysis demonstrated that benefit over placebo was preserved among patients with NYHA class I-II.[108] In contrast, among patients in NYHA class III, treatment with tafamidis resulted in higher rates of hospitalization, reflecting a prolonged overall survival.[108] Treatment with tafamidis has not been studied among patients in NYHA class IV or in case of severe aortic stenosis and in severe chronic kidney disease (eGFR<25 mL/1.73 m2).[36,108,109]

TTR silencers Patisiran is a small interfering RNA (siRNA) encapsulated in lipid nanoparticles whose mechanism of action consists in interfering with transcription of both mutant and wt ATTR.[127–129] In the APOLLO phase 3 study, 225 consecutive patients with mATTR and polyneuropathy were randomized to patisiran (0.3 mg/jg every 3 weeks) or placebo. Patisiran significantly improved neurologic status in mATTR patients.[129] Prespecified subgroup analysis of the APOLLO trial participants with evidence of amyloid cardiac involvement demonstrated that patisiran attenuated the decrease in cardiac output and increase in left ventricular end-diastolic volume. Compared with placebo arm, patients experienced a significant reduction in LV mass index, LV wall thickness, and NT-pro-BNP, suggesting that patisiran could induce reverse myocardial remodeling in ATTR-CA patients.[128]

The antisense oligonucleotide inotersen inhibits the expression of both wt and mutant TTR.[109,130] In the multicentric, double-blind NEURO-TTR trial, 172 patients with mATTR and polyneuropathy were randomized to inotersen (300 mg o.i.d) versus placebo. Almost 63% of the randomized patients showed evidence of cardiac involvement, although the study was not adequately powered to measure the effects on cardiac disease progression.[130] Inotersen improved quality of life and neurologic status in patients with mATTR polyneuropathy. Prespecified subgroup analysis demonstrated that treatment with inotersen was associated to improved 6 minutes walking test and global systolic strain and slowed the increase in LV wall thickness.[130] Treatment was well tolerated, and glomerulonephritis and thrombocythemia were the most relevant adverse reactions.[130]

Diflunisal Diflunisal is a nonselective, nonsteroidal, anti-inflammatory drug which has been demonstrated to stabilize TTR tetramers in vitro, thus preventing amyloid formation.[131–133] In patients with mATTR and polyneuropathy, diflunisal was safe, well tolerated, and improved neurologic status, but there is limited evidence about the potential effects of diflunisal on CA.[132,134] Diflunisal is contraindicated in patients with thrombocytopenia or chronic kidney disease (eGFR<40 mL/1.73 m2) and should be used cautiously in patients taking anticoagulants or with concomitant history of gastrointestinal bleeding.[135]

Orthotopic liver transplantation and heart transplantation Orthotopic liver transplantation has been historically purposed as the first therapy in patients with mATTR and neurologic impairment.[136–138] Although liver transplantation removes the source of mTTR molecules, tissue accumulation of wtTTR can continue after liver transplantation; thus, it could be detrimental in patients with cardiac involvement.[139–141] In particular, carriers of Val30Met mutation showed increased interventricular septal thickness at serial echocardiographic monitoring after liver transplantation, suggesting that mATTR amyloid fibers could promote subsequent deposition of wtATTR in the affected heart.[140] Combined heart and liver transplantation may be considered in young patients with mATTR-CA and advanced heart failure.[138,142] The need for lifelong immunosuppression, exclusion of older patients, and limited organ availability have to be weighted with benefits through an individualized evaluation by heart team. Liver transplantation is not useful in ATTR-CA.[6,36,138]

Table 3
Treatment options in transthyretin cardiac amyloidosis

Treatment	Indication	Phase 3 Trial Eligibility Criteria	Side Effect
Tafamidis	mATTR and wtATTR	End diastolic LV thickness>12 mm, signs and symptoms of HF and plasma circulating levels of NT pro BNP>600 pg/mL Contraindicated in: • Severe CKD (eGFR<25 mL7 min 1.73m2) • Liver transplant • Severe HF (NYHA class IV) • Severe reduction in functional capacity (6MWT<100 m)	Gastrointestinal discomfort
Patisiran	mATTR with polyneuropathy	Documented TTR mutation with polyneuropathy, defined as: • Neuropathy Impairment Score (NIS) 5–130 or • Polyneuropathy disability score (PND)<3b Contraindicated in: • Liver transplantation • NYHA class III and IV symptoms	Infusion-related reactions (premedication with steroids and anti-H1 and H2 drugs is recommended) Vitamin A deficiency (supplementation is recommended) Peripheral edema
Inotersen	mATTR with polyneuropathy	Documented TTR mutation with evidence of stage 1 or stage 2 amyloid familiar polyneuropathy; • NIS 10–130 Contraindicated in: • Mild CKD (eGFR<60 mL/min 1.73 m2) • Liver transplantation • NYHA class III and IV symptoms • Karnofsky performance status score<50 • Concomitant use of tafamidis or diflunisal • Thrombocytopenia	Infusion-related reactions (premedication with steroids and anti-H1 and H2 drugs is recommended Vitamin A deficiency (supplementation is recommended) Thrombocytopenia Glomerulonephritis
Diflunisal	Off label in both wtATTR and mATTR	Confirmed TTR mutation Amyloid familiar polyneuropathy Biopsy proven amyloid deposits Contraindication to tafamidis, inotersen, or patisiran Contraindicated in: • Liver transplantation • Anticoagulation • NYHA class III and IV symptoms • Severe CKD (eGFR<30 mL/min 1.73m2)	Bleeding Gastrointestinal toxicity Fluid retention

CLINICS CARE POINTS

- A clinical history of bilateral carpal tunnel syndrome, lumbar spinal stenosis, or spontaneous biceps tendon rupture can represent an early indicator of ATTR-CA and often precedes cardiac involvement.

- ATTR-CA should be systematically excluded in patients with a clinical history of premature pacemaker implantation or predominant right heart failure, especially if associated to an increased RV wall thickness.

- The absence of low-amplitude QRS complexes should not be considered an exclusion criterion for the diagnosis of ATTR-CA because of its low sensitivity.

- Atrial fibrillation, supraventricular arrhythmias, or conduction disturbances is present in a significant number of patients affected by ATTR-CA.

- Echocardiography is a first-line screening tool in patients with clinically suspected ATTR-CA. Strain parameters are altered to a much greater extent in CA than in other cardiomyopathies, and relative apical sparing is a clinical hallmark of CA.

- Patients with coexisting ATTR-CA and AS are more likely to have low-flow, low-gradient AS or paradoxic low-flow, low-gradient AS.

- CMR with late gadolinium enhancement (LGE) is the gold standard for volume and chamber quantification. CMR should be considered in patients with suspected ATTR to rule out other infiltrative cardiomyopathies.

- No plasma or urinary biomarker can be used for the diagnosis of ATTR-CA. Plasma levels of NT-pro-BNP are often elevated in ATTR-CA, even in patients with mild cardiac involvement or in asymptomatic carriers of a mutation of the *TTR* gene. The disproportion between high levels of plasma NT-pro-BNP and the severity of HF can represent a clinical clue for the diagnosis of CA.

- Up to 5% of the patients older than 65 years have a monoclonal gammopathy of uncertain significance (MGUS), and this could lead to an incorrect diagnosis of AL-CA in patients with coexistence of MGUS and ATTR-CA.

- Biopsy of noninvolved organs (fat pad, bone marrow) should not be considered an option because of low sensitivity both in wtATTR and mATTR (sensitivity 45% and 15%, respectively).

- Regardless of age and familiar history of CA, genetic testing is underscored in patients with confirmed ATTR-CA.

DISCLOSURE

The authors have nothing to disclose.

REFERENCES

1. Merlini G, Bellotti V. Molecular mechanisms of amyloidosis. N Engl J Med 2003;349(6):583–96.
2. Ruberg FL, Berk JL. Transthyretin (TTR) cardiac amyloidosis. Circulation 2012;126(10):1286–300.
3. Blake CCF, Geisow MJ, Oatley SJ, et al. Structure of prealbumin: secondary, tertiary and quaternary interactions determined by Fourier refinement at 1.8 Å. J Mol Biol 1978;121(3):339–56.
4. Monaco HL, Mancia F, Rizzi M, et al. Crystallization of the macromolecular complex transthyretin-retinol-binding protein. J Mol Biol 1994;244(1):110–3.
5. Monaco HL. Three-dimensional structure of the transthyretin-binding protein complex. Clin Chem Lab Med 2002;40(12):1229–36.
6. Ando Y, Coelho T, Berk JL, et al. Guideline of transthyretin-related hereditary amyloidosis for clinicians. Orphanet J Rare Dis 2013;8(1).
7. Tanskanen M, Peuralinna T, Polvikoski T, et al. Senile systemic amyloidosis affects 25% of the very aged and associates with genetic variation in alpha2-macroglobulin and tau: a population-based autopsy study. Ann Med 2008;40(3):232–9.
8. Gillmore JD, Maurer MS, Falk RH, et al. Nonbiopsy diagnosis of cardiac transthyretin amyloidosis. Circulation 2016;133(24):2404–12.
9. Castano A, Haq M, Narotsky DL, et al. Multicenter study of planar technetium 99m pyrophosphate cardiac imaging: predicting survival for patients with ATTR cardiac amyloidosis. JAMA Cardiol 2016;1(8):880–9.
10. Castano A, Narotsky DL, Hamid N, et al. Unveiling transthyretin cardiac amyloidosis and its predictors among elderly patients with severe aortic stenosis undergoing transcatheter aortic valve replacement. Eur Heart J 2017;38(38):2879–87.
11. González-López E, Gallego-Delgado M, Guzzo-Merello G, et al. Wild-type transthyretin amyloidosis as a cause of heart failure with preserved ejection fraction. Eur Heart J 2015;36(38):2585–94.
12. Rosenblum H, Masri A, Narotsky DL, et al. Unveiling outcomes in coexisting severe aortic stenosis and transthyretin cardiac amyloidosis. Eur J Heart Fail 2020. https://doi.org/10.1002/ejhf.1974.
13. Damy T, Costes B, Hagège AA, et al. Prevalence and clinical phenotype of hereditary transthyretin amyloid cardiomyopathy in patients with increased left ventricular wall thickness. Eur Heart J 2016;37(23):1826–34.
14. Longhi S, Guidalotti PL, Quarta CC, et al. Identification of TTR-related subclinical amyloidosis with

99mtc-dpd scintigraphy. JACC Cardiovasc Imaging 2014;7(5):531–2.

15. Mohamed-Salem L, Santos-Mateo JJ, Sanchez-Serna J, et al. Prevalence of wild type ATTR assessed as myocardial uptake in bone scan in the elderly population. Int J Cardiol 2018;270:192–6.

16. Buxbaum JN, Tagoe CE. The genetics of the amyloidoses. Annu Rev Med 2000;51:543–69.

17. Andrade C. A peculiar form of peripheral neuropathy: Familiar atypical generalized amyloidosis with special involvement of the peripheral nerves. Brain 1952;75(3):408–27.

18. Rapezzi C, Quarta CC, Obici L, et al. Disease profile and differential diagnosis of hereditary transthyretin-related amyloidosis with exclusively cardiac phenotype: An Italian perspective. Eur Heart J 2013;34(7):520–8.

19. Parman Y, Adams D, Obici L, et al. Sixty years of transthyretin familial amyloid polyneuropathy (TTR-FAP) in Europe: where are we now? A European network approach to defining the epidemiology and management patterns for TTR-FAP. Curr Opin Neurol 2016;29(Suppl 1):S3–11.

20. Hörnsten R, Pennlert J, Wiklund U, et al. Heart complications in familial transthyretin amyloidosis: impact of age and gender. Amyloid 2010;17(2): 63–8.

21. Suhr OB, Lundgren E, Westermark P. One mutation, two distinct disease variants: unravelling the impact of transthyretin amyloid fibril composition. J Intern Med 2017;281(4):337–47.

22. Rapezzi C, Quarta CC, Riva L, et al. Transthyretin-related amyloidoses and the heart: a clinical overview. Nat Rev Cardiol 2010;7(7):398–408.

23. Quarta CC, Buxbaum JN, Shah AM, et al. The amyloidogenic V122I transthyretin variant in elderly black Americans. N Engl J Med 2015;372(1):21–9.

24. Jacobson DR, Pastore RD, Yaghoubian R, et al. Variant-sequence transthyretin (Isoleucine 122) in late-onset cardiac amyloidosis in black Americans. N Engl J Med 1997;336(7):466–73.

25. Bittencourt PL, Couto CA, Clemente C, et al. Phenotypic expression of familial amyloid polyneuropathy in Brazil. Eur J Neurol 2005;12(4):289–93.

26. Conceição I, De Carvalho M. Clinical variability in type I familial amyloid polyneuropathy (Val30Met): comparison between late- and early-onset cases in Portugal. Muscle Nerve 2007;35(1):116–8.

27. Planté-Bordeneuve V, Lalu T, Misrahi M, et al. Genotypic-phenotypic variations in a series of 65 patients with familial amyloid polyneuropathy. Neurology 1998;51(3):708–14.

28. Almeida MR, Hesse A, Steinmetz A, et al. Transthyretin Leu 68 in a form of cardiac amyloidosis. Basic Res Cardiol 1991;86(6):567–71.

29. Sattianayagam PT, Hahn AF, Whelan CJ, et al. Cardiac phenotype and clinical outcome of familial amyloid polyneuropathy associated with transthyretin alanine 60 variant. Eur Heart J 2012;33(9): 1120–7.

30. Ranløv I, Alves IL, Ranløv PJ, et al. A Danish kindred with familial amyloid cardiomyopathy revisited: identification of a mutant transthyretinmethionine111 variant in serum from patients and carriers. Am J Med 1992;93(1):3–8.

31. Reilly MM, Staunton H, Harding AE. Familial amyloid polyneuropathy (TTR ala 60) in north west Ireland: A clinical, genetic, and epidemiological study. J Neurol Neurosurg Psychiatry 1995;59(1): 45–9.

32. Damy T, Kristen AV, Suhr OB, et al. Transthyretin cardiac amyloidosis in continental Western Europe: an insight through the Transthyretin Amyloidosis Outcomes Survey (THAOS). Eur Heart J 2019; 40(21):1707–15.

33. Maurer MS, Elliott P, Comenzo R, et al. Addressing common questions encountered in the diagnosis and management of cardiac amyloidosis. Circulation 2017;135(14):1357–77.

34. Lousada I, Comenzo RL, Landau H, et al. Light chain amyloidosis: patient experience survey from the amyloidosis research consortium. Adv Ther 2015;32(10):920–8.

35. González-López E, Gagliardi C, Dominguez F, et al. Clinical characteristics of wild-type transthyretin cardiac amyloidosis: disproving myths. Eur Heart J 2017;38(24):1895–904.

36. Kittleson MM, Maurer MS, Ambardekar AV, et al. Cardiac amyloidosis: evolving diagnosis and management: a scientific statement from the American Heart Association. Circulation 2020;142(1):E7–22.

37. Siddiqi OK, Ruberg FL. Cardiac amyloidosis: an update on pathophysiology, diagnosis, and treatment. Trends Cardiovasc Med 2018;28(1):10–21.

38. Connors LH, Sam F, Skinner M, et al. Heart failure resulting from age-related cardiac amyloid disease associated with wild-type transthyretin: a prospective, observational cohort study. Circulation 2016; 133(3):282–90.

39. Pinney JH, Whelan CJ, Petrie A, et al. Senile systemic amyloidosis: clinical features at presentation and outcome. J Am Heart Assoc 2013;2(2). https://doi.org/10.1161/JAHA.113.000098.

40. Witteles RM, Bokhari S, Damy T, et al. Screening for transthyretin amyloid cardiomyopathy in everyday practice. JACC Hear Fail 2019;7(8):709–16.

41. Sperry BW, Reyes BA, Ikram A, et al. Tenosynovial and cardiac amyloidosis in patients undergoing carpal tunnel release. J Am Coll Cardiol 2018; 72(17):2040–50.

42. Fosbøl EL, Rørth R, Leicht BP, et al. Association of carpal tunnel syndrome with amyloidosis, heart failure, and adverse cardiovascular outcomes. J Am Coll Cardiol 2019;74(1):15–23.

43. Sekijima Y, Uchiyama S, Tojo K, et al. High prevalence of wild-type transthyretin deposition in patients with idiopathic carpal tunnel syndrome: a common cause of carpal tunnel syndrome in the elderly. Hum Pathol 2011;42(11):1785–91.

44. Yanagisawa A, Ueda M, Sueyoshi T, et al. Amyloid deposits derived from transthyretin in the ligamentum flavum as related to lumbar spinal canal stenosis. Mod Pathol 2015;28(2):201–7.

45. Westermark P, Westermark GT, Suhr OB, et al. Transthyretin-derived amyloidosis: Probably a common cause of lumbar spinal stenosis. Ups J Med Sci 2014;119(3):223–8.

46. Geller HI, Singh A, Alexander KM, et al. Association between ruptured distal biceps tendon and wild-type transthyretin cardiac amyloidosis. JAMA 2017;318(10):962–3.

47. Falk RH. Diagnosis and management of the cardiac amyloidoses. Circulation 2005;112(13): 2047–60.

48. Pollak A, Falk RH. Left ventricular systolic dysfunction precipitated by verapamil in cardiac amyloidosis. Chest 1993;104(2):618–20.

49. Grogan M, Scott CG, Kyle RA, et al. Natural history of wild-type transthyretin cardiac amyloidosis and risk stratification using a novel staging system. J Am Coll Cardiol 2016;68(10):1014–20.

50. Arvidsson S, Henein MY, Wikström G, et al. Right ventricular involvement in transthyretin amyloidosis. Amyloid 2018;25(3):160–6.

51. Longhi S, Lorenzini M, Gagliardi C, et al. Coexistence of degenerative aortic stenosis and wild-type transthyretin-related cardiac amyloidosis. JACC Cardiovasc Imaging 2016;9(3):325–7.

52. Galat A, Guellich A, Bodez D, et al. Aortic stenosis and transthyretin cardiac amyloidosis: the chicken or the egg? Eur Heart J 2016;37(47):3525–31.

53. Cavalcante JL, Rijal S, Abdelkarim I, et al. Cardiac amyloidosis is prevalent in older patients with aortic stenosis and carries worse prognosis. J Cardiovasc Magn Reson 2017;19(1):98.

54. Cyrille NB, Goldsmith J, Alvarez J, et al. Prevalence and prognostic significance of low QRS voltage among the three main types of cardiac amyloidosis. Am J Cardiol 2014;114(7):1089–93.

55. Quarta CC, Solomon SD, Uraizee I, et al. Left ventricular structure and function in transthyretin-related versus light-chain cardiac amyloidosis. Circulation 2014;129(18):1840–9.

56. Kristen AV, Perz JB, Schonland SO, et al. Non-invasive predictors of survival in cardiac amyloidosis. Eur J Heart Fail 2007;9(6–7):617–24.

57. Orini M, Graham AJ, Martinez-Naharro A, et al. Noninvasive mapping of the electrophysiological substrate in cardiac amyloidosis and its relationship to structural abnormalities. J Am Heart Assoc 2019;8(18):e012097.

58. Valentini F, Anselmi F, Metra M, et al. Diagnostic and prognostic value of low QRS voltages in cardiomyopathies: old but gold. Eur J Prev Cardiol. https://doi.org/10.1093/eurjpc/zwaa027.

59. Carroll JD, Gaasch WH, McAdam KPWJ. Amyloid cardiomyopathy: characterization by a distinctive voltage/mass relation. Am J Cardiol 1982;49(1): 9–13.

60. Sanchis K, Cariou E, Colombat M, et al. Atrial fibrillation and subtype of atrial fibrillation in cardiac amyloidosis: clinical and echocardiographic features, impact on mortality. Amyloid 2019;26(3): 128–38.

61. Feng DL, Edwards WD, Oh JK, et al. Intracardiac thrombosis and embolism in patients with cardiac amyloidosis. Circulation 2007;116(21):2420–6.

62. Longhi S, Quarta CC, Milandri A, et al. Atrial fibrillation in amyloidotic cardiomyopathy: prevalence, incidence, risk factors and prognostic role. Amyloid 2015;22(3):147–55.

63. Mints YY, Doros G, Berk JL, et al. Features of atrial fibrillation in wild-type transthyretin cardiac amyloidosis: a systematic review and clinical experience. ESC Hear Fail 2018;5(5):772–9.

64. Goldsmith YB, Liu J, Chou J, et al. Frequencies and types of arrhythmias in patients with systemic light-chain amyloidosis with cardiac involvement undergoing stem cell transplantation on telemetry monitoring. Am J Cardiol 2009;104(7):990–4.

65. Palladini G, Malamani G, Cò F, et al. Holter monitoring in AL amyloidosis: prognostic implications. Pacing Clin Electrophysiol 2001;24(8):1228–33.

66. Varr BC, Zarafshar S, Coakley T, et al. Implantable cardioverter-defibrillator placement in patients with cardiac amyloidosis. Hear Rhythm 2014;11(1): 158–62.

67. Boldrini M, Salinaro F, Mussinelli R, et al. Prevalence and prognostic value of conduction disturbances at the time of diagnosis of cardiac AL amyloidosis. Ann Noninvasive Electrocardiol 2013;18(4):327–35.

68. Barbhaiya CR, Kumar S, Baldinger SH, et al. Electrophysiologic assessment of conduction abnormalities and atrial arrhythmias associated with amyloid cardiomyopathy. Hear Rhythm 2016; 13(2):383–90.

69. Reisinger J, Dubrey SW, Lavalley M, et al. Electrophysiologic abnormalities in AL (primary) amyloidosis with cardiac involvement. J Am Coll Cardiol 1997;30(4):1046–51.

70. Phelan D, Collier P, Thavendiranathan P, et al. Relative apical sparing of longitudinal strain using two-dimensional speckle-tracking echocardiography is both sensitive and specific for the diagnosis of cardiac amyloidosis. Heart 2012;98(19):1442–8.

71. Ternacle J, Bodez D, Guellich A, et al. Causes and consequences of longitudinal LV dysfunction

assessed by 2D strain echocardiography in cardiac amyloidosis. JACC Cardiovasc Imaging 2016;9(2):126–38.

72. Klein AL, Hatle LK, Burstow DJ, et al. Comprehensive Doppler assessment of right ventricular diastolic function in cardiac amyloidosis. J Am Coll Cardiol 1990;15(1):99–108.

73. Klein AL, Hatle LK, Burstow DJ, et al. Doppler characterization of left ventricular diastolic function in cardiac amyloidosis. J Am Coll Cardiol 1989; 13(5):1017–26.

74. Falk RH, Quarta CC. Echocardiography in cardiac amyloidosis. Heart Fail Rev 2015;20(2):125–31.

75. Feng DL, Syed IS, Martinez M, et al. Intracardiac thrombosis and anticoagulation therapy in cardiac amyloidosis. Circulation 2009;119(18): 2490–7.

76. Liu D, Hu K, Niemann M, et al. Effect of combined systolic and diastolic functional parameter assessment for differentiation of cardiac amyloidosis from other causes of concentric left ventricular hypertrophy. Circ Cardiovasc Imaging 2013;6(6):1066–72.

77. Di Bella G, Minutoli F, Piaggi P, et al. Usefulness of combining electrocardiographic and echocardiographic findings and brain natriuretic peptide in early detection of cardiac amyloidosis in subjects with transthyretin gene mutation. Am J Cardiol 2015;116(7):1122–7.

78. Koyama J, Ikeda S, Ikeda U. Echocardiographic assessment of the cardiac amyloidoses. Circ J 2015;79(4):721–34.

79. Koyama J, Ray-Sequin PA, Falk RH. Longitudinal myocardial function assessed by tissue velocity, strain, and strain rate tissue doppler echocardiography in patients with AL (primary) cardiac amyloidosis. Circulation 2003;107(19):2446–52.

80. Pagourelias ED, Mirea O, Duchenne J, et al. Echo parameters for differential diagnosis in cardiac amyloidosis: a head-to-head comparison of deformation and nondeformation parameters. Circ Cardiovasc Imaging 2017;10(3). https://doi.org/10.1161/CIRCIMAGING.116.005588.

81. Vogelsberg H, Mahrholdt H, Deluigi CC, et al. Cardiovascular magnetic resonance in clinically suspected cardiac amyloidosis. noninvasive imaging compared to endomyocardial biopsy. J Am Coll Cardiol 2008;51(10):1022–30.

82. Karamitsos TD, Piechnik SK, Banypersad SM, et al. Noncontrast T1 mapping for the diagnosis of cardiac amyloidosis. JACC Cardiovasc Imaging 2013;6(4):488–97.

83. Maceira AM, Joshi J, Prasad SK, et al. Cardiovascular magnetic resonance in cardiac amyloidosis. Circulation 2005;111(2):186–93.

84. Martinez-Naharro A, Treibel TA, Abdel-Gadir A, et al. Magnetic resonance in transthyretin cardiac amyloidosis. J Am Coll Cardiol 2017;70(4):466–77.

85. Syed IS, Glockner JF, Feng DL, et al. Role of cardiac magnetic resonance imaging in the detection of cardiac amyloidosis. JACC Cardiovasc Imaging 2010;3(2):155–64.

86. Fontana M, Chung R, Hawkins PN, et al. Cardiovascular magnetic resonance for amyloidosis. Heart Fail Rev 2015;20(2):133–44.

87. Kellman P, Arai AE, McVeigh ER, et al. Phase-sensitive inversion recovery for detecting myocardial infarction using gadolinium-delayed hyperenhancement. Magn Reson Med 2002;47(2):372–83.

88. Martinez-Naharro A, Kotecha T, Norrington K, et al. Native T1 and extracellular volume in transthyretin amyloidosis. JACC Cardiovasc Imaging 2019; 12(5):810–9.

89. Fontana M, Banypersad SM, Treibel TA, et al. Native T1 mapping in transthyretin amyloidosis. JACC Cardiovasc Imaging 2014;7(2):157–65.

90. Dorbala S, Ando Y, Bokhari S, et al. ASNC/AHA/ASE/EANM/HFSA/ISA/SCMR/SNMMI expert consensus recommendations for multimodality imaging in cardiac amyloidosis: Part 1 of 2—evidence base and standardized methods of imaging. J Nucl Cardiol 2019;26(6):2065–123.

91. Damy T, Deux JF, Moutereau S, et al. Role of natriuretic peptide to predict cardiac abnormalities in patients with hereditary transthyretin amyloidosis. Amyloid 2013;20(4):212–20.

92. Perfetto F, Bergesio F, Grifoni E, et al. Different NT-proBNP circulating levels for different types of cardiac amyloidosis. J Cardiovasc Med 2016;17(11): 810–7.

93. Arvanitis M, Koch CM, Chan GG, et al. Identification of transthyretin cardiac amyloidosis using serum retinol-binding protein 4 and a clinical prediction model. JAMA Cardiol 2017;2(3):305–13.

94. Wizenberg TA, Muz J, Sohn YH, et al. Value of positive myocardial technetium-99m-pyrophosphate scintigraphy in the noninvasive diagnosis of cardiac amyloidosis. Am Heart J 1982;103(4 PART 1):468–73.

95. Falk RH, Lee VW, Rubinow A, et al. Sensitivity of technetium-99m-pyrophosphate scintigraphy in diagnosing cardiac amyloidosis. Am J Cardiol 1983;51(5):826–30.

96. Perugini E, Guidalotti PL, Salvi F, et al. Noninvasive etiologic diagnosis of cardiac amyloidosis using 99mTc-3,3-diphosphono-1,2-propanodicarboxylic acid scintigraphy. J Am Coll Cardiol 2005;46(6): 1076–84.

97. Rapezzi C, Quarta CC, Guidalotti PL, et al. Usefulness and limitations of 99mTc-3, 3-diphosphono-1, 2-propanodicarboxylic acid scintigraphy in the aetiological diagnosis of amyloidotic cardiomyopathy. Eur J Nucl Med Mol Imaging 2011;38(3):470–8.

98. Rapezzi C, Guidalotti P, Salvi F, et al. Usefulness of 99mTc-DPD scintigraphy in cardiac amyloidosis. J Am Coll Cardiol 2008;51(15):1509–10.

99. Glaudemans AWJM, Van Rheenen RWJ, Van Den Berg MP, et al. Bone scintigraphy with 99mtechnetium-hydroxymethylene diphosphonate allows early diagnosis of cardiac involvement in patients with transthyretin-derived systemic amyloidosis. Amyloid 2014;21(1):35–44.

100. Bokhari S, Castaño A, Pozniakoff T, et al. 99mTc-pyrophosphate scintigraphy for differentiating light-chain cardiac amyloidosis from the transthyretin-related familial and senile cardiac amyloidoses. Circ Cardiovasc Imaging 2013;6(2): 195–201.

101. Katzmann JA, Abraham RS, Dispenzieri A, et al. Diagnostic performance of quantitative κ and λ free light chain assays in clinical practice. Clin Chem 2005;51(5):878–81.

102. Dispenzieri A, Katzmann JA, Kyle RA, et al. Prevalence and risk of progression of light-chain monoclonal gammopathy of undetermined significance: a retrospective population-based cohort study. Lancet 2010;375(9727):1721–8.

103. Adams D, Suhr OB, Hund E, et al. First european consensus for diagnosis, management, and treatment of transthyretin familial amyloid polyneuropathy. Curr Opin Neurol 2016;29(Suppl 1):S14–26.

104. Quarta CC, Gonzalez-Lopez E, Gilbertson JA, et al. Diagnostic sensitivity of abdominal fat aspiration in cardiac amyloidosis. Eur Heart J 2017;38(24): 1905–8.

105. Buxbaum J, Jacobson DR, Tagoe C, et al. Transthyretin V122I in African Americans with congestive heart failure. J Am Coll Cardiol 2006;47(8):1724–5.

106. Conceição I, Damy T, Romero M, et al. Early diagnosis of ATTR amyloidosis through targeted follow-up of identified carriers of TTR gene mutations*. Amyloid 2019;26(1):3–9.

107. Ponikowski P, Voors AA, Anker SD, et al. 2016 ESC Guidelines for the diagnosis and treatment of acute and chronic heart failure. Eur Heart J 2016;37(27): 2129–200.

108. Maurer MS, Schwartz JH, Gundapaneni B, et al. Tafamidis treatment for patients with transthyretin amyloid cardiomyopathy. N Engl J Med 2018;379(11): 1007–16.

109. Emdin M, Aimo A, Rapezzi C, et al. Treatment of cardiac transthyretin amyloidosis: an update. Eur Heart J 2019;40(45):3699–706.

110. Rubinow A, Skinner M, Cohen AS. Digoxin sensitivity in amyloid cardiomyopathy. Circulation 1981; 63(6 I):1285–8.

111. Vaduganathan M, Mentz RJ, Greene SJ, et al. Combination decongestion therapy in hospitalized heart failure: loop diuretics, mineralocorticoid receptor antagonists and vasopressin antagonists. Expert Rev Cardiovasc Ther 2015;13(7):799–809.

112. Cheng RK, Levy WC, Vasbinder A, et al. Diuretic dose and NYHA functional class are independent predictors of mortality in patients with transthyretin cardiac amyloidosis. JACC CardioOncology 2020; 2(3):414–24.

113. Dubrey S, Pollak A, Skinner M, et al. Atrial thrombi occurring during sinus rhythm in cardiac amyloidosis: Evidence for atrial electromechanical dissociation. Heart 1995;74(5):541–4.

114. El-Am EA, Dispenzieri A, Melduni RM, et al. Direct current cardioversion of atrial arrhythmias in adults with cardiac amyloidosis. J Am Coll Cardiol 2019; 73(5):589–97.

115. Donnellan E, Elshazly MB, Vakamudi S, et al. No association between CHADS-VASc score and left atrial appendage thrombus in patients with transthyretin amyloidosis. JACC Clin Electrophysiol 2019;5(12):1473–4.

116. Hindricks G, Potpara T, Dagres N, et al. 2020 ESC Guidelines for the diagnosis and management of atrial fibrillation developed in collaboration with the European Association of Cardio-Thoracic Surgery (EACTS). Eur Heart J 2020. https://doi.org/ 10.1093/eurheartj/ehaa612.

117. Members AF, Brignole M, Auricchio A, et al. 2013 ESC Guidelines on cardiac pacing and cardiac resynchronization therapy: the task force on cardiac pacing and resynchronization therapy of the European Society of Cardiology (ESC). Developed in collaboration with the European Heart Rhythm Association. EP Eur 2013;15(8):1070–118.

118. Algalarrondo V, Dinanian S, Juin C, et al. Prophylactic pacemaker implantation in familial amyloid polyneuropathy. Hear Rhythm 2012;9(7):1069–75.

119. Donnellan E, Wazni OM, Saliba WI, et al. Cardiac devices in patients with transthyretin amyloidosis: Impact on functional class, left ventricular function, mitral regurgitation, and mortality. J Cardiovasc Electrophysiol 2019;30(11):2427–32.

120. Baumgartner H, Falk V, Bax JJ, et al. 2017 ESC/ EACTS Guidelines for the management of valvular heart disease. Eur Heart J 2017;38(36):2739–91.

121. Treibel TA, Fontana M, Gilbertson JA, et al. Occult transthyretin cardiac amyloid in severe calcific aortic stenosis. Circ Cardiovasc Imaging 2016; 9(8). https://doi.org/10.1161/CIRCIMAGING.116. 005066.

122. Fitzmaurice GJ, Wishart V, Graham ANJ. An unexpected mortality following cardiac surgery: a post-mortem diagnosis of cardiac amyloidosis. Gen Thorac Cardiovasc Surg 2013;61(7):417–21.

123. Sperry BW, Vranian MN, Hachamovitch R, et al. Are classic predictors of voltage valid in cardiac amyloidosis? A contemporary analysis of electrocardiographic findings. Int J Cardiol 2016;214: 477–81.

124. Moreno R, Dobarro D, López De Sá E, et al. Cause of complete atrioventricular block after percutaneous aortic valve implantation: Insights from a

necropsy study. Circulation 2009;120(5). https://doi.org/10.1161/CIRCULATIONAHA.109.849281.

125. Hammarström P, Schneider F, Kelly JW. Trans-suppression of misfolding in an amyloid disease. Science 2001;293(5539):2459–62.

126. Maurer MS, Grogan DR, Judge DP, et al. Tafamidis in transthyretin amyloid cardiomyopathy: effects on transthyretin stabilization and clinical outcomes. Circ Hear Fail 2015;8(3):519–26.

127. Zhang X, Goel V, Robbie GJ. Pharmacokinetics of patisiran, the first approved rna interference therapy in patients with hereditary transthyretin-mediated amyloidosis. J Clin Pharmacol 2019. https://doi.org/10.1002/jcph.1553.

128. Solomon SD, Adams D, Kristen A, et al. Effects of patisiran, an rna interference therapeutic, on cardiac parameters in patients with hereditary transthyretin-mediated amyloidosis: analysis of the APOLLO study. Circulation 2019;139(4):431–43.

129. Adams D, Gonzalez-Duarte A, O'Riordan WD, et al. Patisiran, an RNAi therapeutic, for hereditary transthyretin amyloidosis. N Engl J Med 2018;379(1):11–21.

130. Benson MD, Waddington-Cruz M, Berk JL, et al. Inotersen treatment for patients with hereditary transthyretin amyloidosis. N Engl J Med 2018;379(1):22–31.

131. Sekijima Y, Tojo K, Morita H, et al. Safety and efficacy of long-term diflunisal administration in hereditary transthyretin (ATTR) amyloidosis. Amyloid 2015;22(2):79–83.

132. Castaño A, Helmke S, Alvarez J, et al. Diflunisal for ATTR cardiac amyloidosis. Congest Hear Fail 2012;18(6):315–9.

133. Wixner J, Westermark P, Ihse E, et al. The Swedish open-label diflunisal trial (DFNS01) on hereditary transthyretin amyloidosis and the impact of amyloid fibril composition. Amyloid 2019;26(sup1):39–40.

134. Lohrmann G, Pipilas A, Mussinelli R, et al. Stabilization of cardiac function with diflunisal in transthyretin (ATTR) cardiac amyloidosis. J Card Fail 2020;26(9):753–9.

135. Ikram A, Donnelly JP, Sperry BW, et al. Diflunisal tolerability in transthyretin cardiac amyloidosis: a single center's experience. Amyloid 2018;25(3):197–202.

136. Holmgren G, Steen L, Suhr O, et al. Clinical improvement and amyloid regression after liver transplantation in hereditary transthyretin amyloidosis. Lancet 1993;341(8853):1113–6.

137. Ericzon BG, Wilczek HE, Larsson M, et al. Liver transplantation for hereditary transthyretin amyloidosis: after 20 years still the best therapeutic alternative? Transplantation 2015;99(9):1847–54.

138. Mehra MR, Canter CE, Hannan MM, et al. The 2016 International Society for Heart Lung Transplantation listing criteria for heart transplantation: a 10-year update. J Hear Lung Transpl 2016;35(1):1–23.

139. Liepnieks JJ, Zhang LQ, Benson MD. Progression of transthyretin amyloid neuropathy after liver transplantation. Neurology 2010;75(4):324–7.

140. Okamoto S, Zhao Y, Lindqvist P, et al. Development of cardiomyopathy after liver transplantation in Swedish hereditary transthyretin amyloidosis (ATTR) patients. Amyloid 2011;18(4):200–5.

141. Stangou AJ, Hawkins PN, Heaton ND, et al. Progressive cardiac amyloidosis following liver transplantation for familial amyloid polyneuropathy: implications for amyloid fibrillogenesis. Transplantation 1998;66(2):229–33.

142. Sack FU, Kristen A, Goldschmidt H, et al. Treatment options for severe cardiac amyloidosis: heart transplantation combined with chemotherapy and stem cell transplantation for patients with AL-amyloidosis and heart and liver transplantation for patients with ATTR-amyloidosis. Eur J Cardiothoracic Surg 2008;33(2):257–62.

Clinical and Molecular Aspects of Naxos Disease

Ioannis Protonotarios, MD[a], Angeliki Asimaki, BSc, PhD[b], Zafeirenia Xylouri, MD[a], Alexandros Protonotarios, MD[c], Adalena Tsatsopoulou, MD[d],*

KEYWORDS

- Naxos disease • Arrhythmogenic cardiomyopathy • Woolly hair • Palmoplantar keratoderma
- Plakoglobin • Desmosome • Myocarditis

KEY POINTS

- Naxos disease is an inherited pattern of arrhythmogenic cardiomyopathy with palmoplantar keratoderma and woolly hair.
- The early evident cutaneous features in Naxos disease may serve as a clinical screening tool to spot arrhythmogenic cardiomyopathy in the subclinical stage, in the context of an affected family.
- Episodes mimicking myocarditis may mark the transition from concealed to symptomatic phase of arrhythmogenic cardiomyopathy.
- The causative mutation, identified in the plakoglobin protein gene, indicated the potential role of the desmosomal protein complex as culprit for cardiomyopathy.

INTRODUCTION

Naxos disease (McKusick #601214) is an inherited disorder associating arrhythmogenic right ventricular cardiomyopathy (ARVC) with palmoplantar keratoderma (PPK), as well as peculiar dense, rough, and bristly, resembling steel wire, woolly hair (WH). It was first described in 1986 in patients originating from Naxos, a Greek island in the Aegean Sea, and was named after it by the doctors who made the first description.[1] The first gene responsible for ARVC was identified in Naxos disease in 2000,[2] indicating a potential role of the desmosomal protein complex as culprit for cardiomyopathy.[3] Soon after, mutations in desmosomal genes were identified to cause isolated cardiac and syndromic forms of ARVC[4] (**Table 1**).

This article focuses on the features of Naxos disease and its contribution to the studies of ARVC. Advances in the understanding of the phenotypic spectrum of the latter, particularly in relation to the involvement of the left ventricle (LV) have

led the research and clinical community to replace the descriptive term of ARVC with arrhythmogenic cardiomyopathy (AC), and this is how we are going to refer to it in this article.[5,6]

The description of Naxos disease marked the history of AC (**Fig. 1**), which had started by the clinical and anatomic observations of Giovanni Maria Lancisi at the end of 17th century[7] and was shaped as a clinical entity by Frank Marcus and Guy Fontaine in 1982,[8] whereas the seminal studies by Gaetano Thiene and colleagues, from Padua in 1988, included it in cardiomyopathies and among the causes of juvenile sudden death.[9]

EPIDEMIOLOGY

Following the first description in families originating from Naxos Island, other affected families have been identified in several Aegean islands[10] and the Greek mainland (anecdotal evidence by Dr Tsatsopoulou). The disease prevalence in certain regions of the Greek Aegean islands has

[a] University Hospital Southampton NHS Foundation Trust, Tremona Road, Southampton, Hampshire, SO16 6YD, UK; [b] Molecular & Clinical Sciences Research Institute, St'George's University Hospitals, Blackshaw Road, Tooting, London SW17 0QT, UK; [c] UCL Institute of Cardiovascular Science, 72 Huntley St, London WC1E 6DD, UK; [d] Paediatric Clinic, Hora Naxos 84300, Greece
* Corresponding author.
E-mail address: adalenatsatsop@gmail.com

Heart Failure Clin 18 (2022) 89–99
https://doi.org/10.1016/j.hfc.2021.07.010

Table 1
Desmosomal protein genes causing AC associated or not with PPK and WH

	Protein	Predominant Mode of Inheritance	Ventricular Involvement of AC			PPK	Woolly Hair	Frequency	Remarks
			RV Only	LV Only	Biventricular				
JUP	Plakoglobin	AD	✔		✔			0%–1%	
		AR	✔		✔	✔	✔		
DSP	Desmoplakin	AD		✔	✔	✔	✔	1%–13%	
				✔	✔				
		AR		✔	✔	✔	✔		
PKP2	Plakophilin	AD	✔		✔			20%–45%	Also AR
DSG2	Desmoglein	AD	✔	✔	✔			4%–15%	Also AR
DSC2	Desmocollin	AD	✔		✔	✔	✔	1%–7%	Also AR
			✔		✔				

Abbreviations: AC, arrhythmogenic cardiomyopathy; AD, autosomal dominant; AR, autosomal recessive; LV, left ventricular; PPK, palmoplantar keratoderma; RV, right ventricular.

been estimated to be as high as 1:1000.[11] The same mutation with identical cardiac and cutaneous phenotype has been reported in Turkey.[12] Clinical reports on associations of PPK, WH, and cardiomyopathy followed from several other areas of the world.[13,14] A report by Hamill and colleagues in 1988, on a fatal cardiomyopathy with severe ventricular arrhythmias, alopecia, and PPK in 3 unrelated young toddlers by the age of 18 months, marked the potentially aggressive cardiac phenotype when accompanied by such ectodermal abnormalities.[15,16]

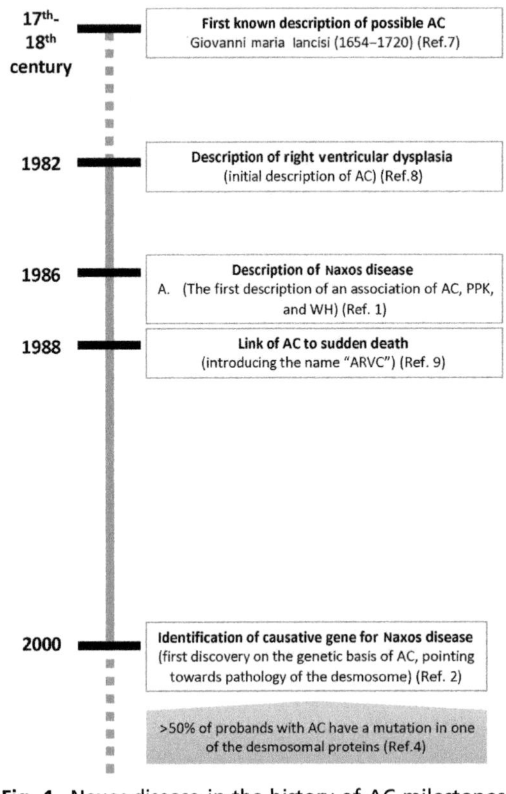

Mutations in *JUP* associating AC with WH or alopecia and PPK or skin fragility have been reported in Turkey, Argentina, and Canada.[17,18] In addition, case reports have related homozygous *JUP* mutations to lethal neonatal epidermolysis, complete absence of scalp hair, and onycholysis.[19,20]

A decade after the first description of Naxos disease in 1986, an association of identical cutaneous characteristics with a type of dilated cardiomyopathy presenting with early arrhythmias was described in families from Ecuador.[21] Subsequently, a mutation in the gene of desmoplakin (*DSP*) was identified as the causative genetic defect.[22] It was given the name of Carvajal syndrome.[23] In the initial description, there was an early presentation of electrocardiographic and echocardiographic phenotype by the age of 7 years. The predominant cardiac phenotype consisted of complex ventricular extrasystoles and episodes of nonsustained ventricular tachycardia with precordial T-wave inversion extending up to V5. Severe left ventricular involvement was present in more than 90% of patients by the second decade of life while 57% of patients developed heart failure and most of them died by adolescence. The phenotype of cardiomyopathy was reported as DCM by Carvajal. Nevertheless, in the first clinical comparison between Naxos ARVC and Carvajal syndrome, it was underscored that the increased arrhythmogenicity and electrocardiographic abnormalities in these patients

17th–18th century	**First known description of possible AC** Giovanni maria Iancisi (1654–1720) (Ref.7)
1982	**Description of right ventricular dysplasia** (initial description of AC) (Ref.8)
1986	**Description of Naxos disease** A. (The first description of an association of AC, PPK, and WH) (Ref. 1)
1988	**Link of AC to sudden death** (introducing the name "ARVC") (Ref. 9)
2000	**Identification of causative gene for Naxos disease** (first discovery on the genetic basis of AC, pointing towards pathology of the desmosome) (Ref. 2)
	>50% of probands with AC have a mutation in one of the desmosomal proteins (Ref.4)

Fig. 1. Naxos disease in the history of AC milestones.

were more consistent with biventricular ARVC than with DCM {*N. Protonotarios, A. Tsatsopoulou. Naxos disease and Carvajal syndrome: cardiocutaneous disorders that highlight the pathogenesis and broaden the spectrum of arrhythmogenic right ventricular cardiomyopathy. Cardiovascular Pathology 2004; 185–194*}.

In 2009, a similar disorder caused by a homozygous mutation in the DSC2 gene was reported.[24] In 2017, the phenotype of Naxos disease was described in 7 unrelated French-Canadian individuals sharing a novel founder *JUP* mutation.[25] In 2020, another unreported *JUP* biallelic mutation was identified in 2 unrelated young individuals from Iran.[26]

GENETIC ASPECTS

Identification of the disease locus in Naxos disease has achieved thanks to the autosomal recessive features of the phenotypic expression within families, where the easy-to-spot cutaneous signs were always accompanied by cardiomyopathy. So, the causative gene was located on chromosome 17q21.[27] Soon after, a 2-base pair (TG) deletion at the 3' end of the plakoglobin gene (*JUP*) was identified as the causative mutation. Specifically, this involves the deletion of nucleotides 2157 and 2158 (*JUP2157del2*), which causes a frameshift and premature termination of translation, altering 5 amino acid residues and truncating the C-terminal domain of the protein.[2]

A similar genotype-phenotype correlation has been reported in 2 adult relatives in a Turkish family who were diagnosed with AC that was associated with WH and alopecia. Molecular genetic investigation revealed homozygosity for a missense mutation in *JUP* (R265H).[28]

Other *JUP* mutations in homozygosity were identified to segregate with PPK, skin fragility, and WH in 3 unrelated Argentinian boys and a Kuwaiti sister and brother with skin fragility, PPK, and sparse WH. Cardiomyopathy was not confirmed at initial assessment as all described patients were in childhood and the authors proposed regular cardiac follow-up for possible detection of early features of AC.[18] In a later report, the eldest patient had developed cardiomyopathy at the age of 19 years.[29]

In an infant girl with generalized epidermolysis, alopecia, and onycholysis who died on day 12 of life because of sepsis and respiratory failure, a homozygous *JUP* nonsense mutation (Q539X) was identified, for which her unaffected first-cousin parents were heterozygous.[20] Complete lack of plakoglobin in her skin was revealed on immunostaining with antibodies to both N-terminal and C-terminal epitopes of plakoglobin and by immunoblotting of skin extracts using the antibody specific to the N-terminal domain of plakoglobin.[20] This resulted in extreme skin fragility and compromised skin barrier formation. The authors suggested that cardiac dysfunction typical of Naxos disease might have developed later in life.

Systematically reviewed up to 2016, mutations in JUP and DSP account for 90.8% of patients presenting with the combination of AC and PPK with hair shaft abnormalities.[30]

In 2017, a homozygous mutation in the exon 5 of the JUP gene (NM_002230.1): c.902A>G (p.Glu301Gly) was identified in a series of 7 unrelated French-Canadian individuals, aged from 12 to 77 years, who had been given the diagnosis of Naxos disease. Interestingly, the youngest patients (12 and 13 years) were ascertained through dermatology clinics because of the cutaneous features of WH and PPK, while the 4 oldest cases (34–77 years) were identified because of symptomatic AC.[25] One patient had cardiac transplantation at the age of 18 years. Four of the oldest patients who fulfilled the 2010 criteria for ARVC diagnosis were at increased arrhythmic risk, so they all received an implantable cardioverter-defibrillator (ICD).[31–33] T-wave inversion in leads V1-V3 was the only suspicious finding in the 13-year-old boy. Four of them also showed abnormal dentition, a feature not observed in the original series of Naxos disease. A cohort of 362 families with skin fragility was recently screened for genetic mutations with next-generation sequencing–based methods.[26] In 2 unrelated probands, 2.5 and 22 year olds, a previously unreported biallelic mutation, JUP: c.201delC; p.Ser68Alafs*92, was identified. The older patient had T-wave inversion in V1-V3, 80 ms prolonged terminal activation duration in V3, and right ventricular enlargement on echocardiogram, diagnosed with a definite ARVC. The younger patient had no evidence of cardiac disease but met possible ARVC diagnosis with one major criterion (the presence of the *JUP* mutation). They both had PPK skin, fragility, and alopecia, while there was a lack of plakoglobin in the epidermis on immunofluorescence studies.

CLINICAL ASPECTS

The families with Naxos disease and the originally described mutation *JUP2156del2* represent more than 90% of the reported individuals carrying a recessive *JUP* mutation.[30] The original series of patients homozygous for *JUP* mutation remains the largest one regularly followed up for up to 35 years.[34,35]

The Cutaneous Phenotype

The peculiar and extremely woolly, mostly dense hair becomes apparent from birth[34] (**Fig. 2**A). It is worth mentioning that observant members of affected families from *JUP* homozygous carriers have reported the hair phenotype in newborn members as a harbinger of severe heart disease. In some patients with *JUP* homozygous mutations (or biallelic), sparse WH or even alopecia has been reported. Alopecia has also been reported with *DSP* mutations.[20,36]

Keratotic lesions generally develop on palms, and soles later, during the first or second year of life, when the child starts to apply pressure on hands and feet and become diffuse later in life[34] (**Fig. 2**B, C). Eczematous lesions, fragile skin, or even erosions and ulcers have been observed on the perioral and sacral areas or dorsal surfaces of the hands and legs in early infancy that improve in later childhood. Diffuse hyperkeratotic palmoplantar plaques that develop later have a well-demarcated erythematous border.[27] In a few cases, less pronounced hyperkeratosis was also present over the flexor and extensor surfaces of the joints and the perianal and interglu-teal folds.[17] Eyebrows and eyelashes are usually curly and dense (see **Fig. 2**A); nevertheless, sparse or absent eyebrows have been occasionally described.[17,26]

The Cardiac Phenotype

The occurrence of cardiomyopathy, according to the revised 2010 diagnostic criteria for ARVC, shows 97% penetrance by adolescence.[31,37] Syncope and/or episodes of sustained ventricular tachycardia of left-bundle branch block configuration are the commonest mode of presentation.[38] One-third of patients become symptomatic before the age of 30 years. Occasionally, the heart disorder may present with sudden death.[11] The age of 13 years was the earliest that a patient with Naxos disease fulfilled the Task Force Criteria (TFC) (**Figs. 3, 4**A, B, **and 5**). However, frequent ventricular extrasystoles of right ventricular origin (>14.000/24 h) have been detected in an asymptomatic 5-year-old girl homozygous for *JUP* mutation, followed up because of the cutaneous phenotype of Naxos disease in the context of family screening. Depolarization changes on her resting 12-lead ECG followed soon, while there was not any functional nor structural abnormality detectable on transthoracic echocardiography.

A

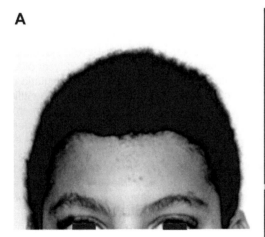

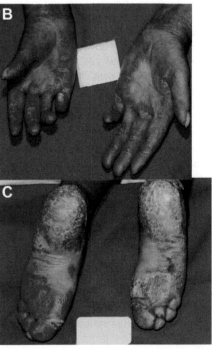

Fig. 2. The cutaneous features of Naxos disease. (*A*) Dense, rough, woolly hair, in a 13-year-old boy; his eyebrows are curly, and the eyelashes are long, dense, and curly. (*B, C*) Diffuse palmoplantar keratoderma in a middle-aged woman. They both had the full triad of AC, WH, and PPK.

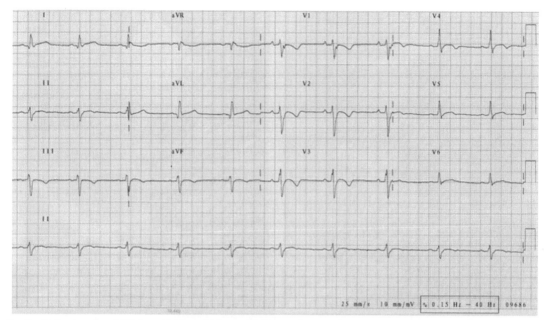

Fig. 3. 12-lead resting ECG, in a 13-year-old boy with Naxos disease, showing sinus rhythm with left QRS axis deviation and terminal activation duration (TAD) > 55 ms in V1-V3 (defined as the duration from the nadir of the S wave until the end of the QRS complex). In addition, T-wave inversion in II, III, aVF, and V1-V5 is noted.

After a noncardiac death at the age of 7 years, expert evaluation of the heart did not reveal any abnormality on gross pathology or regular histology. Abnormalities detected on ultrastructural electron microscopy and immunohistochemistry of myocardium are described in detail in a specific paragraph.[39]

Commonly, when patients develop symptoms, electrocardiographic and structural TFC are met.[38] The great majority of adult patients (92%) exhibit repolarization or depolarization abnormalities on the 12-lead resting electrocardiogram (ECG); T-wave inversion in V1-V3 or across the precordial leads being the most typical finding[34] (see **Fig. 3**). Epsilon waves have been documented in almost 38% of patients.[34] Structural or functional alterations of the right ventricle leading to the diagnosis of ARVC according to the established TFC have been documented on echocardiography or Cardiac Magnetic Resonance (CMR) in all adult patients[34] (**Fig. 4**). Left ventricular structural alterations, localized or diffuse, have also been detected in one-third of patients at presentation.[34] CMR proved to be the most reliable tool for early detection of right ventricular or left ventricular involvement, particularly in young asymptomatic patients with only minor ECG alterations.[40]

Natural History

In the Naxos disease series, 50% of patients become symptomatic from adolescence until the 35th year of life, mostly with syncope.[33] The cardiomyopathy generally progresses with deterioration of right ventricular function, development of new wall motion abnormalities, and emergence or worsening of left ventricular dysfunction. Structural changes have been suggested on 12-lead resting ECG by prolongation of the QRS complex and/or advancing of repolarization changes in contiguous precordial leads.[34] Heart failure symptoms are uncommon at presentation but may develop during time entailing heart transplantation in a minority of patients.[11]

The cardiomyopathy commonly follows a stepwise progression in "hot phases" in some patients, whereas in others, progression is more gradual without significant steps in phenotype deterioration. Each phase is associated with an arrhythmic storm followed by structural deterioration or sudden death.[11,38] Observations on adult patients and children with Naxos disease who presented with episodes of ventricular tachycardia or chest pain and troponin elevation, in the context of normal coronaries, suggest that these "hot steps" may mimic episodes of acute myocarditis.[41] In an adolescent with Naxos disease homozygous for *JUP* mutation, who was followed-up yearly since infancy because of the cutaneous features, it was possible to recognize the newly developed patchy late gadolinium enhancement changes on CMR after an episode of chest pain and cardiac enzyme elevation at the age of 14 years.[42] This

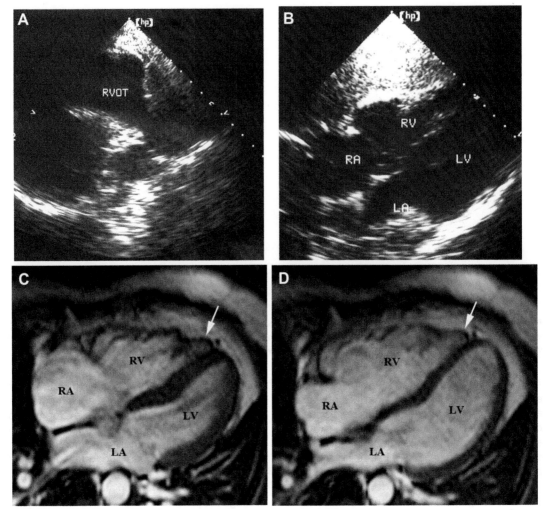

Fig. 4. Kinetic abnormalities of the RV on two-dimensional transthoracic echocardiography and CMR: bulging on RV outflow tract (*A*) and aneurysm of the RV posterior wall (*B*) in a 13-year-old boy with Naxos disease, already fulfilling the TFC for ARVC diagnosis. An aneurysm of the RV apex is revealed on CMR (*arrows*)(*C*: on systole and *D*: diastole) as well as dyskinesia of the RV posterior wall (*C*), in a 32-year-old man with Naxos disease.

episode marked a transition from the concealed to the symptomatic phase of AC, followed by the progression of repolarization changes across the precordial leads. Usually, the development of ventricular ectopics precedes the 12-lead ECG changes, which are followed by structural alterations on 2-dimensional echocardiography.[43] The phenomenon of acute "myocarditis-like" episodes has been increasingly recognized as a presenting mode of AC, mostly on *DSP* variant carriers,[44] and has been chiefly emphasized in children.[45] Myocarditis and cardiomyopathy, although traditionally considered as separate nosologically entities, they appear interconnected under the AC umbrella suggestive that "genetic and inflammatory pathways conspire to cause disease."[46]

In a study of an unselected Naxos disease population with an extensive follow-up, the annual disease-related and sudden death mortality were estimated at 3% and 2.3%, respectively. In patients with the most advanced structural disease that includes biventricular involvement and massive ventricular dilation, a decrease in arrhythmogenicity might be observed.[47]

Management and prevention

Sudden cardiac death (SCD) prevention, whose risk predominates in AC natural history, is the main goal in management strategies. The arrhythmic risk in patients with Naxos disease does not differ from that of dominant AC in PKP2

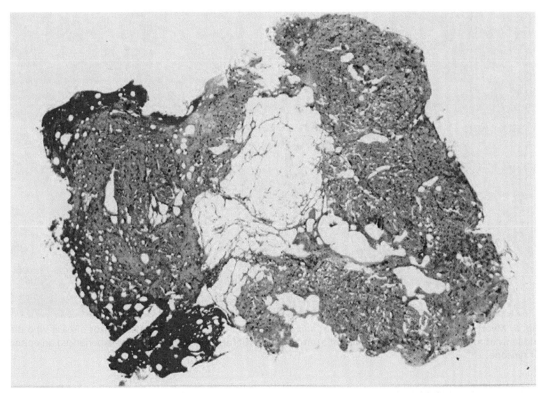

Fig. 5. Endomyocardial biopsy, showing myocyte loss with fibrous and fatty replacement, in an adolescent with Naxos disease.

heterozygotes, although *JUP* homozygous mutation carriers show increased disease penetrance and phenotypic expression as compared with dominant AC[33]; therefore, the same algorithms for SCD prevention are followed. Aborted SCD, sustained ventricular tachycardia, and severe dysfunction of RV and/or LV are absolute indications for ICD implantation.[32] The limited numbers of available cohorts may not allow for risk modeling specifically of Naxos disease patients; however, the similarity of the arrhythmic risk profiles to the other desmosomal gene variants carriers suggests that the generic approach to risk stratification in ARVC can be applied.[33]

In a recent study, even mild LV dysfunction increased arrhythmic risk.[33] This underscores the importance of CMR studies in the evaluation of ventricular structure and function in patients with Naxos disease.

Pharmacologic options include antiarrhythmic agents, β-blockers (class II or III), and heart failure drug therapy, aiming to prevent symptomatic ventricular arrhythmias and improve the quality of life. At end stages, when heart failure might develop, conventional treatment for congestive heart failure is used while heart transplantation might be considered.

To prevent the occurrence of new Naxos disease cases, a screening project of the abnormal gene for parents has been established in Naxos and the Aegean islands.

HISTOPATHOLOGY

Cardiac biopsies in patients with Naxos disease have revealed myocyte loss and fibrofatty replacement of the right ventricular myocardium (see **Fig. 5**). Inflammatory infiltrates have been observed particularly when the biopsy was performed at the time of clinical progression[11] (**Fig. 6**). On examination of a whole heart on postmortem, while the patient was expressing the clinical ARVC phenotype according to diagnostic TFC, the right ventricle showed extensive myocardial atrophy with fibrofatty replacement in the subepicardial and mediomural layers, regionally being transmural, with aneurismal formations (**Fig. 7**). Surviving myocytes in nests surrounded by fibrous tissue appeared as embedded within adiposis. The LV was variably involved, from regional replacement fibrosis[39] to extensive transmural myocardial atrophy and fibrofatty replacement, embedding a few surviving myocytes.[47]

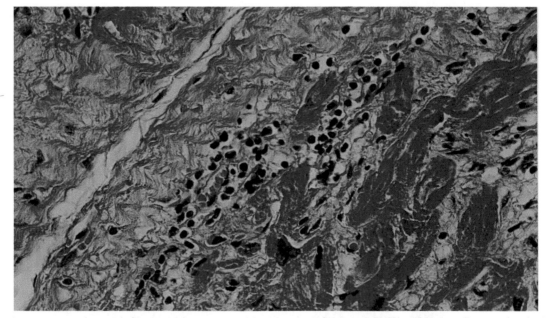

Fig. 6. Myocyte loss with fibrous replacement and lymphocyte infiltrates in a girl with Naxos disease who died suddenly at the age of 20 years, asymptomatic until 2 months before death when she had experienced an episode of syncope.

IMMUNOHISTOCHEMISTRY

Molecular histopathology and electron microscopy of the myocardium provided fundamental insights into the pathophysiology of AC. The study in 2004 on 4 homozygotes for *JUP* mutation with Naxos phenotype was the first to demonstrate that gap junctions are reduced and remodeled in ARVC, a phenomenon that might contribute to its pathogenesis and original presentation with severe ventricular arrhythmias. In 2 of the patients

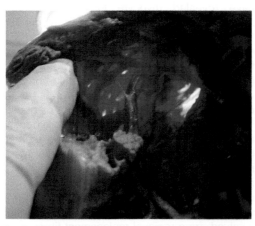

Fig. 7. Paper-thin RV wall, transilluminated, on postmortem. The boy died suddenly at the age of 23 years, after a failure to sense the implanted ICD (the lead is obvious) after an arrhythmic storm.

with advanced disease and in the third one, a 20-year-old girl who died suddenly, connexin-43 expression was significantly reduced in the intercalated disks. This phenomenon was noted not only in affected myocardial areas but also in other areas of both ventricles that otherwise showed no apparent histopathologic abnormalities. Mutant plakoglobin was expressed but failed to localize appropriately in intercalated disks. In addition, the aforementioned findings have been demonstrated in the cardiac tissue of the youngest patient (described in the cardiac phenotype paragraph), the girl who expressed ventricular arrhythmias and died of noncardiac cause at the age of 7 years, whose myocardium was completely normal on regular histopathology.[39]

Similar changes have also been found in buccal mucosa smears obtained from 6 patients with Naxos disease. Most myocardial samples from patients are formalin-fixed, paraffin-embedded tissues, which precludes studies in fresh tissue. Buccal epithelial cells can be easily and safely obtained, and as they express all key junctional proteins may act as a surrogate for the heart. Immunoreactive signal for plakoglobin was absent in all 6 homozygotes for the *JUP* mutation compared to 11 age-matched controls from the island of Naxos. The signal for connexin43 was severely depressed in 5 of 6 patients. Opportunities to characterize molecular pathology in myocardial samples from phenotype-negative gene carriers are limited.

Given the ease of sample preparation, buccal smears were obtained from 12 carriers of the *JUP* mutation. None of these subjects exhibited clinical features of ACM, although some of them had curly hair. Signal for plakoglobin was depressed in 10 of 12 carriers, whereas the signal for Cx43 was reduced in 11 of 12 carriers. The implications of these changes are unclear, but they suggest that redistribution of junctional proteins does not necessarily correlate with the clinical expression of disease. Nonetheless, they question the true recessive nature of the *JUP2157del2* mutation introducing the possibility of a gene dosage effect.[48]

Interestingly, in recent studies of skin molecular histology on electron microscopy, there was a widening of intracellular space and reduced number of desmosomes,[18] while immunofluorescence mapping revealed essentially absent plakoglobin staining.[26] Further studies on desmosomal function and disease mechanisms in the skin from AC patients may provide insights into AC pathogenesis and potential therapeutic strategies.[6]

MOLECULAR ASPECTS

Plakoglobin is a member of the armadillo protein family and a close homolog of β-catenin. It links cell surface cadherin molecules to the cytoskeleton and is the only junctional component found both in desmosomes and adherens junctions. Accordingly, it plays a vital role in maintaining cell-cell adhesion, especially in tissues subjected to increased mechanical stress, such as the heart and the epidermis. In addition to its mechanical role, however, it also has signaling properties. It interacts with components of the Wnt pathway and directly affects gene expression through binding to the LEF/TCF transcription factors.[49]

To gain insights into the molecular mechanisms underlying the pathogenesis of Naxos disease, HEK293 cells were stably transfected to express *JUP* bearing the *2157del2* mutation. Under subconfluent conditions, mutant cells (MUT) showed a greatly reduced degree of clustering compared with cells expressing wildtype *JUP* (WT). This was the first hint that *2157del2* alters cell-cell interactions. To determine the effect of the *JUP* mutation on cell-matrix adhesiveness and cell stiffness, magnetic micromanipulation was used. Briefly, confluent cells were incubated with magnetic beads coated with antibodies against integrin, a major matrix component. The rate of bead detachment was a surrogate for cell-matrix adhesion strength, while the distance of bead displacement in response to magnetic force mirrored cell stiffness. MUT cells were not significantly different from WT cells in either characteristic.

To determine whether the JUP mutation alters cell motility, a wound healing and a single-cell migration assay were used. Wound healing occurred more rapidly in MUT cells without an accompanying increase in cell division rates suggesting that the *JUP* mutation confers enhanced cell motility. To measure the force of cell-cell adhesion, a new method was developed (deform-drag). Briefly, a glass rod was dragged across a field of view, and sequential images were used to detect the smearing of a nuclear label across a field. WT cells were "dragged together," indicating that they were strongly connected to one another. In marked contrast, MUT cells exhibited complete separation immediately adjacent to the wound location, suggesting a dramatically reduced cell-cell adhesion. Finally, to determine the effect of the *JUP* mutation in cellular responses to mechanical perturbation, cells were grown on deformable silicone membranes and subjected to linear, pulsatile stretch. The amount of signal for plakoglobin, N-cadherin, and Cx43 at cell junctions was significantly increased following stretch in WT cells. In contrast, MUT cells showed significantly blunted responses to stretch. Collectively, these observations suggest that cell injury in Naxos disease may arise from loss of cell-cell adhesion and blunted responses to stress.[50]

SUMMARY

The early evident cutaneous features in Naxos disease served as a clinical screening tool to spot the always associated AC, that potentially has an obscure phenotype challenging its diagnosis. Thus, the initial presenting features of AC in children and young adolescents and follow-up of its natural history was made possible. The identification of a mutation in the desmosomal protein plakoglobin as the causative gene for Naxos disease unlocked the current era of desmosomal defects in myocardial disorders.

CLINICS CARE POINTS

- An association of palmoplantar keratoderma and woolly hair warrants a focused history on possible features of arrhythmogenic cardiomyopathy and a detailed family history about similar cutaneous abnormalities, arrhythmogenic cardiomyopathy, or sudden death.

- On documentation of an association of arrhythmogenic cardiomyopathy with palmoplantar keratoderma and woolly hair, a complete molecular genetic investigation for desmosomal genes is indicated.

- In the context of an affected family with Naxos disease, any child with palmoplantar keratoderma and woolly hair, even asymptomatic, should be offered regular cardiological evaluation for the detection of any developed signs of arrhythmogenic cardiomyopathy.

- Infantile wooly hair or alopecia, in association with palmoplantar keratoderma or bullous dermatosis and skin erosions, requires complete molecular genetic investigation for pathogenic mutations in desmosomal genes.

- In an individual with woolly hair and palmoplantar keratoderma, carrier of a pathogenic desmosomal mutation, any symptoms or signs of myocarditis require additional investigations toward arrhythmogenic cardiomyopathy.

DISCLOSURE

The authors have nothing to disclose.

REFERENCES

1. Protonotarios N, Tsatsopoulou A, Patsourakos P, et al. Cardiac abnormalities in familial palmoplantar keratosis. Br Heart J 1986;56(4):321–6.

2. McKoy G, Protonotarios N, Crosby A, et al. Identification of a deletion in plakoglobin in arrhythmogenic right ventricular cardiomyopathy with palmoplantar keratoderma and woolly hair (Naxos disease). Lancet 2000;355(9221):2119–24.

3. Sen-Chowdhry S, McKenna WJ. When rare illuminates common: how cardiocutaneous syndromes transformed our perspective on arrhythmogenic cardiomyopathy. Cell Commun Adhes 2014;21(1):3–11.

4. Patel V, Asatryan B, Siripanthong B, et al. Molecular sciences state of the art review on genetics and precision medicine in arrhythmogenic cardiomyopathy 2020;21(18):6615. Available at. www.mdpi.com/journal/ijms.

5. Protonotarios A, Elliott PM. Arrhythmogenic cardiomyopathies (ACs): diagnosis, risk stratification and management. Heart 2019;105(14):1117–28.

6. Elliott PM, Anastasakis A, Asimaki A, et al. Definition and treatment of arrhythmogenic cardiomyopathy: an updated expert panel report. Eur J Heart Fail 2019;21(8):955–64.

7. Marrone D, Zampieri F, Basso C, et al. History of the discovery of arrhythmogenic cardiomyopathy. Eur Heart J 2019;40(14):1100–4.

8. Marcus FI, Fontaine GH, Guiraudon G, et al. Right ventricular dysplasia: a report of 24 adult cases. Circulation 1982;65(2):384–98.

9. Thiene G, Nava A, Corrado D, et al. Right ventricular cardiomyopathy and sudden death in young people. N Engl J Med 1988;318(3):129–33.

10. Protonotarios N, Tsatsopoulou A. Naxos disease. Indian Pacing Electrophysiol J 2005;5(2):76–80.

11. Protonotarios N, Tsatsopoulou A. Naxos disease: cardiocutaneous syndrome due to cell adhesion defect. Orphanet J Rare Dis 2006;1:4.

12. Narin N, Akcakus M, Gunes T, et al. Arrhythmogenic right ventricular cardiomyopathy (Naxos disease): report of a Turkish boy. Pacing Clin Electrophysiol 2003 Dec;26(12):2326–9.

13. Protonotarios N, Tsatsopoulou A. Advances in genetics: Recessive forms. In: Arrhythmogenic RV Cardiomyopathy/Dysplasia: Recent Advances. Marcus F, Nava A, Thiene G. 2007;15–20. Springer, ISBN 978-88-470-0490-0.

14. Li GL, Saguner AM, Fontaine GH. Naxos disease: from the origin to today. Orphanet J Rare Dis 2018; 13(1):74.

15. Protonotarios N, Tsatsopoulou A, Scampardonis G. Arrhythmogenic cardiomyopathy with ectodermal dysplasia. Am Heart J 1988;116:1651–2.

16. Hammill WW, Fyfe DA, Gillette PC, et al. Cardiomyopathy with arrhythmias and ectodermal dysplasia: a previously unreported association. Am Heart J 1988;115(2):373–7.

17. Winik BC, Asial RA, McGrath JA, et al. Acantholytic ectodermal dysplasia: Clinicopathological study of a new desmosomal disorder. Br J Dermatol 2009; 160(4):868–74.

18. Cabral RM, Liu L, Hogan C, et al. Homozygous mutations in the 5 0 region of the JUP gene result in cutaneous disease but normal heart development in children. J Invest Dermatol 2010;130: 1543–50.

19. Rotemberg V, Garzon M, Lauren C, et al. A novel mutation in junctional plakoglobin causing lethal congenital epidermolysis bullosa. J Pediatr 2017; 191:266–9.e1.

20. Pigors M, Kiritsi D, Krü Mpelmann S, et al. Lack of plakoglobin leads to lethal congenital epidermolysis bullosa: a novel clinico-genetic entity 2011;20(9): 1811–9. Available at: https://academic.oup.com/hmg/article/20/9/1811/882927.

21. Carvajal-Huerta L. Epidermolytic palmoplantar keratoderma with woolly hair and dilated cardiomyopathy. J Am Acad Dermatol 1998;39(3):418–21.

22. Norgett EE, Hatsell SJ, Carvajal-Huerta L, et al. Recessive mutation in desmoplakin disrupts desmoplakin-intermediate filament interactions and causes dilated cardiomyopathy, woolly hair and keratoderma. Hum Mol Genet 2000;9(18): 2761–6.

23. Kaplan SR, Gard JJ, Carvajal-Huerta L, et al. Structural and molecular pathology of the heart in Carvajal syndrome. Cardiovasc Pathol 2004;13(1):26–32.

24. Simpson MA, Mansour S, Ahnood D, et al. Homozygous mutation of desmocollin-2 in arrhythmogenic right ventricular cardiomyopathy with mild palmoplantar keratoderma and woolly hair. Cardiology 2009;113(1):28–34.

25. Marino TC, Maranda B, Leblanc J, et al. Novel founder mutation in French-Canadian families with Naxos disease. Clin Genet 2017;92(4):451–3.

26. Vahidnezhad H, Youssefian L, Faghankhani M, et al. Arrhythmogenic right ventricular cardiomyopathy in patients with biallelic JUP-associated skin fragility. 2020. Available at: https://doi.org/10.1038/s41598-020-78344-9.

27. Coonar AS, Protonotarios N, Tsatsopoulou A, et al. Gene for arrhythmogenic right ventricular cardiomyopathy with diffuse nonepidermolytic palmoplantar keratoderma and woolly hair (Naxos disease) maps to 17q21. Circulation 1998;97(20):2049–58.

28. Erken H, Yariz KO, Duman D, et al. Cardiomyopathy with alopecia and palmoplantar keratoderma (CAPK) is caused by a JUP mutation. Br J Dermatol 2011;165(4):917–21.

29. Boente M del C, Nanda A, Baselaga PA, et al. Cardiomyopathy diagnosed in the eldest child harbouring p.S24X mutation in *JUP*. Br J Dermatol 2016; 175(3):644–6.

30. Polivka L, Bodemer C, Hadj-Rabia S. Combination of palmoplantar keratoderma and hair shaft anomalies, the warning signal of severe arrhythmogenic cardiomyopathy: a systematic review on genetic desmosomal diseases. J Med Genet 2016;53:289–95.

31. Marcus FI, McKenna WJ, Sherrill D, et al. Diagnosis of arrhythmogenic right ventricular cardiomyopathy/dysplasia. Eur Heart J 2010;31(7):806–14.

32. Corrado D, Wichter T, Link MS, et al. Treatment of arrhythmogenic right ventricular cardiomyopathy/dysplasia: an international task force consensus statement. Eur Heart J 2015;36(46):3227–37.

33. Protonotarios A, Anastasakis A, Panagiotakos DB, et al. Arrhythmic risk assessment in genotyped families with arrhythmogenic right ventricular cardiomyopathy. Europace 2016 Apr;18(4):610–6.

34. Protonotarios N, Tsatsopoulou A, Anastasakis A, et al. Genotype-phenotype assessment in autosomal recessive arrhythmogenic right ventricular cardiomyopathy (Naxos Disease) caused by a deletion in plakoglobin. J Am Coll Cardiol 2001;38(5):1477–84.

35. Antoniades L, Tsatsopoulou A, Anastasakis A, et al. Arrhythmogenic right ventricular cardiomyopathy caused by deletions in plakophilin-2 and plakoglobin (Naxos disease) in families from Greece and Cyprus: genotype-phenotype relations, diagnostic features and prognosis. Eur Heart J 2006;27(18):2208–16.

36. Erolu E, Akalın F, Saylan Çevik B, et al. Arrhythmogenic right ventricular dysplasia, cutaneous manifestations and desmoplakin mutation: carvajal syndrome. Pediatr Int 2018;60(10):987–9.

37. Protonotarios N, Anastasakis A, Antoniades L, et al. Arrhythmogenic right ventricular cardiomyopathy/dysplasia on the basis of the revised diagnostic criteria in affected families with desmosomal mutations. Eur Heart J 2011;32(9).

38. Protonotarios NI, Tsatsopoulou AA, Gatzoulis KA. Arrhythmogenic right ventricular cardiomyopathy caused by a deletion in plakoglobin (Naxos disease). Card Electrophysiol Rev 2002;6(1–2):72–80.

39. Kaplan SR, Gard JJ, Protonotarios N, et al. Remodeling of myocyte gap junctions in arrhythmogenic right ventricular cardiomyopathy due to a deletion in plakoglobin (Naxos disease). Hear Rhythm 2004;1(1):3–11.

40. Mavrogeni S, Bratis K, Protonotarios N, et al. Cardiac magnetic resonance can early assess the presence and severity of heart involvement in Naxos disease. Int J Cardiol 2012;154(1):e14–5.

41. Lazaros G, Anastasakis A, Tsiachris D, et al. Naxos disease presenting with ventricular tachycardia and troponin elevation. Heart Vessels 2009;24(1):63–5.

42. Mavrogeni S, Protonotarios N, Tsatsopoulou A, et al. Naxos disease evolution mimicking acute myocarditis: the role of cardiovascular magnetic resonance imaging. Int J Cardiol 2013;166(1).

43. Patrianakos AP, Protonotarios N, Nyktari E, et al. Arrhythmogenic right ventricular cardiomyopathy/dysplasia and troponin release. Myocarditis or the "hot phase" of the disease? Int J Cardiol 2012 May 31;157(2):e26–8.

44. Reichl K, Kreykes SE, Martin CM, et al. Desmoplakin variant-associated arrhythmogenic cardiomyopathy presenting as acute myocarditis circulation: genomic and precision medicine. Circ Genom Precis Med 2018;11:2373.

45. Martins D, Ovaert C, Khraiche D, et al. Myocardial inflammation detected by cardiac MRI in Arrhythmogenic right ventricular cardiomyopathy: a paediatric case series. Int J Cardiol 2018;271:81–6.

46. Protonotarios A, Elliott PM. Arrhythmogenic right ventricular cardiomyopathy as a hidden cause of paediatric myocarditis presentation. Int J Cardiol 2018;271:113–4.

47. Basso C, Tsatsopoulou A, Thiene G, et al. "Petrified" right ventricle in long-standing naxos arrhythmogenic right ventricular cardiomyopathy. Circulation 2001;104(23):E132–3.

48. Asimaki A, Protonotarios A, James CA, et al. Characterizing the molecular pathology of arrhythmogenic cardiomyopathy in patient buccal mucosa cells. Circ Arrhythmia Electrophysiol 2016;9(2):e003688.

49. Swope D, Li J, Radice GL. Beyond cell adhesion: the role of armadillo proteins in the heart. Cell Signal 2013;25(1):93–100.

50. Huang H, Asimaki A, Lo D, et al. Disparate effects of different mutations in plakoglobin on cell mechanical behavior. Cell Motil Cytoskeleton 2008;65(12):964–78.

The Arrhythmic Phenotype in Cardiomyopathy

Marco Merlo, MD[a],[*],[1], Giulia Grilli, MD[a],[1], Chiara Cappelletto, MD[a], Marco Masé, MD[a], Aldostefano Porcari, MD[a], Matteo Dal Ferro, MD[a], Marta Gigli, MD[a], Davide Stolfo, MD[a], Massimo Zecchin, MD[a], Antonio De Luca, MD[a], Luisa Mestroni, MD, FACC, FAHA, FESC[b], Gianfranco Sinagra, MD, FESC[a]

KEYWORDS

• Cardiomyopathies • Sudden cardiac death • Arrhythmic risk stratification

KEY POINTS

- Sudden cardiac death (SCD) and arrhythmia-related events represent a relevant issue in a patient diagnosed with cardiomyopathies.
- A lack of evidence leaves the cardiovascular community with a measure of uncertainty regarding the identification of the highest-risk patients.
- To date, an individualized multiparametric approach associated with a regular follow-up seems the best approach for arrhythmic risk stratification in those patients.

INTRODUCTION

Cardiomyopathies represent a heterogeneous group of disorders in which the heart muscle is structurally and functionally abnormal, in the absence of conditions such as coronary artery disease, hypertension, valvular or congenital heart diseases.[1] Young patients, without comorbidities and with a theoretic long-life expectancy, are usually affected, with the exception of syndromic forms of cardiomyopathies or cardiomyopathies associated with congenital heart diseases, that will not be addressed in this article, among which the rate of noncardiovascular mortality is higher. A genetic basis is frequent, with important clinical consequences on family members.[1] SCD and arrhythmia-related events have always been a matter of concern in these group of patients as they might be the first clinical presentation of the underlying disease and the most important competing risk to heart failure (HF)-related events. In particular, the burden of SCD diverges between different cardiomyopathies. Arrhythmogenic right ventricular cardiomyopathy (ARVC) is recognized as the leading cause, with an annual incidence of SCD of 1% to 1.5% and 30% of patients dying in the fourth decade of life. ARVC mortality rate for fatal arrhythmic events is straight followed by hypertrophic cardiomyopathy (HCM), with an incidence of SCD, implantable cardioverter-defibrillator (ICD) discharge, and resuscitated cardiac arrest estimated to be 1.02% per year, with most of the events occurring in adolescents and young adults. SCD burden is lighter in dilated cardiomyopathies (DCMs) and cardiac amyloidosis (CA) for which HF remains the leading cause of death.[2]

Despite fatal arrhythmic events have been significantly reduced over the last couple of decades as a result of evidence-based pharmacologic and nonpharmacologic therapeutic strategies, arrhythmic risk stratification in cardiomyopathies remains extremely challenging. Globally, we face a lack of definite guidelines because of the absence of clinical trials in this field, with

[a] Cardiovascular Department, Azienda Sanitaria Universitaria Giuliano Isontina (ASUGI), University of Trieste, Italy; [b] Cardiovascular Institute and Adult Medical Genetics Program, University of Colorado Anschutz Medical Campus, Aurora, CO, USA
[1] These authors equally contributed as first authors.
* Corresponding author. Via P. Valdoni 7, Trieste 34100, Italy.
E-mail address: marco.merlo79@gmail.com

Heart Failure Clin 18 (2022) 101–113
https://doi.org/10.1016/j.hfc.2021.07.011
1551-7136/22/© 2021 Elsevier Inc. All rights reserved.

heartfailure.theclinics.com

most of the evidence derived from retrospective data or expert opinions.

The aim of the present review is to describe the arrhythmic expression and to summarize all the current cornerstones of arrhythmic risk stratification in patients with different types of cardiomyopathies to provide practical suggestions in daily clinical management.

DILATED CARDIOMYOPATHY

DCM is a myocardial disease characterized by depressed left ventricular ejection fraction (ie, LVEF <50%),[3] generally (but not invariably) associated with dilatation of the left or both ventricles. Exclusion of secondary cause (ischemic, valvular, or other relevant loading conditions) is mandatory before considering the diagnosis of DCM. Tachyarrhythmias (typically atrial fibrillation), exposure to toxic agents (alcohol, chemotherapy), endocrine disease (ie, thyroid dysfunction, acromegaly), inflammatory involvement (postmyocarditis, sarcoidosis), and genetic causes should be deeply assessed in the work-up of DCM as they carry different prognostic features.[3,4] When no reasonable cause can be found, DCM is labeled as "idiopathic."

Natural history of DCM embraces a broad spectrum of clinical presentations, from asymptomatic or mild forms (ie, early stages of disease diagnosed during structured family screening programs) to more aggressive conditions (such as HF or life-threatening ventricular arrhythmias [VAs]). HF with reduced ejection fraction (HFrEF) is the most common clinical expression, sometimes leading to end-stage HF with necessity of advanced circulatory support (left/biventricular assistant devices) or even cardiac transplant, when indicated. DCM is frequently (up to 30% of cases) burdened by VAs as well, these being very challenging to predict during the course of the disease.[5] The annual incidence of SCD in DCM ranges between 1% and 4%, rarely representing the first manifestation of the disease.[6] If an ICD for secondary prevention after a life-threatening arrhythmic event is strongly recommended by current guidelines,[7] primary prevention of SCD in DCM has recently been questioned by clinical trials. In fact, the DANISH trial failed to identify a statistically significant impact of ICD implantation for the endpoints of overall mortality and cardiovascular death in a broad population of DCM patients, even though the mortality for arrhythmic events was basically halved in the ICD implanted subgroup (4.3% vs 8.2%; hazard ratio [HR], 0.50; $P = .005$).[8] Even though a subgroup analysis of the DANISH trial suggested that younger patients

(aged <59 years) might benefit more from ICD therapy compared with older ones, with a lower overall mortality (HR, 0.51; $P = .02$),[8] further studies are needed to confirm the finding. It appears indeed clear that a better selection of patients, not only driven by the well-known cut off of LVEF $\leq$ 35%, is paramount in the setting of SCD primary prevention in DCM.[9]

Some validated tools are helpful to estimate the proportional risk of SCD compared to the overall mortality in patients with left ventricular (LV) severe systolic dysfunction (ie, Seattle Proportional Risk Model),[9,10] even though no algorithm or score is available to directly calculate the risk of fatal arrhythmic events. To stratify the arrhythmic risk, some "red flags" might be systematically investigated in clinical practice.

Patients' clinical characteristics should be carefully evaluated. Compared to other forms of HFrEF, where comorbidities, NYHA class III-IV, and end-stage HF make the probability of nonarrhythmic death predominant, DCM usually affects younger patients with a lower comorbidity profile, for which SCD represents a more plausible cause of death.[11] Embracing these considerations, current guidelines do not recommend ICD implantation in patients with a life expectancy of less than 1 year and those in NYHA class IV.[7,12] Family history of SCD should be systematically obtained because DCM patients with a threatening background may be carriers of an arrhythmogenic genetic mutation.[13] A study from Stolfo and colleagues[14] showed that history of likely cardiogenic syncope, mostly if in the 6 months before the evaluation, was strongly associated with an arrhythmic outcome during the 12 months after the disease onset. Electrocardiographic (ECG) features might help in VA prediction: QRS characteristics (longer duration and fragmentation) have been linked to a more deranged heart (in terms of fibrotic burden) and hence to SCD.[15,16] Negative T waves might reflect the presence of particularly aggressive genetic mutations that are known to carry a high SCD risk (especially those shared with ARVC—ie, desmosomal mutations, Filamin/C, Lamin A/C)[17] (**Fig. 1**). Recently, together with LVEF and premature ventricular contractions (PVCs) count, the amount of negative T waves and the presence of low-voltage ECG were found to be strong predictors of VA in a population of phospholamban p.Arg14del carriers.[18] In general, the role of frequent PVC (generally with a cutoff >1000/24 h[5]) and nonsustained ventricular tachycardias (NSVTs) for SCD prediction in the DCM population is still unclear and data are contrasting. Some studies linked NSVT to SCD in patients with LVEF greater than 35%[19] and in a

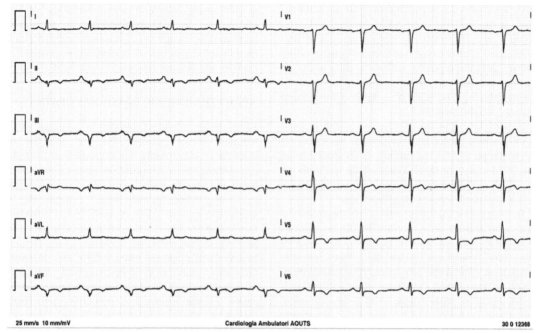

Fig. 1. ECG of a 43-year-old male patient with *FLNC* mutation showing low–voltage QRS complexes in peripheral leads and negative T waves in the inferolateral leads.

subgroup of genetically determined DCM carrying Lamin A/C, phospholamban, or FLNC mutations.[20,21] In this setting, Holter ECG monitoring can unveil an arrhythmic instability that might remain otherwise hidden. Echocardiography, nevertheless remains the cornerstone of SCD prediction in DCM because LVEF (with a cut-off of ≤ 35%) is still crucial in patient selection for ICD implantation in primary prevention, even if more advanced techniques (ie, global longitudinal strain [GLS]) have been proved to further improve arrhythmic risk stratification in DCM.[7,12,22]

In the last decades, cardiac magnetic resonance (CMR) has become the gold standard imaging technique for the assessment of cardiac volumes and LVEF. Furthermore, CMR can provide noninvasive tissue characterization: identification of fibrosis (reported to date in about 30% of DCM) through the late gadolinium enhancement (LGE) technique is strongly associated with hard clinical events, including VA and SCD.[23–25] In a recent study by Di Marco and colleagues, LGE emerged as a strong predictor of the arrhythmic endpoint (HRR, 9.7; P<.001) in a broad population of DCM patients. In the same study, patients with LVEF 21% to 35% but without LGE had a low risk of arrhythmic events (annual event rate 0.7%), suggesting that fibrosis might act as a substrate for VA, favoring reentrant circuits.[26] Similarly, Halliday and colleagues[23] showed that greater LGE

extent, subepicardial and multiple LGE distributions, as well as septal location seemed to confer the greatest risk for SCD. Similar results were obtained in the international DERIVATE registry, in which, together with male gender and LV end-diastolic volume, a >3 segments LGE extent was associated with arrhythmic cardiac events (HR, 1.693; 95% confidence interval, 1.084–2.644; P = .021).[27] The main weakness of LGE is the inability to detect "diffuse" fibrosis, which can be easily identified by targeted techniques such as T1 mapping and quantification of extracellular volume, whose high value is linked to a trend of worst arrhythmic outcomes.[24,28] Strain analysis can be performed on CMR images as well (tissue tracking). As for echocardiography, an impaired GLS can provide additional information for SCD risk stratification in this population.[29,30]

Not to forget genetic testing, which can be crucial in DCM clinical management, especially for what concerns SCD primary prevention. Some genetic mutations (namely pathogenic or likely pathogenic variants in *LMNA, FLNC, RBM20, SCN5A, PLN,* desmosomal genes) have been described as associated with higher arrhythmic burden.[31–34] In 2019, an expert consensus suggested to increase the LVEF cutoff (LVEF <45%) when considering primary prevention ICD implantation in presence of the aforementioned high-risk mutations (class recommendation

IIa).[32] Furthermore, the systematic genetic assessment shed light on a possible overlap between some forms of genetically determined DCM and ARVC, giving birth to a novel comprehensive entity named arrhythmogenic cardiomyopathy (AC),[32] a genetic disorder characterized by a high risk of life-threatening VA, SCD, and, later in the natural history, progressive HF.[35]

In summary, the low accuracy of the current "LVEF-centric" approach in patient selection for prophylactic ICD implantation is undeniable in the DCM scenario; this is particularly true in those forms of cardiomyopathies with a mild dilated LV and a prevalent arrhythmic phenotype.

To overcome this limitation, a multiparametric approach should be endorsed to obtain tailored arrhythmic risk estimation, pursuing the idea of precision medicine. Besides the already mentioned crucial role of genetic characterization, which is immutable over time, some other variables, such as patient age, ECG characteristics, arrhythmic burden, LVEF, and LGE extension may vary over time modifying the patient's individual risk. This highlights the importance of a personal scheduled follow-up with systematic reassessment of patient's risk (**Fig. 2**).

Finally, acute myocarditis (AM) deserves attention because it represents a relatively prevalent cause of DCM. AM is characterized by a polymorphic presentation ranging from asymptomatic or mildly symptomatic onset (ie, chest pain) to sudden cardiac death.[36] Prediction of disease course currently relies on clinical features, systolic function,[37,38] the presence of VAs and LGE at CMR at presentation and during the follow-up.[39,40] Among emerging prognostic tools, GLS appears the most promising, being able to identify subtle systolic dysfunction and providing incremental risk prediction in combination with the aforementioned parameters[41–43] (**Fig. 3**). AM patients with life-threatening arrhythmic presentation represent a challenging scenario where selection of best candidates to ICD implantation is particularly hard as the incidence of future major arrhythmic events in this population is largely unexplored.[44,45] Further studies are required in this field.

ARRHYTHMOGENIC CARDIOMYOPATHY

ARVC is an inherited myocardial disease with a frequent onset between the 3rd and the 5th decade of life, mostly in males (M:F = 3:1). It is characterized by progressive fibro-fatty replacement leading to ventricular dilation, disfunction, and wall motion abnormalities, underpinning the increased risk of SCD and HF.[32,46] Pathogenic mutations (mostly autosomal dominant) are identified in about 60% of patients, with frequent involvement of genes encoding for desmosomes. Of them, plakophilin 2 is the most commonly affected (up to 45% of cases), along with desmoplakin 2, desmoglein 2, desmocollin, and plakoglobin. In the classic form of ARVC, the right ventricle (RV) is predominantly involved. Nevertheless, biventricular involvement is increasingly observed, together with the less common isolated LV form of the disease (the so-called "left-dominant cardiomyopathy") that was recently linked to desmoplakin mutations.[32]

To embrace the whole spectrum of the disease, the multiparametric approach proposed by Marcus and colleagues[47] in 2010, focused on AC with a prevalent RV involvement, has been recently implemented by the Padua Criteria with the introduction of innovative elements (ie, tissue characterization on CMR and myocardial strain measured by echocardiography) for the identification of any form of AC.[48]

Despite ARVD is a rare myocardial disorder, with a prevalence of 1:5000 in the general population, it represents one of the main causes of SCD in young people and athletes. Fatal arrhythmic

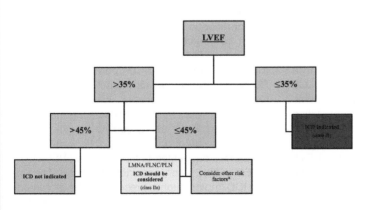

Fig. 2. Modified algorithm for DCM patient selection for ICD implantation based on current ESC guidelines[6] combined with the most recent evidence. [a]Desmosomal mutations, family history of SCD, ECG abnormalities, syncope, NSVT, LGE extension.

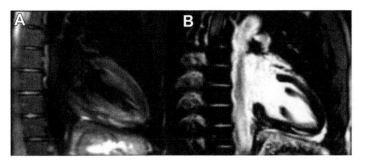

Fig. 3. Acute myocarditis with infarct-like presentation. (*A*) Extensive myocardial edema of the inferior wall; and (*B*) nonischemic LGE matching areas of edema. (*From* Porcari A, De Luca A, Grigoratos C, Biondi F, Faganello G, Vitrella G, Nucifora G, Aquaro GD, Merlo M, Sinagra G. Arrhythmic risk stratification by cardiac magnetic resonance tissue characterization: disclosing the arrhythmic substrate within the heart muscle. Heart Fail Rev. 2020 Jun 20.)

events can occur, in fact, even in asymptomatic patients with apparently normal heart, particularly during vigorous exercise.

Therefore, once the diagnosis is established, the most important goals become management of VAs and SCD prevention. Since sports is widely recognized as a trigger for arrhythmias and disease progression,[49] competitive activities are always contraindicated. Antiarrhythmic drugs (AAD) commonly administrated in AC are beta-blockers, sotalol, and amiodarone. All of them are recommended in patients with arrhythmia-related symptoms or frequent ICD interventions, with only beta-blockers to be considered irrespective of symptoms.[32,46,50]

ICD implantation is the only proven effective strategy to prevent SCD. Indication is well established in the setting of secondary prevention for patients with a history of aborted SCD, sustained VA, and in those with RV/LV severe dysfunction.[32,51] Conversely, patient selection for primary prevention remains controversial in patients with LVEF greater than 35%. Most evidence comes from retrospective studies including only patients fulfilling the 2010 Task Force Criteria.[47] According to available data, clinicians should consider at higher risk patients manifesting syncope, NSVT, or frequent PVCs (>1000/24 h). In addition, several series have identified the inducibility of sustained ventricular tachycardia at electrophysiology study and abnormal substrate with slow conduction at electroanatomic mapping with fragmented/split/late electrograms as markers of electric instability.[52,53]

Extensive tissue abnormalities on CMR are present in ARVC patients at higher risk of major arrhythmic events. In addition, Aquaro and colleagues[54] demonstrated that different CMR presentations are associated with different prognoses: in a well-characterized cohort of 140 ARVC patients, those with LV involvement had a worse prognosis in terms of VAs (**Fig. 4**).

Other clinical characteristics such as younger age, male sex, and proband status are also associated with increased arrhythmic risk in many series, even though they are considered as "minor" risk factors. Genotype has also a prognostic value in risk stratification, with carriers of multiple mutations in the same desmosomal gene or mutations in ≥2 genes related with ARVC at higher arrhythmic risk,[55] similarly to carriers of "highly arrhythmogenic mutations" such as Lamin A/C and Filamin C and TMEM43.[31,32,56,57]

According to the most recent Consensus of Experts, ICD implantation should be considered in patients with 3 major, 2 major and 2 minor or 1 major and 4 minor arrhythmic risk criteria[46] (**Fig. 5**).

Cadrin-Tourigny and colleagues[58] have recently proposed a predictive mathematical model to estimate the risk of major VA at 1, 2, and 5 years. Despite the innovative approach, the limited applicability of the score (only at the first evaluation and for the classic form of the disease fulfilling the 2010 Task Force Criteria[47]) makes it hardly useful in daily clinical practice. Furthermore, some important variables for arrhythmic risk assessment, such as tissue abnormalities on CMR, which must be periodically reassessed, or specific genetic mutations, are not included in the model.[59,60]

HYPERTROPHIC CARDIOMYOPATHY

HCM is the most common inherited myocardial disorder with a prevalence of 1:200 to 1:500 in the general population and is characterized by a left ventricular hypertrophy that is not explained by abnormal loading conditions.[1,61] HCM is frequently transmitted as an autosomal-dominant trait and is mostly related to sarcomeric genes mutation, with genes encoding beta-myosin heavy chain (MYH7) and myosin-binding protein C (MYBPC3) accounting for the majority of cases.[62]

Since 1958, when Donald Teare reported the first 8 cases of young people with asymmetrical cardiac hypertrophy who died suddenly, HCM has been a matter of concern for patients and clinicians worldwide, identified as a common cause

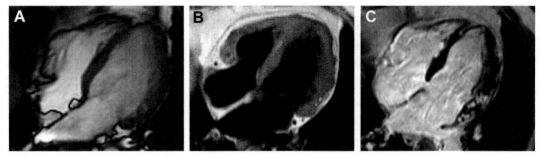

Fig. 4. Cardiac magnetic resonance imaging of AC with biventricular involvement, showing right ventricular free wall aneurysm, irregular epicardial profile of the left ventricle and extensive fibrofatty replacement. (*A*) Cine steady-state free precession imaging, 4-chamber view; areas of "India ink" artifact evident. (*B*) Proton density–weighted black blood imaging, bright areas of the septum and left ventricular wall are evident, consistent with fatty substitution. (*C*) Late gadolinium enhancement imaging, showing extensive fibrotic areas of both ventricles.

of SCD in the young, with no sex- or race-based differences.[63–65]

SCD events are generally related to ventricular sustained arrhythmias, favored by structural myocardial abnormalities, identified as myocyte derangement, microvascular dysfunction, and interstitial/replacement fibrosis, which can facilitate re-entrant circuits.[66]

Several attempts to prevent SCD by prophylactic administration of beta-blockers and AADs (ie, amiodarone or procainamide) failed to demonstrate any efficacy in changing the natural history of the disease.[67]

An effective therapy for treating fatal arrhythmias was unavailable until the introduction of prophylactically inserted ICDs in the 2000s, followed by a 10-fold reduction in overall HCM-related mortality, from 6% per year in the pre-ICD era to 0.5% per year currently.[68]

However, if on one hand ICD efficacy in aborting life-threatening VA is unquestionable, on the other hand, the rate of device-related complications (ie,

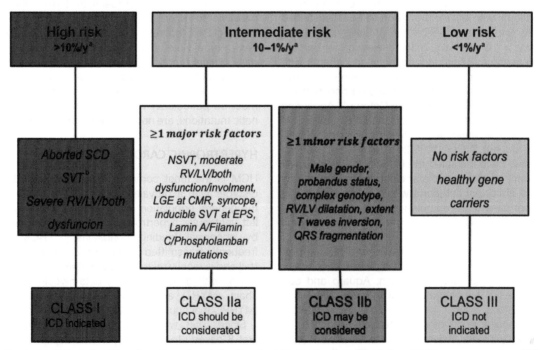

Fig. 5. Modified algorithm for AC patient selection for ICD implantation based on 2019 expert consensus[32,51] combined with the most recent evidence. EPS, electrophysiology study; SVT, sustained ventricular tachycardia. [a]Estimated risk of major ventricular arrhythmias/y; [b]Especially if hemodynamically not tolerated.

inappropriate shocks, infection, thrombosis) is not negligible, especially in consideration of the young age of HCM patients eligible for ICD implantation and the prolonged periods of device dormancy.[69–73]

In light of this, the need for accurate selection of patients for device therapy has arisen over time. Although actual American and European guidelines agree on the strong indication for ICDs implantation for secondary prevention, primary prevention strategies have slightly diverged between the 2 societies over years.[74,75]

The American approach is characterized by a good sensitivity to detect patients at risk, with more lives saved with ICD implantation at a cost of lower specificity overall. In the 2020 American College of Cardiology (ACC)/American Heart Association (AHA) guideline for the diagnosis and treatment of HCM, a class IIa recommendation (ICD reasonable) is made for those with any one of the following risk factors: family history of SCD, recent suspected arrhythmic syncope, maximal left ventricular wall thickness (LVWT) ≥30 mm, LV apical aneurysm, and LV systolic dysfunction (EF <50%). In selected patients in whom the decision to proceed with ICD implantation remains otherwise uncertain, the extension of LGE, assessed by CMR, or the detection of NSVT on ambulatory monitoring may be considered to guide clinicians in the decision making.[74]

In contrast, the European Society of Cardiology (ESC) recommendations are less sensitive but more specific with the results of fewer unnecessary ICD implantations.[63,76,77]

The ESC 2014 guideline recommends a mathematical model for risk stratification of SCD at 5 years, based on a logistic regression formula that comprises 7 continuous or binary variables: age, family history of SCD, maximum LVWT, NSVT, syncope, left atrial diameter, and LV outflow gradient. ICD implantation should be considered (class IIa) in patients with an estimated 5-year risk of ≥ 6% and a life expectancy of more than 1 year, ICD may be considered (IIb) in patients with a risk of between ≥ 4% and less than 6%, and it is not recommended with an estimated risk less than 4%.[75] A pitfall of the ESC algorithm, besides the unproven accuracy for some subgroups of patient (ie, children, elite athletes, and HCM phenocopies) is the exclusion of emerging CMR markers as LGE and apical aneurysm.

In clinical practice, indeed, the use of 15% of LGE as a cut-off to identify patients with the highest arrhythmic risk is already consolidated, while, more recently, an LGE extension greater than 10% of the myocardial mass was shown to be associated with the highest rate of events in patients with a low-intermediate 5-year risk[78,79] (**Fig. 6**).

Despite multicenter registries and studies suggest a more severe clinical phenotype in HCM families carrying multiple gene mutations and a more than 2-fold increased risk for VA and SCD in patients with at least 1 pathogenic or likely pathogenic sarcomeric mutation,[80,81] a prognostic utility of a specific mutation in isolation has not been demonstrated so far.

The genetic profile can also play a major role in identifying nonsarcomeric causes of HCM such as Fabry disease, amyloidosis, or Danon disease, which are characterized by an increased intrinsic risk of threatening VA.[82]

Risk assessment of SCD is critical in children, whose 5-year cumulative proportion of events from diagnosis is presumed to be in the range of 8% to 10%.[83] In this population, risk prediction models have been developed but have not yet been used widely in clinical practice.[83,84] Therefore, at present, a general agreement suggests that ICD therapy for primary prevention in children can be guided by conventional risk markers, where severe LV hypertrophy, unexplained syncope, NSVT, and family history of SCD represent major risk factors, while apical aneurysms, end-stage progression, and diffuse LGE usually develop over extended periods.[85] According to the American and ESC guidelines, implantation of an ICD should be considered in children who have respectively ≥ 1 and ≥ 2 major risk factors, despite the decision must always be based on individual judgment, taking into account strength of the risk factors identified, and the potential complications related to device implants.[74,75]

Few data, instead, support a role for prophylactic ICD implantation in patients after surgical myectomy or alcohol septal ablation, where the residual scar/infarct raises concern on potentially threatening arrhythmias. In this case, the decision should be made on a case-by-case basis.[86,87]

Finally, not to forget as a general recommendation for SCD prevention, the crucial role of a regular follow-up (recommended every 1–2 years) with a systematic risk reassessment.[74,75]

CARDIAC AMYLOIDOSIS

CA is an emerging cause of HF and mortality, mostly resulting from progressive deposition of free light chains (AAL) or transthyretin (ATTR) precursors.[88,89] Cardiac death is among the predominant causes of exitus in these patients, frequently due to end-stage refractory HF.[90] NSVT has been reported in almost 30% of CA patients during routine monitoring and in 75% of those with implanted devices.[91,92]

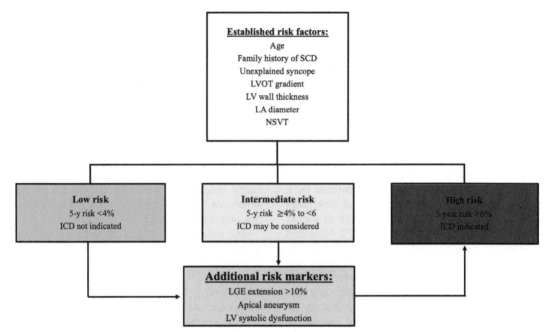

Fig. 6. Modified algorithm for HCM patient selection for ICD implantation based on current ESC guidelines[74] combined with the most recent evidence. LA, left atrial; LVOT, left ventricular outflow tract.

Although the latest studies suggested an association with increased mortality, the prognostic implications of VA in CA are unknown. Recently, a history of NSVT has been proposed as a relevant finding for arrhythmic stratification and candidacy for ICD implantation.[92–94]

According to the latest European and American guidelines, there is insufficient evidence for formal recommendation regarding ICD implantation in primary prevention in patients with CA.[95,96] Although secondary prevention is a recognized indication for ICD implantation in patients with HF and has been translated also to AAL or hereditary ATTR-CA patients (Class IIa Level of Evidence C) with an estimated life expectancy beyond 1 year, the role of prophylactic ICD in CA remains controversial.[7,95–97] Actually, no study clearly demonstrated a survival benefit following ICD implantation for primary or secondary prevention in CA patients.[98,99] Traditionally, CA patients are considered to die predominantly from electro-mechanical dissociation not amenable to defibrillation and effective defibrillation might require delivery of high mean energy in CA.[94,99,100] Finally, preventing SCD might not significantly change the natural history of advanced CA. Recently, Varr and colleagues[92] from the Stanford Amyloid Center proposed an algorithm to orient decision-making. Patients eligible for ICD implantation for primary prevention should be in nonadvanced stages of HF with an NYHA<IV, a life expectancy of more than 1 year, and a history of exertional syncope or documentation of NSVT or VT. However, this algorithm should be tested and validated in dedicated studies giving the small size of the study population used for developing it.

Meanwhile, the selection of candidates for ICD implantation should include age, estimated life expectancy, CA stage based on validated scores, major comorbidities conferring increased risk of noncardiac death (ie, neoplasm), and conditions with recognized indications for SCD prevention (ie, ventricular fibrillation).[88] Noteworthy, ICD implantation for primary prevention might have a role in patients considered for heart transplant as "bridge" strategy or in those with previous myocardial infarction and severe systolic dysfunction.[97]

A critical reappraisal of the natural history of CA is ongoing in the current era characterized by higher diagnostic yields, deeper knowledge of phenotypes, and development of disease-modifying drugs with proven impact on survival, particularly in ATTR-CA.[88] Prognostic stratification of patients and identification of best candidates for initiation of specific treatments are under investigation.

SUMMARY

Over the last decades, cardiomyopathies have been transformed into a contemporary disease with management options that importantly alter clinical course. In this context, many efforts have been made to identify risk factors and improve the accuracy of patient selection for device therapy and prevention of SCD. Although the well-known mathematical models and stated criteria could provide a solid basis for arrhythmic risk stratification, at present patient risk assessment is moving in the direction of a periodic multiparametric evaluation on an individual basis, which cannot prescind from CMR and genetic information.

CLINICS CARE POINTS

- In patients with cardiomyopathies, an ICD for secondary prevention of SCD is always indicated, with the exception of arrhythmic events triggered by a potentially reversible underlying condition (ie, electrolyte imbalance, coronary artery disease, acute myocarditis).

- An LVEF ≤ 35%, associated with a life-expectancy of more than 1 year, represents so far, the main indication for prophylactic ICD implantation in any type of cardiomyopathy.

- When LVEF is greater than 35%, the finding of pathogenic mutation of *LMNA/FLNC/PLN/* desmosomal genes can be crucial in DCM/AC patient selection for prophylactic ICD implantation. Genetic testing could also be pivotal in excluding nonsarcomeric causes of HCM at higher arrhythmic risk.

- LGE burden and location cannot be ignored for an accurate arrhythmic risk stratification in any type of cardiomyopathy.

- Multiparametric evaluation, including family and patient history, arrhythmic burden, ECG and cardiac morphology (beyond LVEF), and characterization must be specifically addressed to different cardiomyopathies and should be periodically reassessed for a fine-grained evaluation of the arrhythmic risk; in this perspective, a scheduled follow-up should be planned on an individual basis.

DISCLOSURE

The authors have nothing to disclose.

REFERENCES

1. Elliott P, Andersson B, Arbustini E, et al. Classification of the cardiomyopathies: a position European Society of Cardiology working group on myocardial and pericardial diseases. Eur Heart J 2008;29: 270–6.

2. Sen-Chowdhry S, McKenna WJ. Sudden death from genetic and acquired cardiomyopathies. Circulation 2012;125(12):1563–76.

3. Pinto YM, Elliott PM, Arbustini E, et al. Proposal for a revised definition of dilated cardiomyopathy, hypokinetic non-dilated cardiomyopathy, and its implications for clinical practice: a position statement of the ESC working group on myocardial and pericardial diseases. Eur Heart J 2016;37(23): 1850–8.

4. Merlo M, Cannatà A, Pio Loco C, et al. Contemporary survival trends and aetiological characterization in non-ischaemic dilated cardiomyopathy. Eur J Heart Fail 2020;22(7):1111–21.

5. Spezzacatene A, Sinagra G, Merlo M, et al. Familial Cardiomyopathy Registry. Arrhythmogenic phenotype in dilated cardiomyopathy: natural history and predictors of life-threatening arrhythmias. J Am Heart Assoc 2015;4(10):e002149.

6. Halliday BP, Cleland JGF, Goldberger JJ, et al. Personalizing risk stratification for sudden death in dilated cardiomyopathy. Circulation 2017; 136(2):215–31.

7. Ponikowski P, Voors AA, Anker SD, et al. 2016 ESC guidelines for the diagnosis and treatment of acute and chronic heart failure: the task force for the diagnosis and treatment of acute and chronic heart failure of the European Society of Cardiology (ESC). Eur Heart J 2016;37(27):2129–200.

8. Køber L, Thune JJ, Nielsen JC, et al. Defibrillator implantation in patients with nonischemic systolic heart failure. N Engl J Med 2016;375:1221–30.

9. Kristensen SL, Levy WC, Shadman R, et al. Risk models for prediction of implantable cardioverter-defibrillator benefit: insights from the DANISH trial. JACC Hear Fail 2019;7(8):717–24.

10. Bilchick KC, Wang Y, Cheng A, et al. Seattle heart failure and proportional risk models predict benefit from implantable cardioverter-defibrillators. J Am Coll Cardiol 2017;69(21):2606–18.

11. Hammersley DJ, Halliday BP. Sudden cardiac death prediction in non-ischemic dilated cardiomyopathy: a multiparametric and dynamic approach. Curr Cardiol Rep 2020;22(9):85.

12. Yancy CW, Jessup M, Bozkurt B, et al. 2017 ACC/AHA/HFSA focused update of the 2013 ACCF/AHA guideline for the management of heart failure: a report of the American College of Cardiology/American Heart Association Task Force on Clinical Practice Guidelines and the Heart Failure Society of Amer. Circulation 2017;136(6):e137–61.

13. Akhtar MM, Elliott PM. Risk stratification for sudden cardiac death in non-ischaemic dilated cardiomyopathy. Curr Cardiol Rep 2019;21(12):155.

14. Stolfo D, Ceschia N, Zecchin M, et al. Arrhythmic risk stratification in patients with idiopathic dilated cardiomyopathy. Am J Cardiol 2018;121(12): 1601–9.

15. Marume K, Noguchi T, Tateishi E, et al. Mortality and sudden cardiac death risk stratification using the noninvasive combination of wide QRS duration and late gadolinium enhancement in idiopathic dilated cardiomyopathy. Circ Arrhythmia Electrophysiol 2018;11(4):e006233.

16. Sha J, Zhang S, Tang M, et al. Fragmented QRS is associated with all-cause mortality and ventricular arrhythmias in patient with idiopathic dilated cardiomyopathy. Ann Noninvasive Electrocardiol 2011;16(3):270–5.

17. Finocchiaro G, Papadakis M, Dhutia H, et al. Electrocardiographic differentiation between "benign T-wave inversion" and arrhythmogenic right ventricular cardiomyopathy. Europace 2019;21(2): 332–8.

18. Van Rijsingen IA, van der Zwaag PA, Groeneweg JA, et al. Outcome in phospholamban R14del carriers: results of a large multicentre cohort study. Circ Cardiovasc Genet 2014;7(4): 455–65.

19. Zecchin M, Di Lenarda A, Gregori D, et al. Are non-sustained ventricular tachycardias predictive of major arrhythmias in patients with dilated cardiomyopathy on optimal medical treatment? Pacing Clin Electrophysiol 2008;31(3):290–9.

20. Van Rijsingen IAW, Arbustini E, Elliott PM, et al. Risk factors for malignant ventricular arrhythmias in lamin A/C mutation carriers. J Am Coll Cardiol 2012;59(5):493–500.

21. Akhtar MM, Lorenzini M, Pavlou M, et al. Association of left ventricular systolic dysfunction among carriers of truncating variants in filamin C with frequent ventricular arrhythmia and end-stage heart failure. JAMA Cardiol 2021;6(8):891–901.

22. Chimura M, Onishi T, Tsukishiro Y, et al. Longitudinal strain combined with delayed-enhancement magnetic resonance improves risk stratification in patients with dilated cardiomyopathy. Heart 2016; 103(9):679–86.

23. Halliday BP, Baksi AJ, Gulati A, et al. Outcome in dilated cardiomyopathy related to the extent, location, and pattern of late gadolinium enhancement. JACC Cardiovasc Imaging 2019;12(8 Pt 2): 1645–55.

24. Alba AC, Gaztañaga J, Foroutan F, et al. Prognostic value of late gadolinium enhancement for the prediction of cardiovascular outcomes in dilated cardiomyopathy: an international, multi-institutional study of the MINICOR Group. Circ Cardiovasc Imaging 2020;13(4):e010105.

25. Bogun FM, Desjardins B, Good E, et al. Delayed-enhanced magnetic resonance imaging in nonischemic cardiomyopathy: utility for identifying the ventricular arrhythmia substrate. J Am Coll Cardiol 2009;53(13):1138–45.

26. Di Marco A, Brown PF, Bradley J, et al. Improved risk stratification for ventricular arrhythmias and sudden death in patients with nonischemic dilated cardiomyopathy. J Am Coll Cardiol 2021;77(23): 2890–905.

27. Guaricci AI, Masci PG, Muscogiuri G, et al. CarDiac magnEtic Resonance for prophylactic implantable-cardioVerter defibrillAtor ThErapy in Non-Ischaemic dilated CardioMyopathy: an international Registry. Europace 2021;23(7):1072–83.

28. Chen Z, Sohal M, Voigt T, et al. Myocardial tissue characterization by cardiac magnetic resonance imaging using T1 mapping predicts ventricular arrhythmia in ischemic and non-ischemic cardiomyopathy patients with implantable cardioverter-defibrillators. Hear Rhythm 2015;12(4):792–801.

29. Van der Bijl P, Delgado V, Bax JJ. Imaging for sudden cardiac death risk stratification: Current perspective and future directions. Prog Cardiovasc Dis 2019;62(3):205–11.

30. Buss SJ, Breuninger K, Lehrke S, et al. Assessment of myocardial deformation with Cardiac magnetic resonance strain imaging improves risk stratification in patients with dilated cardiomyopathy. Eur Heart J Cardiovasc Imaging 2015;16(3):307–15.

31. Gigli M, Merlo M, Graw SL, et al. Genetic risk of arrhythmic phenotypes in patients with dilated cardiomyopathy. J Am Coll Cardiol 2019;74(11): 1480–90.

32. Towbin JA, McKenna WJ, Abrams DJ, et al. 2019 HRS expert consensus statement on evaluation, risk stratification, and management of arrhythmogenic cardiomyopathy. Hear Rhythm 2019;16(11): e301–72.

33. Begay RL, Tharp CA, Martin A, et al. FLNC gene splice mutations cause dilated cardiomyopathy. JACC Basic Transl Sci 2016;1(5):344–59.

34. Smith ED, Lakdawala NK, Papoutsidakis N, et al. Desmoplakin cardiomyopathy, a fibrotic and inflammatory form of cardiomyopathy distinct from typical dilated or arrhythmogenic right ventricular cardiomyopathy. Circulation 2020;141(23): 1872–84.

35. Mestroni L, Sbaizero O. Arrhythmogenic cardiomyopathy: mechanotransduction going wrong. Circulation 2018;137(15):1611–3.

36. Sinagra G, Anzini M, Pereira NL, et al. Myocarditis in clinical practice. Mayo Clin Proc 2016;91: 1256–66.

37. Caforio AL, Pankuweit S, Arbustini E, et al. Current state of knowledge on aetiology, diagnosis, management, and therapy of myocarditis: a position statement of the European Society of Cardiology Working Group on Myocardial and Pericardial

Diseases. Eur Heart J 2013;34(33):2636–48, 2648a–2648d.

38. Anzini M, Merlo M, Sabbadini G, et al. Long-term evolution and prognostic stratification of biopsy-proven active myocarditis. Circulation 2013; 128(22):2384–94.

39. Porcari A, De Luca A, Grigoratos C, et al. Arrhythmic risk stratification by cardiac magnetic resonance tissue characterization: disclosing the arrhythmic substrate within the heart muscle. Heart Fail Rev 2020. https://doi.org/10.1007/s10741-020-09986-0.

40. Aquaro GD, Perfetti M, Camastra G, et al. Cardiac Magnetic Resonance Working Group of the Italian Society of Cardiology. Cardiac MR with late gadolinium enhancement in acute myocarditis with preserved systolic function: ITAMY Study. J Am Coll Cardiol 2017;70(16):1977–87.

41. Merlo M, Porcari A, Sinagra G. The (ultra) sound of a burning heart: a matter of speckles. Int J Cardiol 2018;259:132–3.

42. Porcari A, Merlo M, Crosera L, et al. Strain analysis reveals subtle systolic dysfunction in confirmed and suspected myocarditis with normal LVEF. A cardiac magnetic resonance study. Clin Res Cardiol 2020;109(7):869–80.

43. Fischer K, Obrist SJ, Erne SA, et al. Feature tracking myocardial strain incrementally improves prognostication in myocarditis beyond traditional CMR imaging features. JACC Cardiovasc Imaging 2020;13(9):1891–901.

44. Ammirati E, Veronese G, Brambatti M, et al. Fulminant versus acute nonfulminant myocarditis in patients with left ventricular systolic dysfunction. J Am Coll Cardiol 2019;74(3):299–311.

45. Ammirati E, Cipriani M, Moro C, et al. Registro Lombardo delle Miocarditi. Clinical presentation and outcome in a contemporary cohort of patients with acute myocarditis: multicenter lombardy registry. Circulation 2018;138(11):1088–99.

46. Corrado D, Link MS, Calkins H. Arrhythmogenic right ventricular cardiomyopathy. N Engl J Med 2017;376:1489–90.

47. Marcus FI, McKenna WJ, Sherrill D, et al. Diagnosis of arrhythmogenic right ventricular cardiomyopathy/dysplasia: proposed modification of the task force criteria. Circulation 2010;121:1533–41.

48. Corrado D, Perazzolo Marra M, Zorzi A, et al. Diagnosis of arrhythmogenic cardiomyopathy: the Padua criteria. Int J Cardiol 2020;319:106–14.

49. Finocchiaro G, Papadakis M, Robertus JL, et al. Etiology of sudden death in sports: insights from a United Kingdom regional registry. J Am Coll Cardiol 2016;67:2108–15.

50. Cappelletto C, Gregorio C, Barbati G, et al. Antiarrhythmic therapy and risk of cumulative ventricular arrhythmias in arrhythmogenic right ventricle cardiomyopathy. Int J Cardiol 2021;334:58–64.

51. Calkins H, Corrado D, Marcus F. Risk stratification in arrhythmogenic right ventricular cardiomyopathy. Circulation 2017;136(21):2068–82.

52. Saguner AM, Medeiros-Domingo A, Schwyzer MA, et al. Usefulness of inducible ventricular tachycardia to predict long-term adverse outcomes in arrhythmogenic right ventricular cardiomyopathy. Am J Cardiol 2013;111:250–7.

53. Chahal A, Reza N, Santangeli P. Risk stratification in ARVC/D without an ICD. JACC Clin Electrophysiol 2019.

54. Aquaro GD, De Luca A, Cappelletto C, et al. Prognostic value of magnetic resonance phenotype in patients whit arrhythmogenic right ventricular cardiomyopathy. J Am Coll Cardiol 2020;75(22): 2753–65.

55. Bhonsale A, Groeneweg JA, James CA, et al. Impact of genotype on clinical course in arrhythmogenic right ventricular dysplasia/cardiomyopathy-associated mutation carriers. Eur Heart J 2015; 36:847–55.

56. Merner ND, Hodgkinson KA, Haywood AF, et al. Arrhythmogenic right ventricular cardiomyopathy type 5 is a fully penetrant, lethal arrhythmic disorder caused by a missense mutation in the TMEM43 gene. Am J Hum Genet 2008;82: 809–21.

57. Sinagra G, Merlo M, Pinamonti B, editors. Dilated cardiomyopathy. From genetics to clinical management. Cham: Springer; 2019.

58. Cadrin-Tourigny J, Bosman LP, Nozza A, et al. A new prediction model for ventricular arrhythmias in arrhythmogenic right ventricular cardiomyopathy. Eur Heart J 2019;40:1850–8.

59. Pinamonti B, Dragos AM, Pyxaras SA, et al. Prognostic predictors in arrhythmogenic right ventricular cardiomyopathy: results from a 10-year registry. Eur Heart J 2011;32:1105–13.

60. Cappelletto C, Stolfo D, De Luca A, et al. Lifelong arrhythmic risk stratification in arrhythmogenic right ventricular cardiomyopathy: distribution of events and impact of periodical reassessment. Europace 2018;20:f20–9.

61. Semsarian C, Ingles J, Maron MS, et al. New perspectives on the prevalence of hypertrophic cardiomyopathy. J Am Coll Cardiol 2015;65:1249–54.

62. Lopes LR, Zekavati A, Syrris P, et al. Genetic complexity in hypertrophic cardiomyopathy revealed by high-throughputsequencing. J Med Genet 2013;50:228–39.

63. Maron MS, Rowin EJ, Wessler BS, et al. Enhanced American College of Cardiology/American Heart Association strategy for prevention of sudden cardiac death in high-risk patients with hypertrophic cardiomyopathy. JAMA Cardiol 2019;4:644–57.

64. Dimitrow PP, Chojnowska L, Rudzinski T, et al. Sudden death in hypertrophic cardiomyopathy: old risk

factors reassessed in a new model of maximalized follow-up. Eur Heart J 2010;31:3084–93.

65. Maron BJ, Spirito P, Shen W-K, et al. Implantable cardioverter-defibrillators and prevention of sudden cardiac death in hypertrophic cardiomyopathy. JAMA 2007;298:405–12.

66. Maron BJ, Rowin EJ, Maron MS, et al. Paradigm of sudden death prevention in hypertrophic cardiomyopathy. Circ Res 2019;125:370–8.

67. Melacini P, Maron BJ, Bobbo F, et al. Evidence that pharmacological strategies lack efficacy for the prevention of sudden death in hypertrophic cardiomyopathy. Heart 2007;93:708–10.

68. Maron BJ, Maron MS, Rowin EJ. Perspectives on the overall risk of living with hypertrophic cardiomyopathy. Circulation 2017;135:2317–9.

69. Maron BJ, Casey SA, Olivotto I, et al. Clinical course and quality of life in high risk patients with hypertrophic cardiomyopathy and implantable cardioverter- defibrillators. Circ Arrhythm Electrophysiol 2018;11:e05820.

70. O'Mahony C, Lambiase PD, Quarta G, et al. The long-term survival and the risks and benefits of implantable cardioverter defibrillators in patients with hypertrophic cardiomyopathy. Heart 2012;98:116–25.

71. Woo A, Monakier D, Harris L, et al. Determinants of implantable defibrillator discharges in high risk patients with hypertrophic cardiomyopathy. Heart 2007;93:1044–5.

72. Schinkel AF, Vriesendorp PA, Sijbrands EJ, et al. Outcome and complications after implantable cardioverter-defibrillator therapy in hypertrophic cardiomyopathy: systematic review and meta-analysis. Circ Heart Fail 2012;5:552–9.

73. Maron BJ, Shen W-K, Link MS, et al. Efficacy of implantable cardioverter- defibrillators for the prevention of sudden death in patients with hypertrophic cardiomyopathy. N Engl J Med 2000;342:365–73.

74. Ommen SR, Mital S, Burke MA, et al. 2020 AHA/ACC guideline for the diagnosis and treatment of patients with hypertrophic cardiomyopathy, a report of the American College of Cardiology/American Heart Association Joint Committee on clinical practice guidelines. Circulation 2020;142:e558–631.

75. Elliott PM, Anastasakis A, Borger MA, et al. 2014 ESC guidelines on diagnosis and management of hypertrophic cardiomyopathy. Eur Heart J 2014;35:2733–79.

76. Wang J, Zhang Z, Li Y, et al. Variable and limited predictive value of the European Society of Cardiology hypertrophic cardiomyopathy sudden-death risk model: a meta-analysis. Can J Cardiol 2019;35:1791–9.

77. Choi YJ, Kim HK, Lee SC, et al. Validation of the hypertrophic cardiomyopathy risk-sudden cardiac death calculator in Asians. Heart 2019;105:1892–7.

78. Maron MS, Appelbaum E, Harrigan CJ, et al. Clinical profile and significance of delayed enhancement in hypertrophic cardiomyopathy. Circ Heart Fail 2008;1:184–91.

79. Todiere G, Aquaro GD, Piaggi P, et al. Progression of myocardial fibrosis assessed with cardiac magnetic resonance in hypertrophic cardiomyopathy. J Am Coll Cardiol 2012;60:922–9.

80. Ingles J, Doolan A, Chiu C, et al. Compound and double mutations in patients with hypertrophic cardiomyopathy: implications for genetic testing and counselling. J Med Genet 2005;42(10):e59.

81. Ho CY, Day SM, Ashley EA, et al. Genotype and lifetime burden of disease in hypertrophic cardiomyopathy: insights from the sarcomeric human cardiomyopathy registry (SHaRe). Circulation 2018;138(14):1387–98.

82. Burke MA, Cook SA, Seidman JG, et al. Clinical and mechanistic insights into the genetics of cardiomyopathy. J Am Coll Cardiol 2016;68(25):2871–86.

83. Norrish G, Ding T, Field E, et al. Development of a novel risk prediction model for sudden cardiac death in childhood hypertrophic cardiomyopathy (HCM Risk-Kids). JAMA Cardiol 2019;4:918–27.

84. Miron A, Lafreniere-Roula M, Fan CS, et al. A validated model for sudden cardiac death risk prediction in pediatric hypertrophic cardiomyopathy. Circulation 2020;142:217–29.

85. Decker JA, Rossano JW, Smith EO, et al. Risk factors and mode of death in isolated hypertrophic cardiomyopathy in children. J Am Coll Cardiol 2009;54:250–4.

86. Bytyçi I, Nistri S, Mörner S, et al. Alcohol septal ablation versus septal myectomy treatment of obstructive hypertrophic cardiomyopathy: a systematic review and meta-analysis. J Clin Med 2020;9(10):3062.

87. Maron BJ, Rowin EJ, Maron MS, et al. Evolution of risk stratification and sudden death prevention in hypertrophic cardiomyopathy: twenty years with the implantable cardioverter-defibrillator. Heart Rhythm 2021. https://doi.org/10.1016/j.hrthm.2021.01.019.

88. Porcari A, Merlo M, Rapezzi C, et al. Transthyretin amyloid cardiomyopathy: an uncharted territory awaiting discovery. Eur J Intern Med 2020;82:7–15.

89. Porcari A, Falco L, Lio V, et al. Cardiac amyloidosis: do not forget to look for it. Eur Hear J Suppl 2020;22(Supplement_E):E142–7.

90. Maurer MS, Elliott P, Comenzo R, et al. Addressing common questions encountered in the diagnosis and management of cardiac amyloidosis. Circulation 2017;135(14):1357–77.

91. Dubrey SW, Cha K, Anderson J, et al. The clinical features of immunoglobulin light-chain (AL) amyloidosis with heart involvement. QJM 1998;91(2):141–57.

92. Varr BC, Zarafshar S, Coakley T, et al. Implantable cardioverter-defibrillator placement in patients with cardiac amyloidosis. Hear Rhythm 2014;11(1): 158–62.
93. Palladini G, Malamani G, Cò F, et al. Holter monitoring in AL amyloidosis: prognostic implications. Pacing Clin Electrophysiol 2001;24(8):1228–33.
94. Giancaterino S, Urey MA, Darden D, et al. Management of arrhythmias in cardiac amyloidosis. JACC Clin Electrophysiol 2020;6(4):351–61.
95. Priori SG, Blomström-Lundqvist C, Mazzanti A, et al. 2015 ESC guidelines for the management of patients with ventricular arrhythmias and the prevention of sudden cardiac death. Eur Heart J 2015;36(41):2793–867.
96. Al-Khatib SM, Stevenson WG, Ackerman MJ, et al. 2017 AHA/ACC/HRS guideline for management of patients with ventricular arrhythmias and the prevention of sudden cardiac death: executive summary: a report of the American College of Cardiology/American Heart Association Task Force on Clinical Practice Gu. Hear Rhythm 2018;15(10): e190–252.
97. Hamon D, Algalarrondo V, Gandjbakhch E, et al. Outcome and incidence of appropriate implantable cardioverter-defibrillator therapy in patients with cardiac amyloidosis. Int J Cardiol 2016;222:562–8.
98. Lin G, Dispenzieri A, Kyle R, et al. Implantable cardioverter defibrillators in patients with cardiac amyloidosis. J Cardiovasc Electrophysiol 2013; 24(7):793–8.
99. Kristen AV, Dengler TJ, Hegenbart U, et al. Prophylactic implantation of cardioverter-defibrillator in patients with severe cardiac amyloidosis and high risk for sudden cardiac death. Hear Rhythm 2008;5(2):235–40.
100. Sayed RH, Rogers D, Khan F, et al. A study of implanted cardiac rhythm recorders in advanced cardiac AL amyloidosis. Eur Heart J 2015;36(18): 1098–105.

The Risk of Sudden Unexpected Cardiac Death in Children
Epidemiology, Clinical Causes, and Prevention

Emanuele Monda, MD[a], Michele Lioncino, MD[a], Marta Rubino, MD[a], Martina Caiazza, MD[a], Annapaola Cirillo, MD[a], Adelaide Fusco, MD[a], Roberta Pacileo, MD[a], Fabio Fimiani, MD[a], Federica Amodio, MD[a], Nunzia Borrelli, MD[a], Diego Colonna, MD[a], Barbara D'Onofrio, MD[a], Giulia Frisso, MD, PhD[b], Fabrizio Drago, MD, PhD[c], Silvia Castelletti, MD, PhD[d], Berardo Sarubbi, MD, PhD[a], Paolo Calabrò, MD, PhD[a], Maria Giovanna Russo, MD, PhD[a], Giuseppe Limongelli, MD, PhD[a,e,*]

KEYWORDS

• Sudden cardiac death • Children • Cardiomyopathies • Channelopathies

KEY POINTS

- In children, the main causes of sudden cardiac death (SCD) are inherited cardiac disorders, whereas coronary artery diseases, congenital heart diseases, and myocarditis are rare.
- The identification of inherited cardiac disorders that predispose to SCD is required to prevent future cardiac events both in the proband and affected family members.
- Hypertrophic cardiomyopathy is the major cause of SCD among cardiomyopathies, followed by arrhythmogenic cardiomyopathy.
- Channelopathies represent among the leading cause of sudden arrhythmic death syndrome (sudden unexplained death with negative pathologic and toxicologic assessment).

INTRODUCTION

Sudden unexplained death (SUD) is a tragic event for both the family and community, particularly when it occurs in young individuals. The term SUD is used to refer to an unexpected and sudden death that occurs in an individual older than 1 year.

On the other part, sudden death occurring in the first year of life is defined as sudden unexplained death in infancy.[1]

Sudden cardiac death (SCD) represents the leading form of SUD[2] and is defined as an unexpected event without an obvious extracardiac

[a] Department of Translational Medical Sciences, University of Campania "Luigi Vanvitelli", Via L. Bianchi, 80131 Naples, Italy; [b] Department of Molecular Medicine and Medical Biotechnologies, University of Naples Federico II, Via Pansini 5, 80131 Naples, Italy; [c] Istituto Auxologico Italiano, IRCCS-Center for Cardiac Arrhythmias of Genetic Origin, Via Pier Lombardo 22, 20135 Milan, Italy; [d] Istituto Auxologico Italiano, IRCCS-Center for Cardiac Arrhythmias of Genetic Origin, Milan, Italy; [e] Institute of Cardiovascular Sciences, University College of London and St. Bartholomew's Hospital, Grower Street, London WC1E 6DD, UK
* Corresponding author. Inherited and Rare Cardiovascular Diseases, Department of Translational Medical Sciences, University of Campania "Luigi Vanvitelli", AO Colli - Monaldi Hospital - ERN Guard Heart Member, 80131 Naples, Italy.
E-mail address: limongelligiuseppe@libero.it

Heart Failure Clin 18 (2022) 115–123
https://doi.org/10.1016/j.hfc.2021.07.002

cause, occurring within 1 hour after the onset of symptoms.[3] SCD in children often occurs without warning symptoms, manifesting as the first presentation of an underlying cardiac disease.[4] In children, the main causes of SCD are inherited cardiac disorders,[5–9] whereas coronary artery diseases (congenital or acquired), congenital heart diseases, and myocarditis are rare (**Table 1**). The identification of inherited cardiac disorders that predispose to SCD is a fundamental step to prevent future cardiac events both in the proband and affected family members.[4,10]

The present review examines the current state of knowledge regarding SCD in children, discussing the epidemiology, clinical causes, and prevention strategies.

EPIDEMIOLOGY

SCD is an uncommon event in childhood. Several population-based studies investigated the incidence of SCD in young individuals, reporting an incidence ranging from 0.7 to 7.4 per 100.000 person-years.[5–9,11] Several factors were associated with the variability of the SCD incidence, such as age, sex, country, comorbidities, and participation in athletic activity. The rate of SCD was less than in the adult population and was age dependent, with an initial period of higher risk in infants (<1 year old), a lower rate in children aged 6 to 10 years old, and a progressive increase in risk in children older than 10 years.[6,12,13] Men showed an increased risk, which was twice that of women.[5,14]

CAUSES

Several conditions have been associated with SCD. They can be classified into cardiomyopathies (CMPs), primary arrhythmia syndromes (channelopathies), congenital heart diseases, coronary artery diseases, aortic diseases, and myocarditis. In children who died suddenly, the underlying cardiac cause may be known or in the preclinical phase, and the proportion of the detected risk of SCD varies by age and diagnosis. In the following paragraphs, the authors describe the main causes of SCD in children and the related known risk factors for single cause.

Cardiomyopathies

SCD in children with CMPs depends on age, gender, and phenotype. Male patients and children older than 10 years show a higher risk of SCD. Hypertrophic cardiomyopathy (HCM) is the major cause of SCD among CMPs, followed by arrhythmogenic cardiomyopathy (ACM). SCD due to dilated cardiomyopathy, restrictive cardiomyopathy, or left ventricular (LV) noncompaction is a rare event.[8,15]

Hypertrophic cardiomyopathy

The prevalence of SCD rates in children with HCM varies widely, with reported rates ranging from 1% to 7.2% per year.[16–20] The clinical course of patients with HCM can be extremely variable,[21–28] and the identification of young patients at high risk of SCD is often challenging. Both the European Society of Cardiology and the American Heart Association–American College of Cardiology guidelines recommend implantable cardioverter-defibrillator (ICD) implantation in children with more than 1 risk factor, including unexplained syncope, massive left ventricular hypertrophy (LVH), nonsustained ventricular tachycardia (NSVT), or family history of HCM-related SCD.[29,30] However, a consensus on SCD risk stratification for children with HCM is not currently available. A recent systematic review identified several risk factors for SCD, categorizing them into major and minor risk factors.[31] Major risk factors included previous aborted cardiac arrest or sustained ventricular tachycardia, extreme LVH, syncope, and NSVT, whereas

Table 1
Causes of sudden cardiac death in children categorized into structural and arrhythmogenic causes

	Structural Causes	Arrhythmogenic Causes
Common	Arrhythmogenic cardiomyopathy Hypertrophic cardiomyopathy Myocarditis	Brugada syndrome Catecholaminergic polymorphic ventricular tachycardia Long QT syndrome
Uncommon	Aortic disease Congenital heart disease Coronary artery disease Dilated cardiomyopathy Restrictive cardiomyopathy	Early repolarization syndrome Progressive cardiac conduction disease Short QT syndrome Wolff-Parkinson-White syndrome

minor risk factors included family history of SCD, age at presentation or diagnosis, electrocardiogram (ECG) changes, abnormal blood pressure response to exercise, LV outflow tract obstruction, left atrial size, restrictive physiology, and abnormal 24-hour blood pressure monitoring. Moreover, 2 different risk prediction models for SCD in children with HCM have been recently proposed. Norrish and colleagues[32] developed a 5-year SCD risk prediction model from a retrospective cohort study of 1024 consecutive patients aged 16 years or younger with HCM, with the final model including unexplained syncope, NSVT, left atrial diameter z-score, LV maximal wall thickness z-score, and LV outflow tract gradient. Similarly, Miron and colleagues[33] developed and validated a 5-year SCD prediction model from 572 consecutive patients aged 18 years or younger with HCM. Risk predictors included age at diagnosis, NSVT, unexplained syncope, septal diameter z-score, LV posterior wall diameter z score, left atrial diameter z score, peak LV outflow tract gradient, and presence of a pathogenic variant. Interestingly, both models showed a discrete prediction accuracy, with the potential to improve the application of clinical practice guidelines and shared decision-making for ICD implantation. On the contrary, no ECG abnormalities, either in isolation or combined in the previously described ECG risk score,[34] have been found to be associated with 5-year SCD risk in a large multicenter retrospective cohort of children with HCM.[35]

Arrhythmogenic cardiomyopathy

ACM is a common cause of SCD in children[5,9] and among the most important in young athletes.[36–42] However, there are few studies focused on children with ACM, and, as a consequence, SCD risk factors in those patients are poorly known. Furthermore, no guideline or consensus document provides specific recommendations for risk stratification and ICD implantation in children with ACM. DeWitt and colleagues[43] evaluated 32 children aged 21 years or younger with ACM. Cardiac arrest and ventricular tachycardia occurred in 15% and 31% of patients, and predominant right ventricular disease was significantly associated with both the events. Moreover, they were more likely to occur in probands. Similarly, Riele and colleagues[44] identified 75 patients with pediatric-onset disease (<18 years of age) and found that 15% of pediatric patients presented with SCD and 11% with sudden cardiac arrest (SCA). In most of the patients, SCD occurred during exercise activity. In ACM, participation in high-intensity activity can favor the disease progression

and trigger life-threatening arrhythmias. Therefore, avoidance from competitive sports should be recommended.[45]

Channelopathies

Channelopathies represent among the leading cause of sudden arrhythmic death syndrome (SADS), a term used to describe an individual with SUD who shows negative pathologic and toxicologic assessment (autopsy-negative SUD). In particular, long QT syndrome (LQTS) and catecholaminergic polymorphic ventricular tachycardia (CPVT) are the most common causes of SADS, followed by Brugada syndrome (BrS).[4,46–50]

Long QT syndrome

LQTS is a cause of SUD in up to 20% of victims younger than 30 years.[47,49] Furthermore, about 10% of infants (<1 year) who died suddenly carry a disease-causing mutation in an LQTS-related gene, and a prolonged QT interval in newborns increased the risk of SCD.[50–52] In addition, an episode of SCA during infancy is associated with a very high risk for subsequent SCD during the next 10 years of life.[52]

The risk of SCD in patients with LQTS is influenced by age, gender, genotype, and environmental or genetic modifiers.[53] Men carry an increased risk of SCD during childhood and preadolescence,[54–56] whereas the gender-related risk reverses after childhood, and women show higher risk than men during adolescence and adulthood[56]; the reason of this gender-related risk is unknown. Moreover, other major risk factors in children include the history of syncope, QTc duration greater than 500 ms, and episodes of T wave alternans.[54,57,58] In LQTS there is a strong genotype-phenotype correlation with the most important correlation evidenced for the specific trigger for life-threatening arrhythmias: patients with LQT1 are at increased risk during emotional or physical stresses, conditions characterized by increased sympathetic activity[59]; patients with LQT2 are at increased risk when exposed to sudden noises[59]; patients with LQT3 are at risk during asleep or when they are at rest.

Catecholaminergic polymorphic ventricular tachycardia

CPVT is among the most frequent cause of SADS,[47,60] especially when the death occurred during exertional activity. CPVT can manifest at any age. However, the most common presentation occurs during the first 2 decades of life, with fast palpitations, presyncope, syncope, SCA, or SCD under adrenergic stress.[61] Hayashi and colleagues[62] identified younger at diagnosis, absence of beta-blocking therapy, and history of aborted cardiac arrest as independent predictors for cardiac events. Unfortunately, to date, there is no risk stratification protocol in patients with CPVT.

Brugada syndrome

BrS is a rare cause of SUD. It is mostly diagnosed during adulthood and, given the rarity of BrS in the pediatric population, risk stratification in children and young patients is very difficult. Andorin and colleagues[63] reported that the risk of life-threatening arrhythmias was related to 2 clinical parameters: spontaneous ECG type 1 Brugada pattern and syncope. Subsequently, a clinical score model to predict lethal events in patients younger than or equal to 19 years with BrS was proposed. This model includes 4 main clinical variables: SCD or syncope, spontaneous type 1 ECG pattern, sinus node dysfunction and/or atrial tachycardia, and conduction abnormality.[64] However, an important limitation of these studies was the small sample size of the cohort, which limits the generalization of the results. Indeed, considering the high rate of complication associated with ICD implantation in children, the patient selection requires attention to avoid unnecessary implantation. Interestingly, Mazzanti and colleagues[65] showed that in a cohort of 129 pediatric patients, only 3 of them experienced a life-threatening arrhythmic event and no patients who had presented with syncope experienced a cardiac arrest during follow-up, suggesting that a more conservative approach may be indicated in the pediatric population.

PREVENTION

The prevention of SCD in children can be categorized into 3 different sections: the identification of patients at risk for SCD and the implementation of strategies to prevent the event (primary prevention); the identification of the underlying cause in SCA survivors and the implementation of strategies to prevent further events (secondary prevention); and the identification of family member at risk for SCD.

Identification of Children at Risk for Sudden Cardiac Death

Cardiac arrest is often the first manifestation of an underlying inherited cardiac disease. Thus, cardiovascular screening represents an important prevention strategy to avoid SCD in children. Several screening programs have been proposed for different populations and subgroups, such as athletes, to early detect the patients at risk.[66] Furthermore, children with cardiac inherited disorders can be identified for other reasons, such as family screening (discussed later) or the presence of warning symptoms (eg, syncope or presyncope).[67,68]

In these patients, several interventions should be started, such as lifestyle modification, medical treatment, and ICD implantation in primary prevention for those at high risk.[69,70] The possible lifestyle modification would be avoiding dehydration and electrolyte imbalance for children with channelopathies; avoiding hyperthermia from febrile illnesses for patients with BrS; avoiding strenuous physical activity in patients with HCM, ACM, LQTS, and CPVT; avoiding certain drugs for patients with LQTS or BrS, and so forth.[71] Medical treatment varies according to the underlying cardiac condition.[21,22,69,72–74] For example, beta-blockers play a role in SCD prevention in patients with LQTS and CPVT,[69] whereas their role is uncertain in children with HCM.[70] Finally, in patients considered at high risk for SCD, ICD implantation should be considered. However, as discussed earlier, risk stratification is often difficult in children with CMPs or channelopathies due to the paucity of data in the literature.

Investigations in Sudden Cardiac Arrest Survivors

In children who experienced an SCA, the identification of the underlying cause is mandatory to start appropriate treatment and identify family members at risk. Thus, a comprehensive clinical and instrumental evaluation is required[10] (**Fig. 1**): the information on age, sex, symptoms, and family history activity at the time of SCA. For example, children with BrS or LQT3 generally experience SCA during sleep or at rest, whereas ACM, LQT1, and CPVT during emotional or physical stress.[59,61,63] Baseline investigations should include blood testing, standard 12-lead ECG, high precordial lead ECG, signal-average ECG, echocardiography, and cardiac magnetic resonance (CMR).[75–78] Coronary imaging may be considered in selected cases. Baseline investigation can be helpful to diagnose most overt acquired or genetic cardiac diseases. However, these conditions can be concealed, and provocative maneuvers are sometimes required to obtain a final diagnosis. For example, sodium channel blocker challenge can be useful for the diagnosis of Brugada syndrome,[79] exercise testing may support the diagnosis of CPVT or ACM,[69,80] and so forth. Finally, genetic testing should be considered in patients with a diagnosis or strong suspect for inherited cardiac disease, in particular when the results are likely to

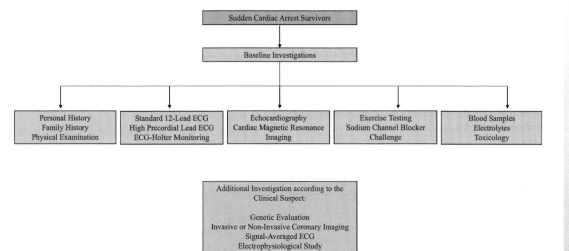

Fig. 1. Investigation of sudden cardiac arrest survivors.

influence the management and to guide family screening.[4,81–84] Of importance, for children who experience an SCA, the prevention of further episodes is mandatory, and, except for selected cases, survivors should undergo ICD implantation.

Identification of Family Members at Risk

Two different strategies can be used to detect family members at risk. If the proband obtained a final diagnosis and showed positive genetic testing for a disease-causing mutation (either obtained in SCA survivors with the genetic testing or in patients who died suddenly with the molecular autopsy), the cascade screening is the best strategy to early identify other family members

who may carry the genetic mutation (**Fig. 2**). Family members who result negative for that implicated variant can be dismissed, whereas those positive will require disease-specific surveillance and therapy.

On the other hand, when the cause of SCD is not identified, either because there was no postmortem examination or because the autopsy was negative, the identification of family members at risk is more difficult and requires a comprehensive screening of first-degree relatives of the SCD victim. Baseline investigations include family history, physical examination, standard 12-lead ECG, high precordial lead ECG, echocardiography, CMR, exercise testing, and sodium channel blocker challenge.[10,85]

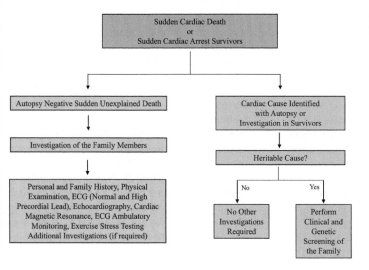

Fig. 2. Identification of family members at risk for sudden cardiac death.

SUMMARY

SCD is a tragic and often unexpected event, especially if it is the sentinel manifestation of the disease in a family. Clinical and genetic evaluation of survivors and family members plays a key role in diagnosing the underlying inherited cardiac disease in the family in order to start appropriate prevention strategies.

CLINICS CARE POINTS

- Cardiovascular screening represents an important prevention strategy to avoid SCD in children. Several screening programs have been proposed for different populations and subgroups, such as athletes, to early detect the patients at risk.

- In children who experienced an SCA, the identification of the underlying cause is mandatory to start appropriate treatment and identify family members at risk.

- In patients considered at high risk for SCD, ICD implantation should be considered. However, risk stratification is often difficult in children with cardiomyopathies or channelopathies due to the paucity of data in the literature.

DISCLOSURE

The authors have nothing to disclose.

REFERENCES

1. Mitchell EA, Krous HF. Sudden unexpected death in infancy: a historical perspective. J Paediatr Child Health 2015;51(1):108–12.
2. Risgaard B, Lynge TH, Wissenberg M, et al. Risk factors and causes of sudden noncardiac death: a nationwide cohort study in Denmark. Heart Rhythm 2015;12(5):968–74.
3. Fishman GI, Chugh SS, Dimarco JP, et al. Sudden cardiac death prediction and prevention: report from a National Heart, Lung, and Blood Institute and Heart Rhythm Society Workshop. Circulation 2010;122(22):2335–48.
4. Monda E, Sarubbi B, Russo MG, et al. Unexplained sudden cardiac arrest in children: clinical and genetic characteristics of survivors. Eur J Prev Cardiol 2020. 2047487320940863.
5. Winkel BG, Holst AG, Theilade J, et al. Nationwide study of sudden cardiac death in persons aged 1-35 years. Eur Heart J 2011;32:983–90.
6. Bagnall RD, Weintraub RG, Ingles J, et al. A prospective study of sudden cardiac death among children and young adults. N Engl J Med 2016;374:2441–52.
7. Winkel BG, Risgaard B, Sadjadieh G, et al. Sudden cardiac death in children (1-18 years): symptoms and causes of death in a nationwide setting. Eur Heart J 2014;35:868–75.
8. Eckart RE, Shry EA, Burke AP, et al. Sudden death in young adults: an autopsy based series of a population undergoing active surveillance. J Am Coll Cardiol 2011;58:1254–61.
9. Wisten A, Krantz P, Stattin EL. Sudden cardiac death among the young in Sweden from 2000 to 2010: an autopsy-based study. Europace 2017;19:1327–34.
10. Stiles MK, Wilde AAM, Abrams DJ, et al. 2020 APHRS/HRS expert consensus statement on the investigation of decedents with sudden unexplained death and patients with sudden cardiac arrest, and of their families. Heart Rhythm 2021;18(1): e1–50.
11. Martens E, Sinner MF, Siebermair J, et al. Incidence of sudden cardiac death in Germany: results from an emergency medical service registry in Lower Saxony. Europace 2014;16(12):1752–8.
12. Mellor G, Raju H, de Noronha SV, et al. Clinical characteristics and circumstances of death in the sudden arrhythmic death syndrome. Circ Arrhythm Electrophysiol 2014;7:1078–83.
13. Papadakis M, Raju H, Behr ER, et al. Sudden cardiac death with autopsy findings of uncertain significance: potential for erroneous interpretation. Circ Arrhythm Electrophysiol 2013;6:588–96.
14. Meyer L, Stubbs B, Fahrenbruch C, et al. Incidence, causes, and survival trends from cardiovascular-related sudden cardiac arrest in children and young adults 0 to 35 years of age: a 30-year review. Circulation 2012;126(11):1363–72.
15. Harmon KG, Asif IM, Klossner D, et al. Incidence of sudden cardiac death in National Collegiate Athletic Association athletes. Circulation 2011;123(15): 1594–600.
16. Kaski J, Tomé Esteban MT, Lowe M, et al. Outcomes after implantable cardioverter-defibrillator treatment in children with hypertrophic cardiomyopathy. Heart 2007;93:372–4.
17. McKenna W, Deanfield J, Faruqui A, et al. Prognosis in hypertrophic cardiomyopathy: role of age and clinical, electrocardiographic and hemodynamic features. Am J Cardiol 1981;47:532–8.
18. McKenna WJ, Deanfield JE. Hypertrophic cardiomyopathy: an important cause of sudden death. Arch Dis Child 1984;59:971–5.
19. Ostman-Smith I, Wettrell G, Keeton B, et al. Age- and gender-specific mortality rates in childhood hypertrophic cardiomyopathy. Eur Heart J 2008;29: 1160–7.

20. Yetman AT, Hamilton RM, Benson LN, et al. Long-term outcome and prognostic determinants in children with hypertrophic cardiomyopathy. J Am Coll Cardiol 1998;32:1943–50.

21. Monda E, Palmiero G, Rubino M, et al. Molecular basis of inflammation in the pathogenesis of cardiomyopathies. Int J Mol Sci 2020;21(18):6462.

22. Monda E, Limongelli G. The hospitalizations in hypertrophic cardiomyopathy: "The dark side of the moon". Int J Cardiol 2020;318:101–2.

23. Limongelli G, Monda E, Tramonte S, et al. Prevalence and clinical significance of red flags in patients with hypertrophic cardiomyopathy. Int J Cardiol 2020;299:186–91.

24. Esposito A, Monda E, Gragnano F, et al. Prevalence and clinical implications of hyperhomocysteinaemia in patients with hypertrophic cardiomyopathy and MTHFR C6777T polymorphism. Eur J Prev Cardiol 2020;27(17):1906–8.

25. Caiazza M, Rubino M, Monda E, et al. Combined PTPN11 and MYBPC3 gene mutations in an adult patient with noonan syndrome and hypertrophic cardiomyopathy. Genes (Basel) 2020;11(8):947.

26. Monda E, Kaski JP, Limongelli G. Editorial: paediatric cardiomyopathies. Front Pediatr 2021;9:696443.

27. Monda E, Rubino M, Lioncino M, et al. Hypertrophic cardiomyopathy in children: pathophysiology, diagnosis, and treatment of non-sarcomeric causes. Front Pediatr 2021;9:632293.

28. Limongelli G, Monda E, D'Aponte A, et al. Combined effect of mediterranean diet and aerobic exercise on weight loss and clinical status in obese symptomatic patients with hypertrophic Cardiomyopathy. Heart Fail Clin 2021;17(2):303–13.

29. Elliott PM, Anastasakis A, Borger MA, et al. 2014 ESC guidelines on diagnosis and management of hypertrophic cardiomyopathy: the task force for the diagnosis and management of hypertrophic cardiomyopathy of the European Society of Cardiology (ESC). Eur Heart J 2014;35(39):2733–79.

30. Ommen SR, Mital S, Burke MA, et al. 2020 AHA/ACC guideline for the diagnosis and treatment of patients with hypertrophic cardiomyopathy: a report of the American College of Cardiology/American Heart Association Joint Committee on Clinical Practice Guidelines [published correction appears in Circulation. 2020 Dec 22;142(25):e633]. Circulation 2020;142(25):e558–631.

31. Norrish G, Cantarutti N, Pissaridou E, et al. Risk factors for sudden cardiac death in childhood hypertrophic cardiomyopathy: a systematic review and meta-analysis. Eur J Prev Cardiol 2017;24(11):1220–30.

32. Norrish G, Ding T, Field E, et al. Development of a novel risk prediction model for sudden cardiac death in childhood hypertrophic cardiomyopathy (HCM Risk-Kids). JAMA Cardiol 2019;4(9):918–27.

33. Miron A, Lafreniere-Roula M, Steve Fan CP, et al. A validated model for sudden cardiac death risk prediction in pediatric hypertrophic cardiomyopathy. Circulation 2020;142(3):217–29.

34. Östman-Smith I, Sjöberg G, Rydberg A, et al. Predictors of risk for sudden death in childhood hypertrophic cardiomyopathy: the importance of the ECG risk score. Open Heart 2017;4(2):e000658.

35. Norrish G, Topriceanu C, Qu C, et al. The role of the electrocardiographic phenotype in risk stratification for sudden cardiac death in childhood hypertrophic cardiomyopathy [published online ahead of print, 2021 Mar 27]. Eur J Prev Cardiol 2021;zwab046.

36. Maron BJ. Sudden death in young athletes. N Engl J Med 2003;349(11):1064–75.

37. Maron BJ, Epstein SE, Roberts WC. Causes of sudden death in competitive athletes. J Am Coll Cardiol 1986;7(1):204–14.

38. Thiene G, Nava A, Corrado D, et al. Right ventricular cardiomyopathy and sudden death in young people. N Engl J Med 1988;318(3):129–33.

39. Barretta F, Mirra B, Monda E, et al. The hidden fragility in the heart of the athletes: a review of genetic biomarkers. Int J Mol Sci 2020;21(18):6682.

40. Monda E, Frisso G, Rubino M, et al. Potential role of imaging markers in predicting future disease expression of arrhythmogenic cardiomyopathy. Future Cardiol 2021;17(4):647–54.

41. Limongelli G, Nunziato M, D'Argenio V, et al. Yield and clinical significance of genetic screening in elite and amateur athletes [published online ahead of print, 2020 Jul 2]. Eur J Prev Cardiol 2020. 2047487320934265.

42. Limongelli G, Nunziato M, Mazzaccara C, et al. Genotype-phenotype correlation: a triple DNA mutational event in a boy entering sport conveys an additional pathogenicity risk. Genes (Basel) 2020;11(5):524.

43. DeWitt ES, Chandler SF, Hylind RJ, et al. Phenotypic manifestations of arrhythmogenic cardiomyopathy in children and adolescents. J Am Coll Cardiol 2019;74(3):346–58.

44. Te Riele ASJM, James CA, Sawant AC, et al. Arrhythmogenic right ventricular dysplasia/cardiomyopathy in the pediatric population: clinical characterization and comparison with adult-onset disease. JACC Clin Electrophysiol 2015;1(6):551–60.

45. Pelliccia A, Solberg EE, Papadakis M, et al. Recommendations for participation in competitive and leisure time sport in athletes with cardiomyopathies, myocarditis, and pericarditis: position statement of the Sport Cardiology Section of the European Association of Preventive Cardiology (EAPC). Eur Heart J 2019;40(1):19–33.

46. Behr ER, Dalageorgou C, Christiansen M, et al. Sudden arrhythmic death syndrome: familial evaluation identifies inheritable heart disease in the majority of families. Eur Heart J 2008;29(13):1670–80.

47. Tester DJ, Medeiros-Domingo A, Will ML, et al. Cardiac channel molecular autopsy: insights from 173 consecutive cases of autopsy-negative sudden unexplained death referred for postmortem genetic testing. Mayo Clin Proc 2012;87(6):524–39.

48. Skinner JR, Crawford J, Smith W, et al. Prospective, population-based long QT molecular autopsy study of postmortem negative sudden death in 1 to 40 year olds. Heart Rhythm 2011;8(3):412–9.

49. Tester DJ, Ackerman MJ. Postmortem long QT syndrome genetic testing for sudden unexplained death in the young. J Am Coll Cardiol 2007;49(2):240–6.

50. Schwartz PJ, Stramba-Badiale M, Crotti L, et al. Prevalence of the congenital long-QT syndrome. Circulation 2009;120(18):1761–7.

51. Schwartz PJ, Stramba-Badiale M, Segantini A, et al. Prolongation of the QT interval and the sudden infant death syndrome. N Engl J Med 1998;338(24):1709–14.

52. Spazzolini C, Mullally J, Moss AJ, et al. Clinical implications for patients with long QT syndrome who experience a cardiac event during infancy. J Am Coll Cardiol 2009;54(9):832–7.

53. Schwartz PJ, Ackerman MJ, Antzelevitch C, et al. Inherited cardiac arrhythmias. Nat Rev Dis Primers 2020;6(1):58.

54. Goldenberg I, Moss AJ, Peterson DR, et al. Risk factors for aborted cardiac arrest and sudden cardiac death in children with the congenital long-QT syndrome. Circulation 2008;117(17):2184–91.

55. Locati EH, Zareba W, Moss AJ, et al. Age- and sex-related differences in clinical manifestations in patients with congenital long-QT syndrome: findings from the International LQTS Registry. Circulation 1998;97(22):2237–44.

56. Zareba W, Moss AJ, Locati EH, et al. Modulating effects of age and gender on the clinical course of long QT syndrome by genotype. J Am Coll Cardiol 2003;42(1):103–9.

57. Priori SG, Schwartz PJ, Napolitano C, et al. Risk stratification in the long-QT syndrome. N Engl J Med 2003;348(19):1866–74.

58. Schwartz PJ, Malliani A. Electrical alternation of the T-wave: clinical and experimental evidence of its relationship with the sympathetic nervous system and with the long Q-T syndrome. Am Heart J 1975;89(1):45–50.

59. Schwartz PJ, Priori SG, Spazzolini C, et al. Genotype-phenotype correlation in the long-QT syndrome: gene-specific triggers for life-threatening arrhythmias. Circulation 2001;103(1):89–95.

60. Tester DJ, Spoon DB, Valdivia HH, et al. Targeted mutational analysis of the RyR2-encoded cardiac ryanodine receptor in sudden unexplained death: a molecular autopsy of 49 medical examiner/coroner's cases. Mayo Clin Proc 2004;79(11):1380–4.

61. Priori SG, Napolitano C, Tiso N, et al. Mutations in the cardiac ryanodine receptor gene (hRyR2) underlie catecholaminergic polymorphic ventricular tachycardia. Circulation 2001;103(2):196–200.

62. Hayashi M, Denjoy I, Extramiana F, et al. Incidence and risk factors of arrhythmic events in catecholaminergic polymorphic ventricular tachycardia. Circulation 2009;119(18):2426–34.

63. Andorin A, Behr ER, Denjoy I, et al. Impact of clinical and genetic findings on the management of young patients with Brugada syndrome. Heart Rhythm 2016;13(6):1274–82.

64. Gonzalez Corcia MC, Sieira J, Pappaert G, et al. A clinical score model to predict lethal events in young patients (≤19 Years) with the brugada syndrome. Am J Cardiol 2017;120(5):797–802.

65. Mazzanti A, Ovics P, Shauer A, et al. Unexpected risk profile of a large pediatric population with brugada syndrome. J Am Coll Cardiol 2019;73(14):1868–9.

66. Mont L, Pelliccia A, Sharma S, et al. Pre-participation cardiovascular evaluation for athletic participants to prevent sudden death: position paper from the EHRA and the EACPR, branches of the ESC. Endorsed by APHRS, HRS, and SOLAECE. Eur J Prev Cardiol 2017;24(1):41–69.

67. Drezner JA, Fudge J, Harmon KG, et al. Warning symptoms and family history in children and young adults with sudden cardiac arrest. J Am Board Fam Med 2012;25(4):408–15.

68. Wisten A, Messner T. Symptoms preceding sudden cardiac death in the young are common but often misinterpreted. Scand Cardiovasc J 2005;39(3):143–9.

69. Priori SG, Blomström-Lundqvist C, Mazzanti A, et al. 2015 ESC Guidelines for the management of patients with ventricular arrhythmias and the prevention of sudden cardiac death: the task force for the management of patients with ventricular arrhythmias and the prevention of sudden cardiac death of the European Society of Cardiology (ESC). Endorsed by: Association for European Paediatric and Congenital Cardiology (AEPC). Eur Heart J 2015;36(41):2793–867.

70. Al-Khatib SM, Stevenson WG, Ackerman MJ, et al. 2017 AHA/ACC/HRS guideline for management of patients with ventricular arrhythmias and the prevention of sudden cardiac death: a report of the American College of Cardiology/American Heart Association Task Force on Clinical Practice Guidelines and the Heart Rhythm Society [published correction appears in Circulation. 2018 Sep 25; 138(13):e419-e420]. Circulation 2018;138(13):e272–391.

71. Ackerman MJ, Zipes DP, Kovacs RJ, et al. American heart association electrocardiography and arrhythmias committee of council on clinical cardiology, council on cardiovascular disease in young, council on cardiovascular and stroke nursing, council on functional genomics and translational biology, and American College of Cardiology. Eligibility and disqualification recommendations for competitive athletes with cardiovascular abnormalities: task force 10: the cardiac channelopathies: a scientific statement from the American Heart Association and American College of Cardiology. Circulation 2015;132(22):e326–9.

72. Antzelevitch C, Yan GX, Ackerman MJ, et al. J-Wave syndromes expert consensus conference report: emerging concepts and gaps in knowledge. J Arrhythm 2016;32(5):315–39.

73. Towbin JA, McKenna WJ, Abrams DJ, et al. 2019 HRS expert consensus statement on evaluation, risk stratification, and management of arrhythmogenic cardiomyopathy. Heart Rhythm 2019;16(11): e301–72.

74. Ammirati E, Contri R, Coppini R, et al. Pharmacological treatment of hypertrophic cardiomyopathy: current practice and novel perspectives. Eur J Heart Fail 2016;18(9):1106–18.

75. Papadakis M, Papatheodorou E, Mellor G, et al. The diagnostic yield of Brugada syndrome after sudden death with normal autopsy. J Am Coll Cardiol 2018; 71:1204–14.

76. Krahn AD, Healey JS, Chauhan V, et al. Systematic assessment of patients with unexplained cardiac arrest: Cardiac Arrest Survivors with Preserved Ejection Fraction Registry (CASPER). Circulation 2009; 120:278–85.

77. White JA, Fine NM, Gula L, et al. Utility of cardiovascular magnetic resonance in identifying substrate for malignant ventricular arrhythmias. Circ Cardiovasc Imaging 2012;5:12–20.

78. Rodrigues P, Joshi A, Williams H, et al. Diagnosis and prognosis in sudden cardiac arrest survivors without coronary artery disease: utility of a clinical approach using cardiac magnetic resonance imaging. Circ Cardiovasc Imaging 2017;10:e006709.

79. Govindan M, Batchvarov VN, Raju H, et al. Utility of high and standard right precordial leads during ajmaline testing for the diagnosis of Brugada syndrome. Heart 2010;96:1904–8.

80. Perrin MJ, Angaran P, Laksman Z, et al. Exercise testing in asymptomatic gene carriers exposes a latent electrical substrate of arrhythmogenic right ventricular cardiomyopathy. J Am Coll Cardiol 2013;62:1772–9.

81. James CA, Bhonsale A, Tichnell C, et al. Exercise increases age-related penetrance and arrhythmic risk in arrhythmogenic right ventricular dysplasia/cardiomyopathy-associated desmosomal mutation carriers. J Am Coll Cardiol 2013;62:1290–7.

82. van Rijsingen IA, van der Zwaag PA, Groeneweg JA, et al. Outcome in phospholamban R14del carriers: results of a large multicentre cohort study. Circ Cardiovasc Genet 2014;7:455–65.

83. van Rijsingen IA, Arbustini E, Elliott PM, et al. Risk factors for malignant ventricular arrhythmias in Lamin A/C mutation carriers: a European cohort study. J Am Coll Cardiol 2012;59:493–500.

84. De Ferrari GM, Dusi V, Spazzolini C, et al. Clinical management of catecholaminergic polymorphic ventricular tachycardia: the role of left cardiac sympathetic denervation. Circulation 2015;131:2185–93.

85. Gray B, Ackerman MJ, Semsarian C, et al. Evaluation after sudden death in the young: a global approach. Circ Arrhythm Electrophysiol 2019;12(8): e007453.

Epidemiology, Pathogenesis, and Clinical Course of Takotsubo Syndrome

Rodolfo Citro, MD, PhD[a],*, Ilaria Radano, MD[a], Michele Bellino, MD[a],
Ciro Mauro, MD[b], Hiroyuky Okura, MD, PhD[c], Eduardo Bossone, MD, PhD[b],
Yoshihiro J. Akashy, MD, PhD[d]

KEYWORDS

• Takotsubo • Cardiomyopathy • Apical ballooning • Acute coronary syndrome • Stress

KEY POINTS

• TTS is an acute and usually reversible heart failure syndrome, most frequently seen in postmenopausal women, often resulting from a stressful emotional or physical triggering event.
• The exact TTS pathophysiology is not yet known. A sudden sympathetic activation and serum catecholamines surge seems to play a key role in the pathophysiology of TTS.
• Initially it was believed to be a benign and self-limiting condition, but a substantial incidence of complications occurring in the acute phase and at long-term follow-up has been demonstrated.
• Multimodality imaging is useful in risk stratification at onset and at follow-up.
• The protective role of some drugs, such as ACEI and β-blockers, in long-term follow-up should be better investigated.

INTRODUCTION

Takotsubo syndrome (TTS) is a recognized clinical entity first diagnosed by Sato and colleagues in 1990. TTS is an acute reversible heart failure syndrome, most frequently seen in postmenopausal women and precipitated generally by significant emotional stress or serious physical illness leading to activation of the sympathetic nervous system.[1–4] It is characterized by a clinical presentation miming acute myocardial infarction (AMI), with chest pain and/or dyspnea, ST segment elevation or depression, and/or T wave inversion on the resting electrocardiogram (ECG), and elevation of serum cardiac troponin.[1]

Two different forms of TTS have been recognized. In primary TTS, generally characterized by an emotional trigger, the related hospitalization arises in a context of relative well-being. However, the secondary form is usually inscribed during the evaluation or treatment of another preexisting critical illness (physical trigger), which often has already required patient hospitalization. The difference between these two settings is relevant because of different management, course, and prognosis.[2,5]

Initially, TTS was believed to represent a benign and self-limiting condition, considering its usual rapid recovery of ejection fraction within days or weeks. However, several studies demonstrated a substantial incidence of life-threatening complications occurring in the acute phase (eg, heart failure, left ventricular [LV] outflow tract obstruction [LVOTO], and mitral regurgitation [MR]) and at long-term follow-up.[6–9]

No conflict of interest to declare.
[a] A.O.U. San Giovanni di Dio e Ruggi d'Aragona, Largo Città d'Ippocrate 1, CAP 84131, Salerno, Italy;
[b] Division of Cardiology, A.O.R.N. Antonio Cardarelli Hospital, Via Antonio cardarelli 9, 80131 Naples, Italy;
[c] Department of Cardiology, Gifu University Graduate School of Medicine, Gifu, Yanagido 1-1, Gifu, Gifu 501-1194, Japan; [d] Division of Cardiology, Department of Internal Medicine, St. Marianna University School of Medicine, 2 Chome-16-1 Sugao, Miyamae Ward, Kawasaki, Kanagawa 216-8511, Japan
* Corresponding author. A.O.U. San Giovanni di Dio e Ruggi d'Aragona. Largo Città d'Ippocrate 1, CAP 84131, Salerno, Italy.
E-mail address: rodolfocitro@gmail.com

Heart Failure Clin 18 (2022) 125–137
https://doi.org/10.1016/j.hfc.2021.08.001
1551-7136/22/© 2021 Elsevier Inc. All rights reserved.

In the literature, there are no clinical trials enrolling patients with TTS, but data from large national and international registers are available: TIN Registry (TakoTsubo Italian Network); Inter-TAK Registry (International Takotsubo registry); GEIST Registry (German, Italian, Spanish Takotsubo registry); RETAKO Registry (Registry on Takotsubo Syndrome), the largest series compiled in Spain; SWEDENHEART Registry; and Japanese registries.

In the present article comprehensive data on epidemiology, pathogenesis, and clinical course of TTS are reviewed.

EPIDEMIOLOGY

Since the initial Japanese description, TTS has been increasingly recognized in different countries. TTS is estimated to represent approximately 1% to 3% of all and 5% to 6% of female patients presenting with suspected ST-segment elevation myocardial infarction (STEMI). However, with increasing awareness and more widespread access to early invasive coronary angiography, TTS is now recognized more frequently.[9–11] Recent studies report in western societies worsening mental health and increasing rates of stress and anxiety, already well-known predisposing factors to developing TTS. Minhas and colleagues[12] reported a significant increase of incidence almost 20 times in the US TTS population. The incidence of primary TTS increased from 2.3 hospitalizations per 100,000 person-years in 2007 to 7.1 in 2012. The corresponding incidence for secondary TTS increased from 3.4 hospitalizations per 100,000 person-years in 2007 to 10.3 in 2012. About 90% of patients with TTS are women with a mean age of 65 to 70 years. Most (80%) are older than 80 years.[9,13] Women older than 55 years have a five-fold greater risk of developing TTS and a 10-fold greater risk than men.[10] However, male patients are diagnosed more often, especially after a physical trigger, such as severe critical medical illnesses.[14] Of note, the TTS prevalence in men seems to be higher in Japan.[15] TTS has also been described in children, the youngest patient reported was a premature neonate born.[16,17]

There are no large-scale data for racial differences, but TTS seems to be uncommon in African-Americans (who experience more in-hospital complications, such as respiratory failure and stroke, and require more frequent mechanical ventilation) and Hispanics, and most of the cases diagnosed in the United States are in Whites.[3,18] A significant chronobiologic variation of TTS occurrence has been reported, characterized by a peak in the summer season, in opposite to AMI pattern.[19]

Pelliccia and colleagues[20] investigated the comorbidities prevalence in 1109 patients with TTS. A relevant prevalence of cardiovascular risk factors and associated comorbidities was found, with a frequency similar in patients with acute coronary syndrome (ACS). Indeed, in a large series of 305 women with acute LV dysfunction, Parodi and colleagues[21] found no difference in the prevalence of hypertension, hypercholesterolemia, and smoking between those with TTS and those with anterior myocardial infarction. In the COUNT study, 17% of patients were obese, 54% had hypertension, 32% had dyslipidemia, 17% had diabetes, and 22% were smokers. These data agree with previous observations of Summer and colleagues.[22] Thus, it might be that a higher prevalence of risk factors leads to premorbid endothelial dysfunction, which, in turn, might be a predisposing factor of TTS. Moreover, a higher prevalence of psychological disorders, pulmonary diseases, malignancy, neurologic diseases, chronic kidney disease, and thyroid diseases was also found. Furthermore, cerebrovascular accidents are correlated with a 10-fold higher odds of TTS. Summers and colleagues[22] demonstrated that women diagnosed with TTS were more likely to have chronic anxiety disorder before the event compared with control subjects and those with AMI. Burgdorf and colleagues[23] reported that patients with TTS more commonly had a previous diagnosis of malignancy or developed malignancies during follow-up, and El-Sayed and colleagues[24] reported an increased prevalence of cancer in these patients.

Tornvall and colleagues[25] enrolled patients from the SCAAR (Swedish Coronary Angiography and Angioplasty Registry, a component of the SWEDE-HEART registry) Registry. The results of the study showed that 15% of patients with TTS had psychiatric disorders. The prevalence of affective and anxiety disorders was higher than in coronary artery disease (CAD) control subjects, which supports findings from previous studies.[25]

Redfors and colleagues[26] investigated 15,348 patients from the prospective SCAAR registry, of whom 302 were confirmed with TTS. The incidence was approximately 2%, similar to those reported previously, and patients with TTS were not older than patients with ACS. Overall, neither baseline characteristics differed more between these two groups of patients. Approximately 14% of the patients diagnosed with TTS had significant concomitant CAD and 4% of them had previously suffered a myocardial infarction, and one patient had previously undergone coronary artery bypass grafting. Thus, these data confirmed that patients with advanced CAD may develop TTS.

PATHOGENESIS

The exact TTS pathophysiology is not yet known. However, significant progress has been made over the last decade, thanks to an increase in laboratory and clinical studies.[27] Several different pathophysiologic pathways may act, individually or synergistically, leading to TTS, but none fully explains all the mechanisms underlying TTS stunning.[28]

A sudden sympathetic activation and serum catecholamines surge seems to play a key role in the pathophysiology of TTS. Indeed, the levels of plasma catecholamine are up to three times elevated in patients with TTS and this syndrome has been reported in many patients diagnosed with pheochromocytoma or subarachnoid hemorrhage.[1,2] Probably, a localized dysregulation of myocardial sympathetic physiology occurs and leads to a variety of regional ballooning patterns.[29] Catecholamines may have a direct or indirect role in myocardial stunning. Macrovascular and microvascular dysfunction with abnormal vasomotor reactivity, through coronary vasoconstriction, could contribute to the pathophysiology in a subset of patients.[30] Epicardial coronary vasospasm was episodically reported during diagnostic angiography in patients with TTS, but vasospasm could be an epiphenomenon because of exposure to high epinephrine and norepinephrine levels.[29,30] However, most patients with TTS do not show any evidence of epicardial spasm, even with the use of provocative agents. Although a reduced microvascular blood flow was reported in the acute phase of TTS, against this microcirculatory hypothesis, Redfors and colleagues[31] demonstrated that contractile dysfunction was not preceded by any alteration in myocardial perfusion, using contrast echocardiography in rat model.

However, there is clinical and preclinical evidence of direct effect of catecholamines on cardiomyocyte function, via calcium overload, reactive oxidative species production, and mitochondrial dysfunction following intense activation of the β-adrenoreceptors (bARs) coupled to the stimulatory Gs protein-adenylyl cyclase-cyclic adenosine monophosphate (cAMP) protein kinase A secondary messenger pathway. The b1AR and b2AR density is highest in the apex, whereas there is an apical-basal gradient of sympathetic nerve density, with the highest sympathetic innervation in the basal LV myocardium and lowest in the apical one, so apical myocardium may be more sensitive to high levels of catecholamines.[32–34] It is now recognized that epinephrine at high levels, paradoxically, exerts a negative inotropic effect, inducing a desensitization process because of

molecular switch of the b2AR from Gs to Gi (inhibitory) protein expression.[35] Moreover, recent studies reported abnormalities in the functional structure and activity in the areas of the brain related to emotions and the sympathetic nervous system. MIBG studies in patients with TTS showed that regional myocardial uptake of MIBG was markedly decreased in the apical akinetic regions of the LV, which suggested disturbances in presynaptic norepinephrine uptake and an increased presynaptic catecholamine discharge. These abnormalities may persist even 12 months after recovery of contractile function.[36]

Another hypothesis proposed is centered on estrogen deprivation. Estrogen has a sympatholytic effect and decreases the number of bARs receptors in cardiac cells.[37] Therefore, reduced estrogen levels during menopause increases sympathetic function and subsequent endothelial dysfunction. Ueyama and colleagues[38] showed, in an experimental study, the prevention of stress-induced LV apical ballooning in rats by pretreatment with estrogen.

Recently, abnormal myocardial metabolism was reported in apical segments during the acute phase in patients with TTS. Particularly, during the TTS acute phase, regional free fatty acid use and extracellular glucose transport were acutely reduced in the affected apical myocardial segments, but not the basal segments. This is explained by the shutdown of mitochondrial metabolism in the hypokinetic or akinetic apical segments.[39]

Evidence is emerging about the possible role of inflammation in the subacute and chronic phases, contributing to long-term cardiac dysfunction and symptoms, because of a systemic inflammatory response syndrome. Despite the macroscopic myocardial recovery, a persistence of microscopic cellular changes has been suggested from recent data. Of note, inflammation pathways involve intramyocardial and systemic inflammation.[40] Recently, several studies showed a prevalence of incomplete recovery of about 16%, highlighting as independent factors elevated C-reactive protein levels at discharge. Moreover, patients with persistent myocardial dysfunction presented a significantly higher incidence of cardiovascular mortality.[41] Neil and colleagues[42] first reported the presence of persistent edema in the affected segments 3 to 4 months after the acute episode, and recently, Scally and colleagues[39] demonstrated abnormalities, including low-grade inflammation at 12 months from the acute TTS episode in some patients.

However, future research is needed to understand myocardial-specific mechanisms, to improve clinical decision-making, the quality of life, and outcomes for patients with TTS.

CLINICAL COURSE
Clinical Presentation

TTS is an acute and usually reversible heart failure syndrome, often resulting from a stressful emotional or physical triggering event. It is the most important differential diagnosis of ACS because of its similar presentation in clinical symptoms, ECG, and cardiac biomarker changes, but with no evidence of culprit atherosclerotic CAD at coronary angiography.[1,2]

ST segment elevation amplitude in TTS is usually lower than in anterior STEMI and after 48 hours in most patients tends to disappear; this evolution might reflect the norepinephrine half-life in stress conditions (8–12 hours). Moreover, the ST segment elevation and troponin I increase magnitude do not correlate with the amount of dysfunctional myocardium at the echocardiographic examination.[2,43]

Specific TTS biomarkers are not described, but troponin I increase is generally detected. Of note, myocardial enzymes rise is lower in patients with TTS than in ACS.[1-3] Moreover, because TTS is characterized by an acute heart failure at onset, plasmatic B-type natriuretic peptide is usually elevated in these patients.[44]

The most common symptoms of TTS are acute chest pain, dyspnea, or syncope, but TTS may be diagnosed incidentally by new ECG changes or a sudden elevation of cardiac biomarkers. Of note, the clinical manifestation of TTS induced by severe physical stress may be dominated by the manifestation of the underlying acute illness.[1,2] Patients with ischemic stroke or seizure-triggered had less frequent chest pain, because of impaired consciousness.[45] However, patients with emotional stress frequently present with chest pain and palpitations.[46] Moreover, a subset of patients with TTS may present with symptoms arising from complications, such as heart failure, pulmonary edema, cardiogenic shock (CS), or cardiac arrest. Most patients with TTS assume dual antiplatelet therapy at admission, but once the diagnosis has been established, only aspirin is continued for 3 months after hospital discharge. There are different types of triggers, physical and emotional. Physical triggers are more common than emotional stressors, particularly in male patients.[9] Of note, precipitating triggers may represent a combination of emotional and physical issues (eg, panic attacks during a medical procedures).[9] However, a specific trigger is not identifiable in about one-third of patients.[47]

Emotional triggers include a range of negative emotions, such as fear, panic, grief (death of a family member, friend), interpersonal conflicts (divorce), and anxiety. Natural disasters are also associated with an increase in TTS events.[6] However, positive emotional events may provoke TTS.[3] Instead, physical stressors may be related to physical activities (sports), medical conditions, or such procedures as cesarean section.[48] Exogenous drugs, such as catecholamines, and sympathomimetic drugs may also act as triggers for TTS including dobutamine stress testing and β-agonists for pulmonary disease.[49] Nervous system conditions (stroke, head trauma, seizures, intracerebral hemorrhage) also represent an important TTS trigger.[50,51] Endogenous catecholamine spillover related to pheochromocytoma represents a distinct physical trigger.[52]

In patients with TTS recruited from the InterTAK Registry,[53] dyspnea was more prevalent than in patients with ACS, whereas chest pain was less frequently reported. ST segment depression occurred less frequently in the TTS group (10.6% vs 28.9%; $P<.001$), whereas T wave inversion was more often noted (35.3% vs 23.4%; $P = .001$). Moreover, QTc prolongation is an ECG hallmark of patients with TTS.[54]

The analysis of 1071 patients enrolled in the multicentric international TTS registry GEIST, showed that dyspnea at hospital admission is present in one-third of patients admitted with TTS.[55] Several cardiac mechanisms could be responsible for dyspnea in the setting of an acute heart failure syndrome including systolic and diastolic dysfunction,[56] mitral insufficiency caused by papillary muscles dysfunction,[57] atrial fibrillation, and heart rate. It is associated with coexisting comorbidities and worse cardiac function during the early phase and is an independent predictor of in-hospital complications and long-term mortality in these patients.[55]

The multicenter Spanish Registry RETAKO is a prospective, voluntary, national registry. The main reason for consulting was chest pain, present in 80.1% of patients, most of whom had good previous functional status. Among these patients, 72.8% reported triggers, such as intense emotional stress, which occurred in 101 patients (50%). On ECG, patients generally showed sinus rhythm (83.7%), and ·anomalies were common (89.1%). The abnormalities seen were mainly in the precordial leads; 61.8% of patients showed ST segment elevation in at least one lead. A negative T wave was seen in 39.5% on the initial test. This finding explained the frequent development of a corrected (lengthened) QT interval (QTc), defined as greater than 450-millisecond duration, which was observed in 78.8% of patients, leading to torsades de pointes. Biomarkers of myocardial necrosis were not high.[57–59]

Data obtained from the SCAAR Registry highlighted an incidence of angina of 73%, dyspnea of 32%, and syncope of 8%. In 38% of cases, a trigger could not be identified, whereas 38% of patients presented an emotional trigger and 22% a physical one.[25] ECG variables and clinical characteristics assessed in this study highlighted two variables that differed significantly between patients with and without in-hospital major adverse cardiac events (MACE). T wave inversions were present at the time of admission in half of our patients with TTS increasing in incidence during hospitalization, and is more common in TTS compared with ACS and is associated with lower risk of MACE, driven by a lower risk of ventricular tachycardia/ventricular fibrillation. This finding is consistent with previous studies. The only other variable that was associated with MACE in this study was sinus rhythm, which was associated with a lower risk of MACE compared with atrial arrhythmias. Other ECG findings that have been reported include ST elevation, fragmented QRS, pathologic Q waves, prolonged QTc, and left bundle branch block. Prolongation of the QTc interval was not significantly more common for patients without versus with MACE.[60]

In a systematic review of 1109 patients from North America, Europe, Asia, and Australia, emotional stressors occurred in 428 patients (39%) and physical stressors in 379 patients (35%), whereas no precipitating event could be identified in 13% of patients. Most patients complained of chest pain (55%), but many patients suffered from dyspnea (26%). Nearly half of patients had ST changes (53%) and Q waves or T changes (49%).[20]

Diagnostic Criteria

Abe and colleagues[61] introduced the first diagnostic criteria for TTS in 2003, later adopted by the Mayo Clinic.[62] In 2014 the Italian group of the Tako-tsubo Italian Network[63] pointed out the possible coexistence of nonsignificant CAD and/or "no culprit" lesions at coronary angiography. Recently, the study group TTS of the Heart Failure Association European Cardiology has defined its diagnostic criteria by developing an algorithm used as a practical guide in the differential diagnosis between TTS and ACS, based on various clinical-instrumental parameters.[1] If the diagnosis has remained uncertain, the diagnostic algorithm precedes the use of imaging methods, such as echocardiography and MRI with late gadolinium enhancement (LGE) in the follow-up, to verify the complete recovery of myocardial function and ventricular morphology, confirming the diagnosis.

Based on the most recent knowledge, the new diagnostic criteria from the experience of the largest international InterTAK registry, have now been adopted, and are also useful in the prognostic stratification of patients with TTS (**Box 1**).[2] The new aspects to underline are the following. The prevalence of significant concomitant CAD is reported in a higher percentage of TTS, ranging from 10% to 29%. In the differential diagnosis, it is important to consider that, unlike myocardial infarction where a territorial regionality of the ischemic myocardium is respected depending on the epicardial coronary artery involved, in TTS the regional kinetics anomalies usually extend beyond the distribution of a single coronary. Furthermore, TTS can coexist with ACS, indeed myocardial infarction can itself trigger TTS.[64] Coronary angiography is fundamental to discriminate between TTS and myocardial infarction with nonobstructive coronary arteries, such as spontaneous coronary dissection, coronary spasm, myocardial bridge, coronary embolism, and so forth.[65] The second innovation is that, albeit rarely, myocardial dysfunction may also be limited of a single coronary territory, in cases of focal TTS involving the anterolateral wall.[63,66]

Another novelty is the creation of the InterTAK diagnostic score, which estimates the presence of TTS with high sensitivity and distinguishes TTS from ACS with high specificity (**Table 1**). An InterTAK score less than or equal to 50 points suggests a medium-low probability of TTS, whereas a score greater than or equal to 50 indicates a high probability.[54] Therefore, patients with low probability should immediately undergo coronary angiography and ventriculography, whereas patients with a high score and who are hemodynamically stable could undergo only transthoracic echocardiography. If a typical pattern for TTS is confirmed, a less invasive method may be useful, such as angiotomography, to rule out ACS.

A differential diagnosis with infectious myocarditis represents another challenging point. More advanced imaging methods, in particular cardiac magnetic resonance (CMR), allow demonstrating myocardial edema, inflammation, and fibrosis thanks to the use of LGE.[66]

Multimodality Imaging

Although echocardiography is the first-line imaging modality in patients with suspicion of TTS, assessment of coronary anatomy by coronary angiography and left ventriculography plays a key role in TTS diagnostic work-up to rule out

Box 1
InterTAK diagnostic criteria

1. Patients show transient left ventricular dysfunction (hypokinesia, akinesia, or dyskinesia) presenting as apical ballooning or midventricular, basal, or focal wall motion abnormalities. Right ventricular involvement can be present. Besides these regional wall motion patterns, transitions between all types can exist. The regional wall motion abnormality usually extends beyond a single epicardial vascular distribution; however, rare cases can exist where the regional wall motion abnormality is present in the subtended myocardial territory of a single coronary artery (focal TTS).

2. An emotional, physical, or combined trigger can precede the TTS event, but this is not obligatory.

3. Neurologic disorders (eg, subarachnoid hemorrhage, stroke/transient ischemic attack, or seizures) and pheochromocytoma may serve as triggers for TTS.

4. New ECG abnormalities are present (ST segment elevation, ST segment depression, T wave inversion, and QTc prolongation); however, rare cases exist without any ECG changes.

5. Levels of cardiac biomarkers (troponin and creatine kinase) are moderately elevated in most cases; significant elevation of brain natriuretic peptide is common.

6. Significant coronary artery disease is not a contradiction in TTS.

7. Patients have no evidence of infectious myocarditis

8. Postmenopausal women are predominantly affected.

From Ghadri JR, Wittstein IS, Prasad A, Sharkey S, Dote K, Akashi YJ, Cammann VL, Crea F, Galiuto L, Desmet W, Yoshida T, Manfredini R, Eitel I, Kosuge M, Nef HM, Deshmukh A, Lerman A, Bossone E, Citro R, Ueyama T, Corrado D, Kurisu S, Ruschitzka F, Winchester D, Lyon AR, Omerovic E, Bax JJ, Meimoun P, Tarantini G, Rihal C, Y-Hassan S, Migliore F, Horowitz JD, Shimokawa H, Lüscher TF, Templin C. International Expert Consensus Document on Takotsubo Syndrome (Part I): Clinical Characteristics, Diagnostic Criteria, and Pathophysiology. Eur Heart J. 2018 Jun 7;39(22):2032-2046.

Table 1
InterTAK diagnostic score

Female sex	25 points
Emotional stress	24 points
Physical stress	13 points
No ST segment depression	12 points
Psychiatric disorders	11 points
Neurologic disorders	9 points
QTc prolongation	6 points
≤50 points: *low/intermediate probability of TTS*	*≥50 points: high probability of TTS*

differentiation of TTS from anterior STEMI,[69] particularly in the presence of the apical nipple sign (a very small zone with preserved contractility of the LV apex), in about 30% of patients with TTS and hawk's beak appearance in patients with the midventricular form.[70] Moreover, conventional angiography is useful for the exclusion of other types of myocardial infarction with nonobstructive coronary arteries, such as plaque rupture or erosion, and spontaneous coronary artery dissection.

The first-line imaging modality for the evaluation of patients suspected for TTS is transthoracic echocardiography, not only for the diagnosis but also to identify patients at higher risk of acute complications and to monitor regression of wall motion abnormalities (WMAs).[71] Transthoracic echocardiography may help to determine the morphologic anatomic variant. Typically, TTS is characterized by apical ballooning in about 60% to 80% of cases (involving the apical and midventricular segments, which seem akinetic or dyskinetic, in contrast to the basal hyperkinetic segments).[72,73] However, other variants have been described: midventricular TTS (akinesis of the midventricular segments, mild hypokinesis, or normal contraction of the apical segments and hypercontractility of the base) and inverted TTS (with apical sparing and severe hypokinesis of the other walls or with basal or reverse TTS, with hypokinesis confined to the basal segments).[73] Another rare variant is the focal form, associated with limited and rapidly reversible WMAs. Right ventricular (RV) involvement also should be assessed and is usually identified by the detection of severe akinesis or dyskinesis, localized at the apical and/or mid-RV segments (biventricular ballooning),[74] configuring the reverse McConnell sign.[75] Its involvement has been associated with adverse in-hospital outcomes.[76]

alternative diagnoses, especially ACS. Obstructive single-vessel coronary lesions are not an exclusion criterion for diagnosis, because myocardial dysfunction usually extends beyond a single epicardial vascular distribution in TTS.[66-68] Biplane left ventriculography allows for the

Spontaneous myocardial function recovery and diastolic indices, namely the E/e′ ratio, should be assessed systematically to identify patients at higher risk for acute adverse events (LVOTO, reversible moderate to severe MR, RV involvement, LV thrombi, and pericardial effusion) and to guide appropriate management. Given that diastolic dysfunction is also transient and reversible, improvement in the E/e′ ratio is used as an additional marker of LV functional recovery.[55,72] Strain imaging by speckle tracking echocardiography allows assessment of global and regional myocardial function in all three layers of the myocardium, highlighting circumferential pattern in patients with TTS.[77,78]

Moreover, evaluation of coronary flow in the distal part of the left anterior descending artery by transthoracic Doppler can differentiate TTS from AMI because of left anterior descending artery occlusion.[79] In patients with poor acoustic window, to better define regional wall motion and the possible presence of intraventricular thrombus contrast echocardiography could be used.[71] Recently, the use of three-dimensional echocardiography is spreading, because it is more accurate to assess myocardial function and RV involvement.[71]

CMR plays a key role in the comprehensive assessment of the functional and structural changes that occur in patients suspected for TTS. During the acute phase, T2-weighted sequences show a high-intensity signal corresponding to myocardial edema of the territory affected by abnormal segmental kinetics on echocardiography. This is a TTS hallmark, whereas the edema distribution follows the distribution territory of the culprit epicardial coronary artery in ACS and the basal and lateral subepicardial segments in myocarditis.[71] Moreover, CMR can rule out ischemic myocardial damage or myocarditis using LGE imaging. LGE in myocarditis reveals patchy myocardial necrosis and fibrosis in 88% of patients. Although the absence of LGE is a common finding in patients with TTS, several studies have reported a subtle focal or patchy LGE also in these patients when using LGE signal intensity threshold of three standard deviations. If signal intensity threshold is five standard deviations, no areas of LGE are detectable in patients with TTS.[80]

In the postacute phase, CMR should be performed within 2 months, especially in case of persisting ECG abnormalities and/or regional WMAs at echocardiography, to definitively confirm the TTS diagnosis.

Cardiac computed tomography also plays an important role in the diagnostic work-up of acute chest pain to exclude conditions, such as pulmonary embolism and aortic dissection, and may be useful in stable patients with a low probability of ACS or in suspected TTS recurrence.[71]

In-hospital Course and Follow-Up

Several studies have demonstrated a substantial incidence of life-threatening complications occurring in the acute phase, with intrahospital mortality ranging from 1% to 4.5%.[81] Although TTS is a reversible condition, hemodynamic and electrical instability during the acute phase expose patients to the risk of serious adverse in-hospital events.

The major clinical complications in the acute phase are: heart failure/pulmonary edema (12%–45%), reversible dynamic LVOTO (10%–25%), CS (6%–20%), major ventricular arrhythmias (ventricular tachycardia/fibrillation 4%–9%), cardiac tamponade (<1%), and wall rupture (<1%).[59,81–83] Therefore, in all patients diagnosed with TTS, risk stratification should be performed by integrating hemodynamic, electrocardiographic (continuous electrocardiographic monitoring for at least 48 hours, including a periodic assessment of the QTc interval), and echocardiographic parameters. Higher risk patients should be monitored for a longer period of time (minimum 72 hours from presentation).[1]

- Acute heart failure complicated by pulmonary congestion/edema, because of severe impairment of LV function, is the most common complication.[1,83]
- LVOTO (defined as an intraventricular gradient >25 mm Hg), results from basal hypercontractility in the small LV cavity with asymmetric hypertrophy of the interventricular septum (**Fig. 1**).[84] It has been described in 10% to 25% of patients with TTS. The reported prevalence in literature is 12%, 7%, and 25% in the TIN registry, RETAKO registry, and El Mahmoud 10,366 patients' series, respectively.[85,86] This complication requires caution in the use of inotrope drugs and close hemodynamic and echocardiographic monitoring to verify their effectiveness. The cautious administration of fluids associated with intravenous short-half-life β-blockers (especially esmolol), improving cardiac filling, and reducing basal segments hypercontractility, have proven effective in reducing LVOTO.[87]
- CS is a potentially fatal complication. It is important to assess whether reduced cardiac output leading to hypotension is caused by LVOTO or by severe LV dysfunction, because the management of these two conditions is different.[1,9,57]
- Arrhythmias, atrial and ventricular, are a common complication during the acute phase of

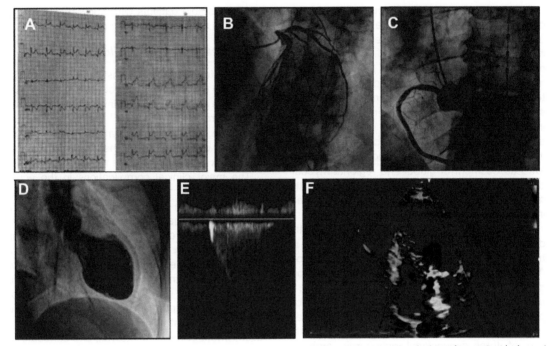

Fig. 1. (*A–F*) TTS clinical case. (*From* Mauro C, Vriz O, Romano L, Citro R, Russo V, Ranieri B, Alamro B, Aladmawi M, Granata R, Galzerano D, Bellino M, Cocchia R, Mehta RM, Dellegrottaglie S, Alsergani H, Mehta RH, Bossone E. Imaging Cardiovascular Emergencies: Real World Clinical Cases. Heart Fail Clin. 2020 Jul;16(3):331-346.)

TTS, occurring in 20% to 25% of cases. The predisposing factors for ventricular arrhythmias are: younger age, male sex, severe reduced LV ejection fraction (LVEF), higher troponin level, and QTc interval greater than 510 milliseconds, with the consequent risk of torsade de pointes. However, ventricular arrhythmias in TTS are generally limited to the acute phase, therefore the defibrillator implant is generally not indicated.[88]

- TTS may be associated with systemic hypercoagulability, because of sympathetic hyperactivation, so during the acute phase, patients are potentially at risk of arterial and venous thromboembolic disease. In patients with reduced ejection fraction less than 35% and apical ballooning pattern, the risk of ventricular thrombi formation and systemic embolism was documented in 2% to 12% of cases.[82]
- Mild pericardial effusions have been documented in approximately 40% of patients with TTS. Acute pericarditis to be treated with colchicine and pericardial tamponade requiring pericardiocentesis were both rare (<1%).[89]
- Rupture of the free wall of the left ventricle or perforation of the interventricular septum, often preceded by persistent elevation of the ST segment, occur in less than 1% of patients.[89]

Multicenter registers experience
Recent data from the InterTAK Registry revealed that short- and long-term outcomes of patients with TTS are similar to those of patients with ACS.[9–23,25] Advanced age, hypotension at hospital admission, severe LV systolic (LVEF <35%) and diastolic dysfunction, and significant MR are all conditions associated with increased risk of early adverse events. Other parameters predicting adverse in-hospital outcomes are: physical trigger, acute neurologic or psychiatric diseases, and troponin greater than 10 upper reference limit.[9,57]

Of note, patients with a severe reduction in LVEF (<35%), compared with those with less impaired systolic function, more frequently experienced an adverse outcome not only in the acute phase but also at long-term follow-up.[90] Furthermore, in the InterTAK Registry, patients with TTS complicated by CS present an increased risk of mortality in the short term and at 5 years of follow-up. These clinical observations suggest that more extensive myocardial stunning because of catecholamine release leads not only to more severe acute systolic dysfunction but also to greater long-term cardiac functional and structural changes. This incomplete recovery is consistent with the persistence of newly diagnosed cardiac symptoms, including angina, exertional dyspnea, palpitations, dizziness, and anxiety.[91]

Moreover, RV involvement has been shown to be a negative prognostic factor for acute heart failure, CS, and in-hospital death. Its prevalence is low, about 13.4%, but these patients should undergo close clinical and echocardiographic monitoring.[75,76]

In the RETAKO Registry experience, the common acute complications include acute heart failure (8.9%), arrhythmias (28%, mainly supraventricular), renal failure, iatrogenic complications, and others derived from comorbidities. Despite the short follow-up of this study (3.2 months), a generally favorable outcome following hospital discharge was observed.[58] Almendro-Delia and colleagues[92] demonstrated that out of a total of 711 patients, 11.4% developed CS and in-hospital complication rates, including mortality, were significantly higher in this subgroup. At long-term follow-up, CS was the strongest independent predictor of all-cause mortality, cardiovascular, and noncardiovascular death, whereas no significant difference in the recurrence rate was observed between groups. Male sex, QTc interval prolongation, lower LVEF at admission, physical triggers, and presence of LVOTO were associated with CS. Uribarri and colleagues[59] also confirmed that patients with TTS related to physical stress present a worse short- and long-term prognosis in terms of mortality, also in cardiovascular mortality. Recently, in patients enrolled in InterTAK, stratified according to the trigger event, it was also shown that patients presenting with emotional triggers had a better short- and long-term prognosis, whereas patients with secondary TTS caused by neurologic diseases experienced the absolute worst prognosis.[91]

In a prognostic study on 1007 patients enrolled in GEIST registry, in-hospital complications among patients with TTS mainly consisted of acute heart failure, including CS and pulmonary edema, with an incidence ranging from 12% to 45%. The in-hospital mortality rate for TTS was approximately 4.2%, with a higher rate among male patients and patients with secondary TTS. Acute complications may be associated with a worse outcome at long-term follow-up.[93] Patients with TTS with in-hospital complications had higher mortality rates at 2.6 ± 2 years follow-up. From this analysis derived a clinical score based on four clinical and echocardiographic variables (male sex, neurologic disorders, right ventricle involvement, and LVEF), useful in early risk stratification of TTS.[93] Moreover, in this registry population has been demonstrated that the presence of dyspnea at admission is independently associated with complicated in-hospital course and worse long-term prognosis.[55]

Analyzing the patients enrolled in the Swedish SCAAR and RIKS-HIA registries, Redfors and colleagues[26] highlighted that the risk of CS was higher in TTS than in those with non-STEMI. Thirty-day mortality in patients with TTS was 4.1% and was comparable with ACS. Thus, TTS is not as a benign syndrome as was once believed. Ghadri and colleagues[91] also recently confirmed these Swedish data.

Several observations could explain why patients with TTS remain at high risk long after the index hospitalization. For example, the recidivism rate may be as high as 14% and may be associated with potentially lethal arrhythmias.

Recurrence

The incidence of recurrence varies from 3.5% to 10%. Both the triggering event and the ballooning pattern may differ during recurrent TTS. Although many patients have been treated with β-blockers because of their antiadrenergic action, these drugs have not shown an effective protective action and there are also conflicting results regarding the role of angiotensin-converting enzyme inhibitors (ACEI) and angiotensin receptor blockers.[6,9] However, in the InterTAK observational register, the ACEI or angiotensin receptor blockers assumption was associated with an improvement in survival at 1-year follow-up, unlike β-blockers.[9]

To date, it is difficult to provide specific recommendations because of the lack of randomized controlled clinical trials. Psychological support and estrogen implementation may be helpful.

SUMMARY

TTS syndrome is a pathology still partly unknown. From the pathophysiologic point of view, several complex mechanisms involving the central nervous system, peripheral nerves, receptor systems, inflammatory markers, chemical, and hormonal mediators seem to be involved in the appearance of a common phenotype of reversible myocardial dysfunction. Why there are categories predisposed to develop TTS, such as postmenopausal women, patients with mood disorders, thyroid disorders, asthmatic crisis, malignancies, and so forth remains a mystery to be clarified. It is still unclear how and why myocardial stunning most often involves the apex and why there are variant forms involving other parts of the left ventricle and the right ventricle. Unresolved issues remain the possible persistence of myocardial damage because of incomplete recovery and its impact on prognosis. A knowledge gap regarding the identification of specific biomarkers, the selection of patients at risk, the duration of hospitalization, the management of mechanical and arrhythmic complications during the acute phase, and the modalities and timing of follow-up needs to be addressed. The application of multimodality imaging should be encouraged, not only for diagnostic purpose but also for in-hospital and long-term prognostic stratification. The protective role of some drugs, such as ACEI and β-blockers, in long-term follow-up and the impact of this disease on quality of life and its medical-legal implications should be deeply investigated.

CLINICS CARE POINTS

- Although about 90% of patients with TTS are women with a mean age of 65 to 70 years, male patients are diagnosed more often, especially after a physical trigger, and experience worse outcomes.

- The prevalence of significant concomitant CAD in patients with TTS ranges from 10% to 29%, so CAD evidence at coronary angiography should not rule out TTS diagnosis.

- Some categories, such as patients with mood disorders, thyroid disorders, and malignancies, are predisposed to develop TTS.

- Although TTS was believed to represent a benign and self-limiting condition, several studies have demonstrated in-hospital mortality ranging from 1% to 4.5%, comparable with ACS and adverse long-term outcomes, compared with the general population.

- Echocardiography should be used early at hospital admission, to identify higher-risk patients and to adopt adequate therapeutic management.

- Multimodality imaging, including CMR, could be useful in the diagnostic work-up to rule out other clinical conditions, such as myocarditis, ACS, and myocardial infarction with nonobstructive coronary arteries.

REFERENCES

1. Lyon AR, Bossone E, Schneider B, et al. Current state of knowledge on Takotsubo syndrome: a position statement from the Taskforce on Takotsubo Syndrome of the Heart Failure Association of the European Society of Cardiology. Eur J Heart Fail 2016;18:8–27.
2. Ghadri JR, Wittstein IS, Prasad A, et al. International expert consensus document on Takotsubo syndrome (Part I): clinical characteristics, diagnostic criteria, and pathophysiology. Eur Heart J 2018;39: 2032–46.
3. Ghadri JR, Sarcon A, Diekmann J, et al. Happy heart syndrome: role of positive emotional stress in Takotsubo syndrome. Eur Heart J 2016;37:2823–9.
4. Kato K, Lyon AR, Ghadri JR, et al. Takotsubo syndrome: aetiology, presentation and treatment. Heart 2017;103:1461–9.
5. Medina de Chazal H, Del Buono MG, Keyser-Marcus L, et al. Stress cardiomyopathy diagnosis and treatment: JACC state-of-the-art review. J Am Coll Cardiol 2018;72:1955–71.
6. Sharkey SW, Windenburg DC, Lesser JR, et al. Natural history and expansive clinical profile of stress (takotsubo) cardiomyopathy. J Am Coll Cardiol 2010;55:333–41.
7. Akashi YJ, Goldstein DS, Barbaro G, et al. Takotsubo cardiomyopathy: a new form of acute, reversible heart failure. Circulation 2008;118:2754–62.
8. Citro R, Rigo F, Previtali M, et al. Differences in clinical features and in-hospital outcomes of older adults with takotsubo cardiomyopathy. J Am Geriatr Soc 2012;60:93–8.
9. Templin C, Ghadri JR, Diekmann J, et al. Clinical features and outcomes of takotsubo (stress) cardiomyopathy. N Engl J Med 2015;373:929–38.
10. Deshmukh A, Kumar G, Pant S, et al. Prevalence of Takotsubo cardiomyopathy in the United States. Am Heart J 2012;164:66–71.
11. Brinjikji W, El-Sayed AM, Salka S. In-hospital mortality among patients with takotsubo cardiomyopathy: a study of the National Inpatient Sample 2008 to 2009. Am Heart J 2012;164:215–21.
12. Minhas AS, Hughey AB, Kolias TJ. Nationwide trends in reported incidence of takotsubo cardiomyopathy from 2006 to 2012. Am J Cardiol 2015;116: 1128–31.
13. Schneider B, Athanasiadis A, Stollberger C, et al. Gender differences in the manifestation of takotsubo cardiomyopathy. Int J Cardiol 2013;166:584–8.
14. Park JH, Kang SJ, Song JK, et al. Left ventricular apical ballooning due to severe physical stress in patients admitted to the medical ICU. Chest 2005; 128:296–302.
15. Aizawa K, Suzuki T. Takotsubo cardiomyopathy: Japanese perspective. Heart Fail Clin 2013;9:243–7.
16. Otillio JK, Harris JK, Tuuri R. A 6-year-old girl with undiagnosed hemophagocytic lymphohistiocytosis and takotsubo cardiomyopathy: a case report and review of the literature. Pediatr Emerg Care 2014;30:561–5.
17. Rozema T, Klein LR. Takotsubo cardiomyopathy: a case report and literature review. Cardiol Young 2016;26:406–9.
18. Nascimento FO, Larrauri-Reyes MC, Santana O, et al. Comparison of stress cardiomyopathy in Hispanic and non-Hispanic patients. Rev Esp Cardiol (Engl Ed) 2013;66:67–8.
19. Citro R, Previtali M, Bovelli D, et al. Chronobiological patterns of onset of Takotsubo cardiomyopathy: a

multicenter Italian study. J Am Coll Cardiol 2009; 54(2):180–1.

20. Pelliccia F, Parodi G, Greco C, et al. Comorbidities frequency in Takotsubo syndrome: an international collaborative systematic review including 1,109 patients. Am J Med 2015;128(6):654.e11-9.

21. Parodi G, Del Pace S, Carrabba N, et al. Incidence, clinical findings, and outcome of women with left ventricular apical ballooning syndrome. Am J Cardiol 2007;99(2):182–5.

22. Summers MR, Lennon RJ, Prasad A. Premorbid psychiatric and cardiovascular diseases in apical ballooning syndrome (takotsubo/stress-induced cardiomyopathy): potential pre-disposing factors? J Am Coll Cardiol 2010;55(7):700–1.

23. Burgdorf C, Kurowski V, Bonnemeier H, et al. Long-term prognosis of the transient left ventricular dysfunction syndrome (Takotsubo cardiomyopathy): focus on malignancies. Eur J Heart Fail 2008;10(10):1015–9.

24. El-Sayed AM, Brinjikji W, Salka S. Demographic and co-morbid predictors of stress (Takotsubo) cardiomyopathy. Am J Cardiol. 2012;110(9):1368–72.

25. Tornvall P, Collste O, Ehrenborg E, et al. A case-control study of risk markers and mortality in Takotsubo stress cardiomyopathy. J Am Coll Cardiol 2016; 67(16):1931–6.

26. Redfors B, Vedad R, Angeras O, et al. Mortality in takotsubo syndrome is similar to mortality in myocardial infarction: a report from the SWEDEHEART registry. Int J Cardiol 2015;185:282–9.

27. Akashi YJ, Nef HM, Lyon AR. Epidemiology and pathophysiology of Takotsubo syndrome. Nat Rev Cardiol 2015;12:387–97.

28. Lyon AR, Citro R, Schneider B, et al. Pathophysiology of takotsubo syndrome: JACC state-of-the-art review. J Am Coll Cardiol 2021;77(7):902–21.

29. Wittstein IS, Thiemann DR, Lima JA, et al. Neurohumoral features of myocardial stunning due to sudden emotional stress. N Engl J Med 2005;352:539–48.

30. Fiol M, Carrillo A, Rodriguez A, et al. Left ventricular ballooning syndrome due to vasospasm of the middle portion of the left anterior descending coronary artery. Cardiol J 2012;19:314–6.

31. Redfors B, Shao Y, Wikstrom J, et al. Contrast echocardiography reveals apparently normal coronary perfusion in a rat model of stress-induced (Takotsubo) cardiomyopathy. Eur Heart J Cardiovasc Imaging 2014;15:152–7.

32. Kawano H, Okada R, Yano K. Histological study on the distribution of autonomic nerves in the human heart. Heart Vessels 2003;18:32–9.

33. Lyon AR, Rees PSC, Prasad S, et al. Stress (Takotsubo) cardiomyopathy: a novel pathophysiological hypothesis to explain catecholamine-induced acute myocardial stunning. Nat Clin Pract Cardiovasc Med 2008;5:22–9.

34. Mori H, Ishikawa S, Kojima S, et al. Increased responsiveness of left-ventricular apical myocardium to adrenergic stimuli. Cardiovasc Res 1993;27:192–8.

35. Paur H, Wright PT, Sikkel MB, et al. High levels of circulating epinephrine trigger apical cardiodepression in a beta2-adrenergic receptor/Gi-dependent manner: a new model of Takotsubo cardiomyopathy. Circulation 2012;126:697–706.

36. Madias JE. Do we need MIBG in the evaluation of patients with suspected Takotsubo syndrome? Diagnostic, prognostic, and pathophysiologic connotations. Int J Cardiol 2016;203:783–4.

37. Machuki JO, Zhang HY, Harding SE, et al. Molecular pathways of oestrogen receptors and b-adrenergic receptors in cardiac cells: recognition of their similarities, interactions and therapeutic value. Acta Physiol (Oxf) 2018;222:e12978.

38. Ueyama T, Kasamatsu K, Hano T, et al. Catecholamines and estrogen are involved in the pathogenesis of emotional stress-induced acute heart attack. Ann N Y Acad Sci 2008;1148:479–85.

39. Scally C, Rudd A, Mezincescu A, et al. Persistent long-term structural, functional, and metabolic changes after stress-induced (Takotsubo) cardiomyopathy. Circulation 2018;137:1039–48.

40. Yoneyama K, Akashi YJ. Myocardial contractile function recovery, systemic inflammation, and prognosis in Takotsubo syndrome. Circ J 2021. Online ahead of print.

41. Matsushita K, Lachmet-Thébaud L, Marchandot B, et al. Incomplete recovery from Takotsubo syndrome is a major determinant of cardiovascular mortality. Circ J 2021.

42. Neil C, Nguyen TH, Kucia A, et al. Slowly resolving global myocardial inflammation/oedema in Takotsubo cardiomyopathy: evidence from T2-weighted cardiac MRI. Heart 2012;98:1278–84.

43. Santoro F, Stiermaier T, Tarantino N, et al. ST-elevation magnitude and evolution in Takotsubo syndrome. Int J Cardiol 2018;257:39.

44. Nguyen TH, Neil CJ, Sverdlov AL, et al. N-terminal pro-brain natriuretic protein levels in Takotsubo cardiomyopathy. Am J Cardiol 2011;108(9):1316–21.

45. Jung JM, Kim JG, Kim JB, et al. Takotsubo-like myocardial dysfunction in ischemic stroke: a hospital-based registry and systematic literature review. Stroke 2016;47:2729–36.

46. Song BG, Yang HS, Hwang HK, et al. The impact of stressor patterns on clinical features in patients with takotsubo cardiomyopathy: experiences of two tertiary cardiovascular centers. Clin Cardiol 2012;35:E6–13.

47. Gianni M, Dentali F, Grandi AM, et al. Apical ballooning syndrome or takotsubo cardiomyopathy: a systematic review. Eur Heart J 2006;27:1523–9.

48. Citro R, Lyon A, Arbustini E, et al. Takotsubo syndrome after cesarean section: rare but possible. J Am Coll Cardiol 2018;71(16):1838–9.

49. Abraham J, Mudd JO, Kapur NK, et al. Stress cardiomyopathy after intravenous administration of catecholamines and beta-receptor agonists. J Am Coll Cardiol 2009;53:1320–5.

50. Scheitz JF, Mochmann HC, Witzenbichler B, et al. Takotsubo cardiomyopathy following ischemic stroke: a cause of troponin elevation. J Neurol 2012;259:188–90.

51. Stollberger C, Wegner C, Finsterer J. Seizure-associated Takotsubo cardiomyopathy. Epilepsia 2011; 52:e160–7.

52. Y-Hassan S, Falhammar H. Clinical features, complications, and outcomes of exogenous and endogenous catecholamine-triggered Takotsubo syndrome: a systematic review and meta-analysis of 156 published cases. Clin Cardiol 2020;43(5):459–67.

53. Ghadri JR, Cammann VL, Templin C. The International Takotsubo Registry: rationale, design, objectives, and first results. Heart Fail Clin 2016;12: 597–603.

54. Ghadri JR, Cammann VL, Jurisic S, et al. A novel clinical score (InterTAK Diagnostic Score) to differentiate takotsubo syndrome from acute coronary syndrome: results from the International Takotsubo Registry. Eur J Heart Fail 2016;19(8):1036–42.

55. Arcari L, Musumeci MB, Stiermaier T. Incidence, determinants and prognostic relevance of dyspnea at admission in patients with Takotsubo syndrome: results from the international multicenter GEIST registry. Sci Rep 2020;10(1):13603.

56. Medeiros K, O Connor MJ, Baicu CF, et al. Systolic and diastolic mechanics in stress cardiomyopathy. Circulation 2014;129:1659–67.

57. Citro R, Rigo F, D'Andrea A, et al. Echocardiographic correlates of acute heart failure, cardiogenic shock, and in-hospital mortality in Takotsubo cardiomyopathy. JACC Cardiovasc Imaging 2014;7: 119–29.

58. Nunez Gil IJ, Andrés M, Almendro Delia M, et al. Characterization of Takotsubo cardiomyopathy in Spain: results from the RETAKO National Registry. Rev Esp Cardiol 2015;68(6):505–12.

59. Uribarri A, Nunez-Gil IJ, Conty A, et al. Short- and long-term prognosis of patients with Takotsubo syndrome based on different triggers: importance of the physical nature. J Am Heart Assoc 2019;8:e013701.

60. Jha S, Zeijlon R, Enabtawi I, et al. Electrocardiographic predictors of adverse in-hospital outcomes in the Takotsubo syndrome. Int J Cardiol 2020;299: 43–8.

61. Abe Y, Kondo M, Matsuoka R, et al. Assessment of clinical features in transient left ventricular apical ballooning. J Am Coll Cardiol 2003;41:737–42.

62. Prasad A, Lerman A, Rihal CS. Apical ballooning syndrome (Takotsubo or stress cardiomyopathy): a mimic of acute myocardial infarction. Am Heart J 2008;155:408–17.

63. Parodi G, Citro R, Bellandi B, et al. Revised clinical diagnostic criteria for Takotsubo syndrome: the Takotsubo Italian Network proposal. Int J Cardiol 2014;172:282–3.

64. Y-Hassan S. Clinical features and outcome of pheochromocytoma-induced takotsubo syndrome: analysis of 80 published cases. Am J Cardiol 2016;117:1836–44.

65. Thygesen K, Alpert JS, Jaffe AS, et al. Fourth universal definition of myocardial infarction (2018). Circulation 2018;138:e618–51.

66. Kato K, Kitahara H, Fujimoto Y, et al. Prevalence and clinical features of focal takotsubo cardiomyopathy. Circ J 2016;80:1824–9.

67. Ghadri JR, Wittstein IS, Prasad A, et al. International expert consensus document on Takotsubo syndrome (Part II): diagnostic workup, outcome, and management. Eur Heart J 2018;39:2047–62.

68. Parodi G, Citro R, Bellandi B, et al. Takotsubo cardiomyopathy and coronary artery disease: a possible association. Coron Artery Dis 2013;24: 527–33.

69. Patel SM, Lennon RJ, Prasad A. Regional wall motion abnormality in apical ballooning syndrome (Takotsubo/stress cardiomyopathy): importance of biplane left ventriculography for differentiating from spontaneously aborted anterior myocardial infarction. Int J Cardiovasc Imaging 2012;28:687–94.

70. Desmet W, Bennett J, Ferdinande B, et al. The apical nipple sign: a useful tool for discriminating between anterior infarction and transient left ventricular ballooning syndrome. Eur Heart J Acute Cardiovasc Care 2014;3:264–7.

71. Citro R, Okura H, Ghadri JR, et al. Multimodality imaging in takotsubo syndrome: a joint consensus document of the European Association of Cardiovascular Imaging (EACVI) and the Japanese Society of Echocardiography (JSE). J Echocardiogr 2020; 18:199–224.

72. Citro R, Rigo F, Ciampi Q, et al. Echocardiographic assessment of regional left ventricular wall motion abnormalities in patients with takotsubo cardiomyopathy: comparison with anterior myocardial infarction. Eur J Echocardiogr 2011;12:542–9.

73. Citro R, Lyon AR, Meimoun P. Standard and advanced echocardiography in takotsubo (stress) cardiomyopathy: clinical and prognostic implications. J Am Soc Echocardiogr 2015;28(1):57–74.

74. Citro R, Caso I, Provenza G, et al. Right ventricular involvement and pulmonary hypertension in an elderly woman with takotsubo cardiomyopathy. Chest 2010;137:973–5.

75. Liu K, Carhart R. "Reverse McConnell's sign?": a unique right ventricular feature of Takotsubo cardiomyopathy. Am J Cardiol 2013;111:1232–5.

76. Citro R, Bossone E, Parodi G, et al. Independent impact of RV involvement on in-hospital outcome

of patients with takotsubo syndrome. JACC Cardio-vasc Imaging 2016;9:894–5.

77. Pilgrim TM, Wyss TR. Takotsubo cardiomyopathy or transient left ventricular apical ballooning syndrome: a systematic review. Int J Cardiol 2008;124:283–92.

78. Kobayashi Y, Okura H, Kobayashi Y, et al. Left ven-tricular myocardial function assessed by three-dimensional speckle tracking echocardiography in Takotsubo cardiomyopathy. Echocardiography 2017;34:523–9.

79. Watanabe N. Noninvasive assessment of coronary blood flow by transthoracic Doppler echocardiogra-phy: basic to practical use in the emergency room. J Echocardiogr 2017;15:49–56.

80. Eitel I, von Knobelsdorff-Brenkenhoff F, Bernhardt P, et al. Clinical characteristics and cardiovascular magnetic resonance findings in stress (takotsubo) cardiomyopathy. JAMA 2011;306:277–86.

81. Citro R, Bossone E, Parodi G, et al. Clinical profile and in-hospital outcome of caucasian patients with takotsubo syndrome and right ventricular involve-ment. Int J Cardiol 2016;219:455–61.

82. Schneider B, Athanasiadis A, Schwab J, et al. Com-plications in the clinical course of takotsubo cardio-myopathy. Int J Cardiol 2014;176:199–205.

83. Madhavan M, Rihal CS, Lerman A, et al. Acute heart failure in apical ballooning syndrome (TakoTsubo/stress cardiomyopathy): clinical correlates and Mayo Clinic risk score. J Am Coll Cardiol 2011;57:1400–1.

84. Mauro C, Vriz O, Romano L, et al. Imaging cardio-vascular emergencies: real world clinical cases. Heart Fail Clin 2020;16(3):331–46.

85. Yoshioka T, Hashimoto A, Tsuchihashi K, et al. Clin-ical implications of midventricular obstruction and intravenous propranolol use in transient left

ventricular apical ballooning (Takotsubo cardiomy-opathy). Am Heart J 2008;155(3):526.e1-7.

86. Mahmoud EI, Mensencal N, Pilliere R, et al. Preva-lence and characteristics of left ventricular outflow tract obstruction in Takotsubo syndrome. Am Heart J 2008;156(3):543–8.

87. Santoro F, Ieva R, Ferraretti A, et al. Hemodynamic effects, safety, and feasibility of intravenous esmolol infusion during takotsubo cardiomyopathy with left ventricular outflow tract obstruction: results from a multicenter registry. Cardiovasc Ther 2016;34:161–6.

88. Pant S, Deshmukh A, Mehta K, et al. Burden of ar-rhythmias in patients with Takotsubo cardiomyopa-thy (apical ballooning syndrome). Int J Cardiol 2013;170:64–8.

89. Parodi G, Scudiero F, Citro R, et al. Risk stratification using the CHA(2)DS(2)-VASc Score in Takotsubo syndrome: data from the Takotsubo Italian Network, Takotsubo Italian Network (TIN). J Am Heart Assoc 2017;6(9):e006065.

90. Citro R, Radano I, Parodi G, et al. Long-term outcome in patients with Takotsubo syndrome pre-senting with severely reduced left ventricular ejec-tion fraction. Eur J Heart Fail 2019;21(6):781–9.

91. Ghadri JR, Kato K, Camman VL, et al. Long-term prognosis of patients with Takotsubo syndrome. J Am Coll Cardiol 2018;72(8):874–82.

92. Almendro-Delia M, Nunze-Gil IJ, Lobo M, et al. Short- and long-term prognostic relevance of cardio-genic shock in Takotsubo syndrome. JACC Heart Fail 2018;6(11):928–36.

93. Santoro F, Núñez Gil IJ. Assessment of the German and Italian stress cardiomyopathy score for risk stratification for in-hospital complications in patients with Takotsubo syndrome. JAMA Cardiol 2019;4(9):892–9.

Genetics in Congenital Heart Diseases

Unraveling the Link Between Cardiac Morphogenesis, Heart Muscle Disease, and Electrical Disorders

Anwar Baban, MD, PhD[a],*, Valentina Lodato, MD[a],
Giovanni Parlapiano, MD[b], Fabrizio Drago, MD[a]

KEYWORDS

- Congenital heart diseases (CHDs) • Progressive aspect • Cardiomyopathies (CMPs) • Arrhythmias
- Genotype-phenotype correlation

KEY POINTS

- Potential progressivity in cardiac phenotype secondary to genetically determined variants.
- Genes known to be causative for congenital heart diseases (CHDs) can predispose to cardiomyopathies (CMPs) or major arrhythmic events.
- Clinicians must be aware of underestimated progressive cardiac phenotype in some of the genetically determined CHDs. Stratification of risk is required in certain CHDs.
- Potential red flags for genetically determined and potentially progressive conditions in CHDs include familial CHDs, progressive arrhythmic events, and myocardial dysfunction unexplained by hemodynamic factors. The identification of etiologic factors can be an example of conducting a personalized medicine care and tailored patient management.
- Left ventricular noncompaction (LVNC) in CHDs can be a risk factor for perioperative complications and increased morbidity and mortality.

BACKGROUND

Congenital heart diseases (CHDs) represent about 0.8% to 1% livebirths.[1] This value is progressively changing with the rapid advances in tools applied in prenatal diagnosis. CHDs are caused by several mechanisms where most are multifactorial.[2] Most CHDs are isolated with no evidence of other affected organ systems. Incidence is similar in both sexes, but males are more affected by severe lesions. Ancestry and ethnicity can sometimes modify the incidence of specific abnormalities.[3] The origin of CHDs is majorly unknown. However,

a classification according to etiologic basis can be observed in different literature data. CHDs in chromosomal abnormalities represent ~8% to 10% of all CHDs. In approximately 30% a monogenic/digenic involvement is reported.[4] In fact, wide genetic heterogeneity including incomplete penetrance and variable expressivity is the rule in CHDs.

INSIGHT IN PATHOGENESIS

About 400 genes coding for transcription factors, cell signaling transducers, and chromatin

---

[a] Department of Pediatric Cardiology and Cardiac Surgery, Bambino Gesù Children Hospital and Research Institute, IRCCS, Piazza Sant'Onofrio 4, 00165 Rome, Italy; [b] Laboratory of Medical Genetics, Bambino Gesù Children Hospital and Research Institute, IRCCS, Piazza Sant'Onofrio 4, 00165 Rome, Italy
* Corresponding author. Department of Pediatric Cardiology and Cardiac Surgery, Bambino Gesù Children Hospital and Research Institute, Piazza Sant'Onofrio 4, 00165 Rome, Italy.
E-mail addresses: anwar.baban@opbg.net; cardiogenetica@opbg.net

Heart Failure Clin 18 (2022) 139–153
https://doi.org/10.1016/j.hfc.2021.07.016
1551-7136/22/© 2021 Elsevier Inc. All rights reserved.

modifiers are associated with CHD pathogenesis. Many of these protein products collaborate synergistically and in specific pathways determining cell type specification, differentiation, and development of cardiac structure and function. Among the principal genes implicated in CHDs there are transcription factors such as *NKX2-5, GATA* family, *T-Box* family, *Forkhead Box* family, nuclear receptors family, and *HAND* family. Also a lot of signaling pathways such as Nodal signaling, Notch signaling and others, myofilament and extracellular matrix proteins, chromatin modifiers, cilia and cilia-transduced cell signaling, and RAS/MAPK cascade may be involved in the pathogenesis of CHDs. CHDs are classified according to various criteria. The phenotype is generally divided into main categories: right-sided lesions, left-sided lesions, conotruncal defects, laterality defects, and isolated septal defects.[2]

Comparative transcriptome studies have highlighted the possible involvement in the formation of the cardiac atrial septum, cardiomyocyte proliferation, and heart muscle development not only of known specific cardiac transcription factors (such *GATA4* and *NKX2-5*) and extracellular signal molecules (*VEGFA* and *BMP10*) but also of cardiac sarcomeric proteins like *MYL2, MYL3, MYH7, TNNT1,* and *TNNT3*. Wang and colleagues[5] demonstrated their dysregulation in atrial septal defect (ASD), one of the most common CHD subtype. Among these, proteins belonging to the cell cycle pathway also play a role.[5] All these data reflect the potential synergy of genes as a continuity in predisposition to the complete spectrum of malformative, functional, and arrhythmic changes.

Is There a Link Among Congenital Heart Diseases and Potentially Progressive Heart Diseases (Cardiomyopathies and Arrhythmias)?

Rapidly growing studies in literature are bringing light into a new era in understanding not only the origin of CHDs but also the pathophysiology and potential clinical risk stratification and implications in clinical management.

Understanding the genetic background of CHDs can lead to a potential modification in the risk stratification of patients undergoing clinical and surgical management in terms of perioperative management: risk of heart failure, anesthetic complications, length of stay in intensive care unit, respiratory problems, pulmonary vascular resistance, infectious risk, and predisposition to lymphatic complications such as chylothorax, bleeding, and thrombotic risk.[6–8]

CHDs, cardiomyopathies (CMPs), and arrhythmias were previously thought to be separate entities. This aspect is slowly vanishing, and determined lines separating these 3 major groups seem to be inconsistent when deep genotyping and even phenotyping is undertaken. In fact with advanced technologies (conclusion of human genome project and rapid diffusion of next-generation sequencing [NGS]) and growing clinical observations, it has been shown that the same gene can predispose to CHDs, CMPs, and/or progressive arrhythmic events within one family or within the same individual. The aim of this review is to delineate this aspect through increasingly reported evidences in the literature. We try to exchange views on the potential progressive nature of certain genetic disorders classically known to be causative of "static" cardiac events. We try to bring examples of different genetic causes starting from chromosomal, copy number variants (CNVs) and ending up with examples from monogenic disorders.

CMPs have been classified as primary or secondary by the American Heart Association (AHA). In the first case the disease involves only the myocardium, whereas secondary CMP is part of a systemic condition. However, the 2 conditions sometimes overlap.

Primary CMPs may have genetic, acquired, or mixed etiology. Genetics of childhood CMPs is complex, potentially underestimated, and underdiagnosed due to complexity, rarity, and above all heterogeneity. CHDs in association with genetically determined CMP is a rapidly expanding issue because of the potential complications and importance of perioperative preparation. Determining whether congestive heart failure in a child is due to anatomic/hemodynamic causes rather than "endogenic"/primary CMP might completely change the prognostic issue.[9]

On the other hand, CHDs can be associated to arrhythmic conditions, which can be primary or secondary in nature. CHDs might be caused by sinus node or atrioventricular (AV) conduction system abnormalities, abnormal hemodynamics, primary myocardial disease, hypoxic tissue damage, or residual or postoperative sequelae. Sinus node abnormalities can be congenitally totally or partially absent (left atrial [LA] isomerism), displaced (hearts with juxtaposition of the LA appendages or with sinus venous defects of superior vena cava [SVC] type), doubled (right isomerism), or dysfunctional (absent right SVC). Atrioventricular block (AVB) can be due to conduction system displacement with abnormal development of the central fibrous body in congenitally corrected transposition of the great arteries (CC-TGA) (2% per year) or in individuals with isomeric derangement of the atrial appendages.[10] We can observe in heart defects with AV discordance 2 distinct AV nodes ("twin AV nodes"). Accessory AV connections may be present in patients with Ebstein anomaly. Multiple accessory pathways are often found in other conditions like heterotaxy syndromes, CC-TGA, atrioventricular canal (AVC) defects (AVCDs), and univentricular physiology. Regarding tachyarrhythmias, a relatively high percentage of all adult patients with CHD develop supraventricular tachycardia (SVT) such as intra-atrial reentry tachycardias and atrial flutter over the course of their lives and also other rarer forms. Ventricular ectopy and nonsustained ventricular tachycardias (VTs <30 s; NSVT) are common. Sustained ventricular arrhythmias (monomorphic VT, polymorphic VT, and ventricular fibrillation [VF]) can be observed in tetralogy of Fallot (TOF), complex forms of dextrotransposition of the great arteries (d-TGA), systemic right ventricles, and left ventricular (LV) outflow tract obstructive lesions.[11]

Bradyarrhythmia in CHD can be due to complete heart block (CC-TGA, atrioventricular septal defect [AVSD], heterotaxy syndrome, L-looped single ventricle).[11]

A surprisingly mixed form of bradyarrhythmia and tachyarrhythmia due to sinus node dysfunction can be associated with LA isomerism.[10–12]

Deciphering the Cause of Certain Congenital Heart Diseases from Progressive Point of View

In the following sections we decipher some of the genetic conditions that are related to CHDs but with potential progressive aspects including myocardial dysfunction (CMPs), progressive arrhythmic events (both in tachyarrhythmia and bradyarrhythmia), or vascular involvement. We selected specific conditions (chromosomal aneuploidies, CNVs, and monogenic disorders) in which phenotypic overlap of a wide spectrum of cardiac manifestations is still underestimated but rapidly emerging. This relatively new vision might change the way a clinician can manage a CHD in terms of risk stratification and clinically oriented prevention/delay of complications.

Chromosomal Aneuploidies

Down syndrome

As originally described by Garrod in 1894, Down syndrome (DS) (MIM # 190685), the commonest chromosomal aneuploidy (prevalence: 1–5 in 10,000), is often associated with CHD (44%–58%), with a relatively fixed pattern of defects: AVSDs (17%–43%), ventricular septal defects (VSDs, 11%–33%), ASDs (7%–11%), and patent ductus arteriosus (PDA, 2%–6%), followed by TOF (2%–6%).

CMPs are rarely reported in DS.[6,13–15] We revised the literature in this term and identified 13 patients with primary myocardial disease (5 hypertrophic, 2 unspecified, 1 arrhythmogenic cardiomyopathy, 3 endocardial fibroelastosis, 1 left ventricular noncompaction [LVNC], and 1 myocardial fibrosis). In our published cohort, we found 1 patient with infantile-onset dilated cardiomyopathy (DCM) and 2 patients with hypertrophic cardiomyopathy (HCM) and AVSD. The latter showed marked LV hypertrophy without any specific loading or hemodynamic factors that could account for this condition. Both of them were successfully corrected for AVSD. The patient with DCM is on regular heart failure treatment.

Regarding major arrhythmic abnormalities, in our cohort, we noticed AVB in 27 patients, mainly subjected to AVSD repair (18 of 27, 66.7%). AVBs requiring pacemaker implantation (14; 51.9%) were observed postoperatively in those operated in the late 1990s and the early 2000s (range 1991–2004).

Trisomy 18

Trisomy 18 was described for the first time by Edwards in 1960, and it is the second most common autosomal trisomy syndrome after trisomy 21 (overall prevalence 1 in 6000 live births). The main clinical signs are prenatal intrauterine growth restriction (IUGR), specific craniofacial features, major malformations and significant intellectual disability, and other minor anomalies. CHDs like ASD, VSD, PDA, and polyvalvular disease are present in more than 90% of children.[16]

However, myocardial involvement is reported in a variable spectrum even if it is still considered an unusual condition in trisomy 18. Among these, 2 patients with biventricular HCM have been reported by Limongelli and colleagues[17] and by Banka and colleagues,[18] in the latter case in a mosaicism condition. In 2011, LVNC was described in a newborn with trisomy 18.[19] In an older report (1968), a case of postmortem extensive myocardial fibrosis in a 5-month-old female infant with trisomy 18 syndrome was described by Kurien and Duke.[20]

Specific arrhythmic spectrum is not largely observed in trisomy 18. However, it is majorly associated to the structural abnormalities.

Turner syndrome

Turner syndrome (TS) is one of the commonest chromosomal abnormalities in 1 to 5 of 10,000. CHDs occur in 23% to 50% of individuals with TS and are mainly divided into 2 groups: left ventricular outflow anomalies (LVOTA) and vascular abnormalities. LVOTA are most common, with a prevalence of 15% to 30% for bicuspid aortic valve (BAV) and 7% to 18% for aortic coarctation (CoA). Additional, but less frequent, anomalies include hypoplastic left heart syndrome (HLHS) and mitral valve anomalies. Variable degree of congenital coronary arterial anomalies is prevalent in TS.[21–23]

A variety of other cardiovascular conditions are emerging in association with TS, including early-onset hypertension, ischemic heart disease, and stroke.[22] For instance, hypertension is one of the most important modifiable risk factors in TS: leading to increased aortic diameter, myocardial hypertrophy, stroke, and myocardial infarction. Although hypertension is a recognizable morbidity in TS, little is documented about its measurement, definitions, and management.[24]

The association of TS and CMP is rarely reported (5 times in literature, including one patient published in our series). The major phenotype included LVNC (3 patients were morphologically diagnosed without functional impact, whereas the other 2 developed heart failure that needed medical treatment).[25,26]

Copy Number Variants

Genomic microarrangement (CNV) syndromes are also frequently associated with CHD. Large de novo CNVs (present in the probands but absent in both parents) have been reported in sporadic CHD. Previous studies estimate that 5% to 10% of sporadic, nonsyndromic CHD in patients with normal karyotype is secondary to a rare (≤1% population frequency) CNV. Some CNVs encompass genes with important role in heart development including basic science studies of model organisms.[27]

22q11.2 deletion syndrome
The 22q11.2 deletion syndrome (22q11.2DS) (MIM # 192430 # 188400) is the most frequent chromosomal microdeletion syndrome of varying sizes (0.7–3 Mb), but most frequently ∼3 Mb, resulting in a highly variable clinical presentation. The estimated prevalence ranges from 1:3000 to 1:6000 live births. 22q11.2DS has been identified in most patients with DiGeorge syndrome, velocardiofacial syndrome, and conotruncal anomaly face syndrome.[28]

CHDs are present in 75% to 80% of patients with 22q11.2DS, and they represent the main cause of mortality. Commonly, CHDs comprise outflow tracts defects, including TOF; pulmonary atresia with VSD; interruption of aortic arch (13%), mainly type B; truncus arteriosus (6%);

and VSD. Aortic arch anomalies, either in association with intracardiac anomalies or isolated, are also commonly seen: cervical aortic arch, double aortic arch, right-sided aortic arch, and abnormal origin of the subclavian arteries.

The association of CMP in 22q11.2DS is rarely reported. An interesting report from 2006 described 2 neonates with ventricular dysfunction who had restoration of normal ejection fraction after medical treatment and appropriate management of severe hypocalcemia. Other sporadic reports of LVNC in 22q11.2DS are also described almost always in association with CHDs.[26–29] Another potential progressive aspect in microdeletion 22q11.2 includes aortic root dilatation[30] where clinical management and wider clinical observations need to be collected at multicentric level.

Williams syndrome
In Williams syndrome (WS) (MIM # 194050) cardiovascular involvement includes both malformative aspect, progressive elastin arteriopathy, and "dynamic/functional" abnormalities in terms of arterial hypertension. WS is a relatively frequent microdeletion syndrome with estimated prevalence of approximately 1 in 7500.

Elastin arteriopathy is estimated in 75% to 80% of affected individuals and may affect any artery.[31–34] LVOT anomalies are the commonest mainly due to supravalvar aortic stenosis, but they can affect any part of the aorta.[35] HCM in WS has been previously reported.[36] However, it is really difficult to determine whether it is a primary manifestation or secondary to hemodynamic aspects related to LVOTO.

Arrhythmias, mainly QTc prolongation, are described in more than one report in WS.[34,37,38] The cause is difficult to be determined because it can be secondary to anatomic/hemodynamic background or it can be an independent factor secondary to double hit of 2 genetically determined conditions probably due to the common prevalence of both diseases (channelopathies causing long QT syndrome [LQTS] and WS). Multicentric studies are needed to determine this peculiar association.

1p36 deletion syndrome
1p36 deletion is the most common subtelomeric microdeletion observed in humans with an estimated incidence of 1 in 5000 to 1 in 10,000 live births. 1p36 deletion (MIM # 607872) results in a contiguous gene syndrome characterized mainly by multiple congenital anomalies and intellectual disability.[39] The most common CHDs are ASD and VSD, PDA, valvular anomalies, TOF, and CoA.[40] Progressive cardiac involvement includes

an underestimated aortic dilatation[40,41] and relatively more known myocardial changes including LVNC in terms of morphologic involvement down to severe end-stage heart failure.[26,40,42] Genes that may contribute to the development of CMP associated with 1p36 deletions include *SKI, PRKCZ, PRDM16, RERE, UBE4B,* and *MASP2.* Several lines of evidence show that *PRDM16* haploinsufficiency contributes to LVNC and CMD. *PRDM16* is located in the critical region for CMP defined by Gajecka and colleagues,[43] and multiple animal models show that its haploinsufficiency leads to ventricular hypoplasia and abnormal ventricular morphology. Literature revision reports that variants in *PRDM16* can be causative to isolated DCM showing potential indication of including this gene in clinical panels.[44]

6q25.1 deletion syndrome

6q25.1 deletion syndrome (MIM # 612863) is an increasingly acknowledged syndrome with a major cardiac involvement; it includes a contiguous gene syndrome with a major component involving *TAB2* (OMIM # 605101) encoding the 3K7 binding protein activated by TGF-β/MAP 3K7 (TAB2), which plays an essential role in the activation of IL-1-induced JNK/NF-K signaling. TAB2 is expressed in the endothelial lining of the developing human heart including major cytoplasmic expression in ventricular trabeculae, conotruncal cushions of outflow tract, and in developing aortic valves.[45] Haploinsufficiency of *TAB2* causes a wide spectrum of defects including variable cardiac manifestations: hypoplastic aortic arch, CoA, septal defects, valvular heart disease, premature ventricular contraction (PVC), PDA, and tachycarrhythmias[45] in addition to rare cases of HLHS[46] and TOF.[47] Indeed, a recurrent 6q25.1 deletion syndrome is characterized by cardiomyopathy, congenital heart defects, and other minor anomalies. Cheng and colleagues[48] in 2017 also described patients with CMP, dilated in some cases and nondilated (without giving explanation of the subtype) in others, with significant myocardial dysfunction not justified by their structural cardiac abnormalities. In a similar manner, *TAB2* variants can be causative to CMP with biventricular failure, as in the family described by Caulfield and colleagues[49] (p.Arg347Ter).

The extracardiac phenotype spectrum related to 6q25.1 deletion syndrome and abnormalities in *TAB2* locus is highly variable. In fact it can include facial dysmorphism, IUGR, short stature, hypotonia, connective tissue abnormalities such as joint laxity or hypermobility, and developmental delay and possible intellectual disability.[48]

This rapidly emerging phenotype might be taken into consideration in conditions of syndromic CHDs and overlapping CMP spectrum.

Monogenic Conditions

Monogenic disorders in CHDs are a relatively infrequent group but considered a rapidly growing category through increased molecular knowledge and possibility to undertake massive genomic sequencing. This highly heterogenous group includes several examples, but we opted to select the most frequent ones paying major attention to the phenotypic variability that they can cause; the panel of disorders is summarized in **Table 1** and **Fig. 1**.

Sarcomeric protein genes (MYH7)

MYH7 (myosin heavy chain 7) (MIM # 160760) encodes a sarcomeric protein. Sarcomere is the contractile unit of skeletal and cardiac striated muscle tissue. *MYH7* encompasses 23-kb genomic DNA and is composed of 41 exons, 38 of which encode a protein of 1935 amino acids. *MYH7* has 3 main regions, the head, which contains binding sites with actin and ATP; a neck, which interacts with essential light chains/regulatory light chains; and a last (rod) coil-coiled region.[50]

The role of *MYH7* is well known in several pathways ranging from heart morphogenesis and development, regulation of heart and striated muscle contractions, adult heart development, and actin-myosin filament sliding.[5] Pathogenic variants in *MYH7* are known to cause different types of CMPs such as HCM (hotspots: surface spanning the converter domain and the myosin mesa, the flat surface of the myosin catalytic domain); DCM, including peripartum; and LVNC (hotspots: segment 1 domain and the crucial functional domains of the ATP binding domain).[51] Rarely, it can be associated with skeletal myopathies. Several pathogenic *MYH7* variants show a high frequency in specific populations.[1]

As mentioned earlier, *MYH7* functional effect is not only observed in heart muscle contraction and adult heart development but also well observed in heart morphogenesis and development. This observation guided certain studies to search for *MYH7* variants in CHDs (**Fig. 2**A). The results were confirmed especially when CHDs were associated with LVNC morphology. In fact, *MYH7* variants have been described in Ebstein anomaly.[52] Less frequently it was associated with BAV[53] and VSD, ASD, pulmonary artery hypoplasia demonstrating pleiotropism, and reduced *MYH7* penetrance in the pathogenesis of CHD.[50] Often these anatomic changes were in association with CMP (typically LVNC).[1] A proposal for

Table 1
Monogenic disorders and associated phenotypic spectrum

Gene	CHDs	Cardiomyopathies	Arrhythmias	Other Manifestations/ Associated Syndrome
MYH7	ASD, VSD, Ebstein anomaly, BAV, PA hypoplasia, CoA	HCM, DCM, LVNC	Tachyarrhythmias: AF, WPW, VF, NSVT, VT	SM
GATA4	TOF, ASD, VSD, AVSD, heterotaxy spectrum	DCM, HCM	Tachyarrhythmias: AF	GUD, CDH, ID
NKX2-5	ASD, VSD, TOF, HLHS, TGA, VD	DCM, LVNC	Bradyarrhythmias: progressive CCD; tachyarrhythmias: AF, VT	
TBX5	ASD, VSD, PDA, TOF, AVCD, HLHS, TAPVR, TA	DCM, LVNC	Bradyarrhythmias: progressive CCD; tachyarrhythmias: both supraventricular (AF) and ventricular (VT, NSVT), LQTS, BrS	HOS, ULD
TBX20	ASD, DORV, TOF, TA, BAV, TAAs, VD	DCM, LVNC	Bradyarrhythmias: progressive CCD; tachyarrhythmias: PVC	

Abbreviations: AF, atrial fibrillation; BrS, Brugada syndrome; CCD, cardiac conduction defects; CDH, congenital diaphragmatic hernia; DORV, double outlet right ventricle; GUD, genitourinary defects; HOS, Holt-Oram syndrome; ID, intellectual disability; PA, pulmonary artery; SM, skeletal myopathies; TAAs, thoracic aortic aneurysms; TAPVR, total anomalous pulmonary venous return; TA, truncus arteriosus; ULD, upper-limb defects; VD, valvular dysplasia; WPW, Wolff-Parkinson-White.

genotype-phenotype correlation of CHDs in *MYH7* fails to be met because these variants scattered along the gene from head and rod (p.Met362Arg; p.Tyr283Asp; p.Tyr350Asn, p.Leu390Pro, p.Met439Arg, and p.Glu1220del; Lys1459Asn; p.Glu1573Lys; p.Asn1918Lys) of the gene have been described as associated with CHD.[50–53]

One of the described variant considered a Dutch *MYH7* founder variant p.Asn1918Lys in the tail domain (terminal region of the rod) was associated to a predisposition to childhood-onset CMP and CHDs, mainly BAV (6.3% compared with 1.4% in general population), CoA, and Ebstein anomaly. This variant was described in a rather benign course with considerable variable expressivity in terms of manifestation of either CMP or CHD.[1]

The description of sarcomeric genes in CMP, which is part of CHD, is a rapidly emerging genotype-phenotype correlation; this is not only specific to *MYH7* but also to troponin-codifying genes. In a recent description, we observed an unexplained systolic dysfunction in a patient with CHD (CoAo), which was hiding a genetic background of troponin-codifying gene *TNNT2*. In other words, unexplained CMP within CHD might be the tip of an iceberg for a misdiagnosed genetic background.[54]

Recently, Hirono and colleagues[51] analyzed potential genetic predisposition to heart failure in patients undergoing corrective surgery within CHD. The investigators identified 8 *MYH7* variants from 30 patients with LVNC and CHDs; they concluded that an association between CHD and CMP (specifically LVNC) seems to be an additional surgical risk factor. A correct prediction of the phenotype

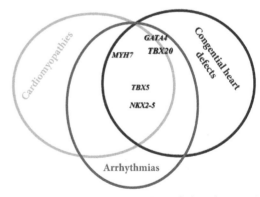

Fig. 1. Schematic representation of the phenotypic overlap of the discussed examples in monogenic disorders. Clinical characteristics include a variable degree of congenital heart defects, cardiomyopathies, and arrhythmias.

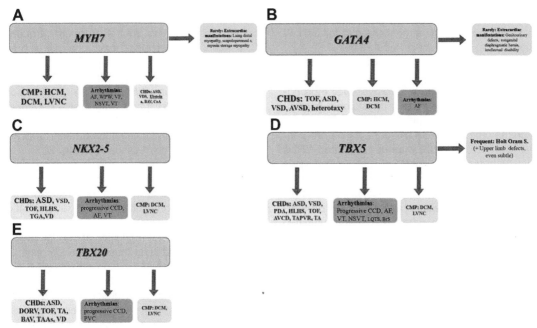

Fig. 2. Phenotypic spectrum of the discussed monogenic disorders in order of their reported frequency in literature: (*A*) *MYH7*, (*B*) *GATA4*, (*C*) *NKX2-5*, (*D*) *TBX5*, (*E*) *TBX20*. a, anomaly; BrS, Brugada syndrome; CCD, cardiac conduction defects; DORV, double outlet right ventricle; S, syndrome; TA, truncus arteriosus; TAA, thoracic aortic aneurysms; TAPVR, total anomalous pulmonary venous return; VD, valvular dysplasia; VSD, ventricular septal defect; WPW, Wolff-Parkinson-White.

therefore seems important for risk stratification in treatment planning.[51]

Previous studies show a wide spectrum of arrhythmic changes in patients with *MYH7* variants mainly in HCM phenotyping; this is explained mainly by hemodynamic consequences of LV hypertrophy, outflow obstruction, and increased LA pressure and volume, with atrial fibrillation (AF) occurring as a secondary phenomenon. Atrial dilation has also been noted in patients with *MYH7* variants and mild to moderate LV hypertrophy. On the other hand, ventricular arrhythmias are often explained in HCM-*MYH7* base due to progressive apoptotic changes, fibrosis, and cardiomyocyte damage leading to progressive arrhythmic changes.[55,56] However, progressively increasing evidence in literature described wide arrhythmic variability even independently from the degree of myocardial involvement. Some of these studies suggest that arrhythmic changes (AF, idiopathic VF) can anticipate major myocardial changes and might be a red flag for identifying the potential progressive nature of the disease especially in the presence of other factors including familial condition and unusual young age at presentation.[57,58]

Transcription Factors

Transcription factor GATA4

GATA4 (MIM #600576) encodes a zinc finger transcription factor GATA4 that interacts with several genes involved in cardiogenesis. *GATA4* consists of 442 amino acids, which determine the following conserved domains: transcription activation domain 1 (TAD1, amino acid [aa] 1–74), transcription activation domain 2 (TAD2, aa 130–177), N-terminal zinc finger (N-Znf, aa 217–241), C-terminal zinc finger (C-Znf, aa 271–295), and the nuclear localization signal (NLS, aa 271–325).[59]

In humans and animal models, *GATA4* has been demonstrated to be essential for normal cardiogenesis because it is highly expressed in cardiomyocytes at different developmental stages and continues expression in the adult cardiac myocytes, where it regulates the transcription of several key structural and regulatory genes including atrial natriuretic factor, brain natriuretic factor, carnitine palmitoyltransferase Ib, troponin I, troponin C, and a- and b-myosin heavy chain. Moreover, it forms complexes with other transcriptional factors, including *NKX2-5, TBX5, SRF, SMAD1, SMAD4,* and *JARID2.*[60–62]

Variants in *GATA4* are generally associated with CHDs such as TOF, ASD, and VSD.[63] *GATA4* variants in CHDs are scattered along the gene. However, literature revision showed that VSD-associated *GATA4* variants are mainly observed to fall mainly in the 3′ and 5′ terminals.[64]

Rarely, *GATA4* variants can be causative to complex syndromic CHDs context in association to genitourinary abnormalities even if isolated nonsyndromic CHD is almost the rule for *GATA4* variants.[65]

Over time *GATA4* is progressively reported in DCM and HCM.[63–66] This evidence confers to *GATA4* a probable role in cardiovascular morphogenesis and maintenance of physiologic homeostatic remodeling in adult hearts (**Fig. 2**B).

On the other hand, *GATA4* variants are progressively reported in DCM without associated CHDs p.Val291Leu and p.Cys271Ser.[67,68] *GATA4* plays an important role not only in cardiovascular morphogenesis but also in maintaining physiologic homeostatic remodeling in adult hearts by promoting cell survival and regeneration and inhibiting apoptosis.[69–74] *GATA4* interacts with multiple partners involved in causing CMP (including *NKX2-5* or *TBX20*, alfa-actin, alfa myosin heavy chain, troponin C, troponin I). It is therefore hypothesized that its impairment gives susceptibility to DCM by downregulating expressions of the target genes.[68–75] *GATA4* variant p.Ala343Thr has been associated with HCM and is involved in its phenotypic heterogeneity.

It was thought that the variants might impair mRNA structure as well as phosphorylation and activation of downstream target promoters by interaction with other transcription factors such as GATA6 and MEF2. In the same study, Alonso-Montes and colleagues[66] also suggest a polymorphism, T allele for p.Asn352, located in exon 6 of *GATA4*, in subjects whose age-adjusted LV mass was in the upper percentile for sex-specific distribution.

In a single study, Kwon and colleagues[70] demonstrated experimental studies involving ERRγ (estrogen-related receptor gamma)/GATA4 signal pathway in cardiac hypertrophy suggesting that these signal cascades deserve attention as potential novel therapeutic agents to prevent cardiac hypertrophy and fibrosis and that an inverse agonist of ERRγ (GSK-5182) could be considered a molecular component for the investigation of novel HCM drugs.

Transcription factor NKX2-5

NKX2-5 (MIM # 600584) is an important transcription factor for cardiac development and homeostasis. The gene is located on chromosome 5q34, is composed of 2 exons, and encodes a protein containing the homeodomain of 324 amino acids.[76] The protein is composed of 3 functional domains: the tinman domain (TN), the homeodomain (HD), and the NK2-specific domain (NK2-SD). The HD domain can either bind to the highly conserved sequence of targeted DNA fragment or undergo complex formation with other transcription factors, including GATA4, TBX5, and TBX20. Subsequently it can synergistically regulate the expression of multiple critical genes, such as troponin I, troponin C, α-actin, and α-myosin heavy chain, which are important substrates for normal myocardial functional aspect. All these data show that pathogenetic variants in *NKX2-5* can have both developmental (CHD) and progressive degenerative consequences on the heart (both arrhythmic and myocardial dysfunction) in addition to lack of adaptation of the heart tissue[64–77] (**Fig. 2**C).

NKX2-5 is involved in cardiac morphogenesis/embryogenesis including looping/tube, atrial, ventricular, and septal formations; positive regulation of cell proliferation; antiapoptosis; differentiation and development of global heart muscle cells; adult cardiac development; regulation of cardiac muscle contraction; and striated muscle development.[5]

Pathogenetic loss-of-function variants in *NKX2-5* determine relatively variable cardiac phenotype. NKX2-5 is the first transcription factor that was linked to familial ASD that includes a complex spectrum influencing trabeculation, compaction and septation, and the development of conduction system myocytes, including ASD, VSD, TOF, HLHS, TGA, and valvular abnormalities. In fact, *NKX2-5* variants can predispose to progressive cardiac arrhythmias including both bradyarrhythmias (cardiac conduction defect) and tachyarrhythmias (both supraventricular [AF] and ventricular, including VT).[64] Su and colleagues[64] summarized *NKX2-5* variants in an attempt to underline genotype-phenotype correlation. In that study they concluded that variants in TN and HD domains are those related to CHD, and specifically those of HD are correlated with ASD and AVB subtypes.

In the last few years, increasing evidence shows the role of *NKX2-5* in causing CMP (+/− LVNC). To the best of our knowledge, 8 *NKX2-5* variants have been reported in association to CMP: p.Ile184-Met, p.Ser146Trp, p.Ile184Phe, p.Arg139Trp, p.Glu167Ter, p.Phe145Leu, p.Tyr248Ter, and p.Asp226AlafsTer5[76–81] with a variable degree of penetrance. Literature report does not include genotype-phenotype correlation, although it can be observed that 6 of 8 reported variants lie in the HD domain (from 138 to 197 aa), whereas the last 2 reported by Ross and colleagues[81] lie in the NK and COOH carboxyl terminus. Haploinsufficiency and a downregulation of target genes (mainly sarcomeric) or a dominant negative effect secondary to *NKX2-5* variants could be the pathologic mechanism underlying DCM.

The cardiac phenotype in the reported DCM family was almost always associated to the "classic *NKX2-5* phenotype." In other words, a potential red flag that can help clinicians in suspecting *NKX2-5* variants includes DCM in association with progressive conduction abnormalities and ASD.

Literature reports mention a complex multisystemic involvement related to 5q34-q35.2 deletion majorly caused by contiguous gene deletion involving *NKX2-5*. The phenotype in most patients includes malformative spectrum with intellectual disability. The cardiac manifestation was within the aforementioned context including CHD, progressive conduction defects, and less frequently DCM.[82]

Transcription factor TBX5

TBX5 (MIM #601620) is T-box transcription factor 5. The gene located on 12q24.21 chromosomal region contains 9 exons and encodes for a protein of 518 amino acids. This factor is a member of T-box proteins that are involved in the regulation of cell-type mainly cardiomyocyte differentiation, morphogenesis, and organogenesis.[83] The *T-box domain* contained in these proteins is highly conserved throughout members of this family and across species. T-box 5 is a transcription factor implicated in 2 major systems: cardiac differentiation by synergistically acting with *NKX2-5, GATA4,* and TBX20 and in upper limb embryogenesis. Preferential and inconstant expression of *TBX5* in heart tissue is well established in literature. In later embryologic stages it is known to be expressed in endocardium and myocardium of the inflow region, the atria, the AVC, and the left ventricle.[84]

TBX5 is associated in 70% of cases with Holt-Oram syndrome (HOS) also known as the *heart-hand syndrome* (OMIM # 142900). This autosomal dominant condition is characterized by variable degrees of association of upper-limb defects (ULDs) and cardiac abnormalities (CHDs, arrhythmias, and recent reports of DCM). The heart-hand association is decoupled progressively in different studies showing importance of considering *TBX5* variants even in apparently isolated CHDs or ULDs[85] (**Fig. 2**D).

ULDs may be unilateral or bilateral, symmetric or asymmetric (mainly radial defects), and with variable expression: triphalangeal or absent thumbs, phocomelia, fusion or anomalous development of the carpal and thenar bones, abnormal pronation and supination, abnormal opposition of the thumb, and sloping shoulders and restriction of shoulder joint movement.[85–87] Genotype-phenotype correlation is rather difficult, and it was previously reported that variants in exons 3, 4, 5, and 7 are highly associated with the HOS subtype.[64]

The most common CHDs in *TBX5* variants are ASD, VSD, or PDA. However, complex CHDs are also described including HLHS, total anomalous pulmonary venous return, and TA. Other conotruncal association was reviews by our group including the association of *TBX5* pathogenic variants in TOF and AVCD.[85–87]

Arrhythmias are variable in *TBX5* variants wherein it was traditionally reported as progressive AVB. However, recent studies included evidence of possible predisposition to tachyarrhyhthmias (both supraventricular and ventricular ones). These data are well established in experimental studies, in sporadic reports in literature,[88,89] and from our personal observation (unpublished data, Baban, 2019).

In the past months, emerging studies have demonstrated the *TBX5* variants in channelopathies. Markunas and colleagues[90] reported a missense variant (p.Thr223Met) that cosegregates with LQTS in a family with otherwise genotype-negative LQTS and sudden death. The investigators suggested pathogenicity of the variant due to deleterious in silico scores and highly conserved region of *TBX5*.[90] In a similar manner, Nieto-Marin and colleagues[91] described other 2 variants (p.Asp111Tyr and p.Phe206Leu), related, respectively, to LQTS and Brugada syndrome (BrS), in 2 unrelated patients with structurally normal hearts. Functional studies on these variants demonstrated abnormalities in regulation of repolarization in cardiomyocytes, through a modulation of *SCN5A* transcription suggesting *TBX5* variants as a modulator for the intensity of the electrical phenotype in patients with LQTS and BrS.[91]

Regarding potential causative role of *TBX5* in DCM, loss-of-function variants in multiple transcriptional factors that synergistically act with *TBX5 (GATA4, NKX2-5, GATA6,* and *TBX20)* are well described in DCM in humans. Therefore functional defects in *TBX5* increase susceptibility to DCM by reducing functional integrity of target genes.[92] In a single study, Rathjens and colleagues[89] demonstrated in experimental studies reestablishment of normal myocardial function and rhythm in *TBX5* knockout mice by the application of *TBX5*-dependent transcriptome systemic adeno-associated virus (AAV) 9. Moreover, since 2008, Zhu and colleagues[93] have demonstrated that *TBX5* haploinsufficient mice show a significant diastolic dysfunction, a remarkable degree, and suggested an evidence for the role of *TBX5* in ventricular relaxation, which represents a major component for heart failure pathogenesis. In the same study they showed diastolic dysfunction on Doppler echocardiography in 8 patients with HOS who had normal heart structure (no CHD). In a similar manner, we have observed these data in 2 patients with HOS who showed diastolic dysfunction in the absence of hemodynamic cause that could justify it (unpublished data, Baban, 2019). These data support the association of *TBX5* variants in cardiac dysfunction independently from heart failure secondary to CHDs.[93]

Previously reported *TBX5* variants in DCM included both those with full-blown picture of HOS (associated with CHDs, arrhythmias, and ULDs) and those reported as an isolated DCM even if the detailed multisystemic phenotyping was not reported in all studies. These variants were scattered along the gene: p.Ser154Ala, p.Ala143Thr, p.Arg279Ter; p.Arg237Gln, c.363-1G>A, c.510+5G>T, p.Gln218Glu.[81,92,94–96]

Transcription factor TBX20

TBX20 (MIM #606061), located on 7p.14.2 chromosomal region, contains 8 exons and encodes for T-Box transcription factor 20, another member of the T-Box family. This protein of 447 amino acids is involved in cardiovascular development, through cardiomyocyte proliferation, and in cardiac remodeling in response to pathophysiological stress.[97] In fact, *TBX20* cardiac modulation was widely studied in murine model, demonstrating the expression in endocardium and myocardium and in the precursor structures of ventricles, cardiac valves, and AV septum.[98–100] In a recent study, Fang and colleagues[101] demonstrated that *TBX20* induction in zebrafish can promote heart regeneration by inducing cardiomyocyte dedifferentiation and endocardial expansion.

An interesting aspect of *TBX20*, as for *TBX5*, is the extreme variability of the cardiac phenotype to which it can predispose ranging from CHDs, arrhythmias, to DCM (**Fig. 2**E).

TBX20 variants are implicated in variable CHDs: ASD, aortic and mitral valve defects,[102] double outlet right ventricle,[103] TOF and TA,[104] BAV, and thoracic aortic aneurysms.[105] To the best of our knowledge genotype-phenotype correlation is unknown.

TBX20 is essential not only in heart development but also in adult heart function, homeostasis, and physiologic and pathophysiological adaptation.[99] The predisposition to DCM seems to be due to abnormalities in interaction between *TBX20* and Castor Zinc Finger Protein 1, encoded by *CASZ1*.[106] In fact *TBX20* variants can determine LV dilatation, systolic, and diastolic dysfunction.[107]

Previously described *TBX20* variants related to DCM included p.Phe256Ile, p.Glu143Ter, and p.Phe256Ile.[106,108,109] In most cases, the variants were fully penetrant in family members, and were occasionally associated to CHDs (ASD) and arrhythmias (both in bradyarrhythmia [AVB] and tachyarrhythmia [PVC]).

TBX20 was described also in association with LVNC. In 2018 it was reported in a 9-year-old girl with LVNC and restrictive physiology. The patient's mother was diagnosed to have arrhythmias, LVNC, and DCM at the age of 18 years, and she had an implantable cardioverter-defibrillator (ICD) implanted. The maternal grandmother died suddenly at age 45 years. In this family a novel *TBX20* variant (p.Met224Val) was identified.[110]

The rarity of this condition might be related to the recent focused search for variants within this gene. With time, NGS tests will determine the real frequency and phenotypic spectrum related to this condition.

SUMMARY

CHDs are a common morbidity in children. Genetic heterogeneity reigns in this field. However, rapidly growing molecular tools will progressively "purify" and stratify this group of diseases on the basis of possibly identifiable genetic background. The cause can be determined in less than half of patients. However, certain "red flags" must be taken in consideration to conditions that might be the point for an iceberg that can lead to potentially progressive dynamic condition (arrhythmic and dysfunctional substrate) that apparently seems to be static (CHDs). In other words, by reviewing previous sections, particular attention must be paid and genetic investigations can be of great help in the subtypes of CHDs with familial condition, syndromic (multiorgan) context, and progressive (both arrhythmic and myocardial/especially LVNC) association. These associations seem to be at higher risk for genetic background and subsequent need for relatively different risk stratification and patient-tailored specific management in terms of application of diagnostic tools and therapeutic measures (preoperative management, expectation for perioperative stay, postoperative ventilation period, increased risk for specific complications [arrhythmic, infectious, or dysfunctional, including PMK/ICD implant ± anti–heart failure treatment]). This management can be an example of personalized medicine care in the genomic era. More knowledge means more awareness, risk stratification, prevention, and potential search for therapeutic approaches whether in pharmacologic or interventistic terms.

CLINICS CARE POINTS

- Genetic screening in CHDs that coexist with arrhythmias and cardiomyopathy (that cannot be explained at hemodynamic level) is a promising approach; specifically, it adds prognostic information to standard risk factors for predicting new-onset heart failure, providing additional arrhythmic risk stratification; however, there is still no evidence of

- cost-effectiveness to justify its adoption at a large scale.
- Genetic evaluation and multidisciplinary management are strongly recommended in the diagnostic process of CHDs especially when a combination of structural and functional abnormalities (CMPs and arrhythmias) coexists.
- Identifying the association between CHDs, CMPs, and arrhythmias allows for risk stratification and specific management planning.
- Positive family history of CHDs, idiopathic CMP, and arrhythmias can have the same origin (variable expressivity).
- The most active research topic in the genetic field is the identification of genetic background able to identify patients with a potential worse outcome. Even if this aspect has not yet entered into clinical practice especially due to rarity, heterogeneity, and cost in applying genetic test, it warrants further discussion.
- The presence of LVNC within CHD context can represent a red flag that needs specific follow-up due to higher risk for developing CMP and arrhythmia.
- Recently, research studies are focused on the possibility of identifying specific genotype for specific cardiac phenotypes. Indeed, the possibility to identify pathophysiological pathways mostly involved in the different structural-functional phenotypes would allow a better tailoring of management and treatment.

DISCLOSURE

The authors have nothing to disclose.

ACKNOWLEDGMENTS

The authors acknowledge that the program "Cardiogenetic pathway for children with heart diseases" is part of good clinical practice project from Bambino Gesù health directorate. The authors thank Dr Federica Calì and Daniela Corbo for logistic support.

FINANCIAL CONFLICTS OF INTEREST AND FUNDING

The authors declare no conflict of interest, and funding was not obtained for producing the article.

REFERENCES

1. Van der Linde IHM, Hiemstra YL, Bökenkamp R, et al. A Dutch MYH7 founder mutation, p. (Asn1918Lys), is associated with early onset cardiomyopathy and congenital heart defects. Neth Heart J 2017;25(12):675–81.
2. Williams K, Carson J, Lo C. Genetics of congenital heart disease. Biomolecules 2019;9(12):879.
3. Nees SN, Chung WK. The genetics of isolated congenital heart disease. Am J Med Genet C Semin Med Genet 2020;184(1):97–106.
4. Geddes GC, Przybylowski LF 3rd, Ware SM. Variants of significance: medical genetics and surgical outcomes in congenital heart disease. Curr Opin Pediatr 2020;32(6):730–8.
5. Wang W, Niu Z, Wang Y, et al. Comparative transcriptome analysis of atrial septal defect identifies dysregulated genes during heart septum morphogenesis. Gene 2016;575(2 Pt 1):303–12.
6. Baban A, Olivini N, Cantarutti N, et al. Differences in morbidity and mortality in Down syndrome are related to the type of congenital heart defect. Am J Med Genet A 2020;182(6):1342–50.
7. Calcagni G, Unolt M, Digilio MC, et al. Congenital heart disease and genetic syndromes: new insights into molecular mechanisms. Expert Rev Mol Diagn 2017;17(9):861–70.
8. Baban A, Iodice FG, Di Molfetta A, et al. Deciphering genetic variants of warfarin metabolism in children with ventricular assist devices. Pediatr Cardiol 2021. https://doi.org/10.1007/s00246-021-02585-2. 10.1007/s00246-021-02585-2.
9. Brieler J, Breeden MA, Tucker J, et al. Cardiomyopathy: an overview. Am Fam Physician 2017;96(10):640–6.
10. Baban A, Cantarutti N, Adorisio R, et al. Long-term survival and phenotypic spectrum in heterotaxy syndrome: a 25-year follow-up experience. Int J Cardiol 2018;268:100–5.
11. Hernández-Madrid A, Paul T, Abrams D, et al. Arrhythmias in congenital heart disease: a position paper of the European Heart Rhythm Association (EHRA), Association for European Paediatric and Congenital Cardiology (AEPC), and the European Society of Cardiology (ESC) Working Group on Grown-up Congenital heart disease, endorsed by HRS, PACES, APHRS, and SOLAECE. Europace 2018;20(11):1719–53.
12. Di Mambro C, Calvieri C, Silvetti MS, et al. Bradyarrhythmias in repaired atrioventricular septal defects: single-center experience based on 34 years of follow-up of 522 patients. Pediatr Cardiol 2018;39(8):1590–7.
13. Assenza GE, Autore C, Marino B. Hypertrophic cardiomyopathy in a patient with Down's syndrome. J Cardiovasc Med (Hagerstown) 2007;8(6):463–4.
14. Hoe TS, Chan KC, Boo NY. Cardiovascular malformations in Malaysian neonates with Down's syndrome. Singapore Med J 1990;31(5):474–6.

15. Körten MA, Helm PC, Abdul-Khaliq H, et al. Eisen-menger syndrome and long-term survival in pa-tients with Down syndrome and congenital heart disease. Heart 2016;102(19):1552–7.

16. Cereda A, Carey JC. The trisomy 18 syndrome. Or-phanet J Rare Dis 2012;7:81.

17. Limongelli G, Pacileo G, Melis D, et al. Trisomy 18 and hypertrophy cardiomyopathy in an 18-year-old woman. Am J Med Genet A 2008;146A(3):327–9.

18. Banka S, Metcalfe K, Clayton-Smith J. Trisomy 18 mosaicism: report of two cases. World J Pediatr 2013;9(2):179–81.

19. Beken S, Cevik A, Turan O, et al. A neonatal case of left ventricular noncompaction associated with tri-somy 18. Genet Couns 2011;22(2):161–4.

20. Kurien VA, Duke M. Trisomy 17-18 syndrome. Report of a case with diffuse myocardial fibrosis and review of cardiovascular abnormalities. Am J Cardiol 1968;21(3):431–5.

21. Völkl TM, Degenhardt K, Koch A, et al. Cardiovas-cular anomalies in children and young adults with Ullrich-Turner syndrome the Erlangen experience. Clin Cardiol 2005;28(2):88–92.

22. Silberbach M, Roos-Hesselink JW, Andersen NH, et al. Cardiovascular health in turner syndrome: a scientific statement from the American Heart Asso-ciation. Circ Genom Precis Med 2018;11(10):e000048.

23. Viuff MH, Trolle C, Wen J, et al. Coronary artery anomalies in Turner Syndrome. J Cardiovasc Com-put Tomogr 2016;10(6):480–4.

24. De Groote K, Demulier L, De Backer J, et al. Arterial hypertension in Turner syndrome: a review of the literature and a practical approach for diagnosis and treatment. J Hypertens 2015;33(7):1342–51.

25. Bhatia S, Qasim A, Almasri M, et al. Left ventricular noncompaction in a child with turner syndrome. Case Rep Pediatr 2019;2019:6824321.

26. Digilio MC, Bernardini L, Gagliardi MG, et al. Syn-dromic non-compaction of the left ventricle: associ-ated chromosomal anomalies. Clin Genet 2013;84(4):362–7.

27. Fahed AC, Gelb BD, Seidman JG, et al. Genetics of congenital heart disease: the glass half empty. Circ Res 2013;112(4):707–20 [published correction appears in Circ Res 2013;112(12):e182].

28. Botto LD, May K, Fernhoff PM, et al. A population-based study of the 22q11.2 deletion: phenotype, incidence, and contribution to major birth defects in the population. Pediatrics 2003;112(1 Pt 1):101–7.

29. Branton H, Warren AE, Penney LS. Left ventricular noncompaction and coronary artery fistula in an in-fant with deletion 22q11.2. Pediatr Cardiol 2011;32(2):208–10.

30. John AS, McDonald-McGinn DM, Zackai EH, et al. Aortic root dilation in patients with 22q11.2 deletion

31. Morris CA, Demsey SA, Leonard CO, et al. Natural history of Williams syndrome: physical characteris-tics. J Pediatr 1988;113(2):318–26.

32. Pober BR, Johnson M, Urban Z. Mechanisms and treatment of cardiovascular disease in Williams-Beuren syndrome. J Clin Invest 2008;118(5):1606–15.

33. Del Pasqua A, Rinelli G, Toscano A, et al. New find-ings concerning cardiovascular manifestations emerging from long-term follow-up of 150 patients with the Williams-Beuren-Beuren syndrome. Car-diol Young 2009;19(6):563–7.

34. Collins RT 2nd, Kaplan P, Somes GW, et al. Cardio-vascular abnormalities, interventions, and long-term outcomes in infantile Williams syndrome. J Pediatr 2010;156(2):253–8.e1.

35. Radford DJ, Pohlner PG. The middle aortic syn-drome: an important feature of Williams' syndrome. Cardiol Young 2000;10(6):597–602.

36. Das KM, Momenah TS, Larsson SG, et al. Williams-Beuren syndrome: computed tomography imaging review. Pediatr Cardiol 2014;35(8):1309–20.

37. Twite MD, Stenquist S, Ing RJ. Williams syndrome. Paediatr Anaesth 2019;29(5):483–90.

38. Collins RT 2nd. Clinical significance of prolonged QTc interval in Williams syndrome. Am J Cardiol 2011;108(3):471–3.

39. 1 p36 deletion syndrome. Available at: https://www.orpha.net/consor/cgi-bin/OC_Exp.php?Lng=IT&Expert=1606.

40. Zaveri HP, Beck TF, Hernández-García A, et al. Identification of critical regions and candidate genes for cardiovascular malformations and car-diomyopathy associated with deletions of chromo-some 1p36. PLoS One 2014;9(1):e85600.

41. Brazil A, Stanford K, Smolarek T, et al. Delineating the phenotype of 1p36 deletion in adolescents and adults. Am J Med Genet A 2014;164A(10):2496–503.

42. Jordan VK, Zaveri HP, Scott DA. 1p36 deletion syn-drome: an update. Appl Clin Genet 2015;8:189–200.

43. Gajecka M, Mackay KL, Shaffer LG. Monosomy 1p36 deletion syndrome. Am J Med Genet C Semin Med Genet 2007;145C(4):346–56.

44. Delplancq G, Tarris G, Vitobello A, et al. Cardiomy-opathy due to PRDM16 mutation: first description of a fetal presentation, with possible modifier genes. Am J Med Genet C Semin Med Genet 2020;184(1):129–35.

45. Thienpont B, Zhang L, Postma AV, et al. Haploin-sufficiency of TAB2 causes congenital heart de-fects in humans. Am J Hum Genet 2010;86(6):839–49.

46. Cheng A, Neufeld-Kaiser W, Byers PH, et al. 6q25.1 (TAB2) microdeletion is a risk factor for

hypoplastic left heart: a case report that expands the phenotype. BMC Cardiovasc Disord 2020; 20(1):137.

47. Weiss K, Applegate C, Wang T, et al. Familial TAB2 microdeletion and congenital heart defects including unusual valve dysplasia and tetralogy of fallot. Am J Med Genet A 2015;167A(11):2702–6. https://doi.org/10.1002/ajmg.a.37210.

48. Cheng A, Dinulos MBP, Neufeld-Kaiser W, et al. 6q25.1 (TAB2) microdeletion syndrome: congenital heart defects and cardiomyopathy. Am J Med Genet A 2017;173(7):1848–57. https://doi.org/10.1002/ajmg.a.38254.

49. Caulfield TR, Richter JE Jr, Brown EE, et al. Protein molecular modeling techniques investigating novel TAB2 variant R347X causing cardiomyopathy and congenital heart defects in multigenerational family. Mol Genet Genomic Med 2018;6(4):666–72.

50. Postma AV, van Engelen K, van de Meerakker J, et al. Mutations in the sarcomere gene MYH7 in Ebstein anomaly. Circ Cardiovasc Genet 2011;4(1): 43–50.

51. Hirono K, Hata Y, Miyao N, et al. Left ventricular noncompaction and congenital heart disease increases the risk of congestive heart failure. J Clin Med 2020;9(3):785.

52. Bettinelli AL, Mulder TJ, Funke BH, et al. Familial ebstein anomaly, left ventricular hypertrabeculation, and ventricular septal defect associated with a MYH7 mutation. Am J Med Genet A 2013; 161A(12):3187–90.

53. Basu R, Hazra S, Shanks M, et al. Novel mutation in exon 14 of the sarcomere gene MYH7 in familial left ventricular noncompaction with bicuspid aortic valve. Circ Heart Fail 2014;7(6):1059–62.

54. Caiazza M, Lioncino M, Monda E, et al. Troponin T mutation as a cause of left ventricular systolic dysfunction in a young patient with previous surgical correction of aortic coarctation. Biomolecules 2021;11(5):696.

55. Norrish G, Ding T, Field E, et al. Development of a novel risk prediction model for sudden cardiac death in childhood hypertrophic cardiomyopathy (HCM Risk-Kids). JAMA Cardiol 2019;4(9):918–27.

56. Blair E, Redwood C, de Jesus Oliveira M, et al. Mutations of the light meromyosin domain of the beta-myosin heavy chain rod in hypertrophic cardiomyopathy. Circ Res 2002;90(3):263–9.

57. Zhang S, Wilson J, Madani M, et al. Atrial arrhythmias and extensive left atrial fibrosis as the initial presentation of MYH7 gene mutation. JACC Clin Electrophysiol 2018;4(11):1488–90.

58. Frontera A, Vlachos K, Kitamura T, et al. Long-term follow-up of idiopathic ventricular fibrillation in a pediatric population: clinical characteristics, management, and complications. J Am Heart Assoc 2019; 8(9):e011172.

59. Reamon-Buettner SM, Borlak J. GATA4 zinc finger mutations as a molecular rationale for septation defects of the human heart. J Med Genet 2005;42(5): e32.

60. Pikkarainen S, Tokola H, Kerkelä R, et al. GATA transcription factors in the developing and adult heart. Cardiovasc Res 2004;63(2):196–207.

61. Perrino C, Rockman HA. GATA4 and the two sides of gene expression reprogramming. Circ Res 2006; 98(6):715–6.

62. Brody MJ, Cho E, Mysliwiec MR, et al. Lrrc10 is a novel cardiac-specific target gene of Nkx2-5 and GATA4. J Mol Cell Cardiol 2013;62:237–46.

63. Chen J, Qi B, Zhao J, et al. A novel mutation of GATA4 (K300T) associated with familial atrial septal defect. Gene 2016;575(2 Pt 2):473–7.

64. Su W, Zhu P, Wang R, et al. Congenital heart diseases and their association with the variant distribution features on susceptibility genes. Clin Genet 2017;91(3):349–54.

65. GATA-BINDING PROTEIN 4; GATA4. Available at: https://www.omim.org/entry/600576.

66. Alonso-Montes C, Rodríguez-Reguero J, Martín M, et al. Rare genetic variants in GATA transcription factors in patients with hypertrophic cardiomyopathy. J Investig Med 2017;65(5):926–34.

67. Zhao L, Xu JH, Xu WJ, et al. A novel GATA4 loss-of-function mutation responsible for familial dilated cardiomyopathy. Int J Mol Med 2014;33(3):654–60.

68. Li RG, Li L, Qiu XB, et al. GATA4 loss-of-function mutation underlies familial dilated cardiomyopathy. Biochem Biophys Res Commun 2013;439(4): 591–6.

69. Kikuchi K, Holdway JE, Werdich AA, et al. Primary contribution to zebrafish heart regeneration by gata4(+) cardiomyocytes. Nature 2010; 464(7288):601–5.

70. Kwon DH, Eom GH, Kee HJ, et al. Estrogen-related receptor gamma induces cardiac hypertrophy by activating GATA4. J Mol Cell Cardiol 2013;65: 88–97.

71. Qian L, Huang Y, Spencer CI, et al. In vivo reprogramming of murine cardiac fibroblasts into induced cardiomyocytes. Nature 2012;485(7400):593–8.

72. Song K, Nam YJ, Luo X, et al. Heart repair by reprogramming non-myocytes with cardiac transcription factors. Nature 2012;485(7400):599–604.

73. Suzuki YJ, Evans T. Regulation of cardiac myocyte apoptosis by the GATA-4 transcription factor. Life Sci 2004;74(15):1829–38.

74. Xu X, Zhang L, Liang J. Rosuvastatin prevents pressure overload induced myocardial hypertrophy via inactivation of the Akt, ERK1/2 and GATA4 signaling pathways in rats. Mol Med Rep 2013;8(2):385–92.

75. Li J, Liu WD, Yang ZL, et al. Prevalence and spectrum of GATA4 mutations associated with sporadic

dilated cardiomyopathy. Gene 2014;548(2): 174–81.

76. Hanley A, Walsh KA, Joyce C, et al. Mutation of a common amino acid in NKX2.5 results in dilated cardiomyopathy in two large families. BMC Med Genet 2016;17(1):83.

77. Xu JH, Gu JY, Guo YH, et al. Prevalence and spectrum of NKX2-5 mutations associated with sporadic adult-onset dilated cardiomyopathy. Int Heart J 2017;58(4):521–9.

78. Costa MW, Guo G, Wolstein O, et al. Functional characterization of a novel mutation in NKX2-5 associated with congenital heart disease and adult-onset cardiomyopathy. Circ Cardiovasc Genet 2013;6(3):238–47.

79. Yuan F, Qiu XB, Li RG, et al. A novel NKX2-5 loss-of-function mutation predisposes to familial dilated cardiomyopathy and arrhythmias. Int J Mol Med 2015;35(2):478–86.

80. Sveinbjornsson G, Olafsdottir EF, Thorolfsdottir RB, et al. Variants in NKX2-5 and FLNC cause dilated cardiomyopathy and sudden cardiac death. Circ Genom Precis Med 2018;11(8):e002151.

81. Ross SB, Singer ES, Driscoll E, et al. Genetic architecture of left ventricular noncompaction in adults. Hum Genome Var 2020;7:33.

82. Arya P, Wilson TE, Parent JJ, et al. An adult female with 5q34-q35.2 deletion: a rare syndromic presentation of left ventricular non-compaction and congenital heart disease. Eur J Med Genet 2020; 63(4):103797.

83. Varela D, Conceição N, Cancela ML. Transcriptional regulation of human T-box 5 gene (TBX5) by bone- and cardiac-related transcription factors. Gene 2021;768:145322.

84. Greulich F, Rudat C, Kispert A. Mechanisms of T-box gene function in the developing heart. Cardiovasc Res 2011;91(2):212–22.

85. Baban A, Postma AV, Marini M, et al. Identification of TBX5 mutations in a series of 94 patients with Tetralogy of Fallot. Am J Med Genet A 2014; 164A(12):3100–7.

86. McDermott DA, Fong JC, Basson CT. Holt-Oram syndrome. In: Adam MP, Ardinger HH, Pagon RA, et al, editors. GeneReviews®. Seattle (WA): University of Washington, Seattle; 2004. p. 1–16. Available at: https://www.ncbi.nlm.nih.gov/books/NBK1111/.

87. Baban A, Pitto L, Pulignani S, et al. Holt-Oram syndrome with intermediate atrioventricular canal defect, and aortic coarctation: functional characterization of a de novo TBX5 mutation. Am J Med Genet A 2014;164A(6):1419–24.

88. Burnicka-Turek O, Broman MT, Steimle JD, et al. Transcriptional patterning of the ventricular cardiac conduction system. Circ Res 2020;127(3):e94–106.

89. Rathjens FS, Blenkle A, Iyer LM, et al. Preclinical evidence for the therapeutic value of TBX5 normalization in arrhythmia control. Cardiovasc Res 2020;cvaa239. https://doi.org/10.1093/cvr/cvaa239.

90. Markunas AM, Manivannan PKR, Ezekian JE, et al. TBX5-encoded T-box transcription factor 5 variant T223M is associated with long QT syndrome and pediatric sudden cardiac death. Am J Med Genet A 2021;185(3):923–9.

91. Nieto-Marín P, Tinaquero D, Utrilla RG, et al. Tbx5 variants disrupt Nav1.5 function differently in patients diagnosed with Brugada or Long QT Syndrome. Cardiovasc Res 2021;cvab045. https://doi.org/10.1093/cvr/cvab045.

92. Zhang XL, Qiu XB, Yuan F, et al. TBX5 loss-of-function mutation contributes to familial dilated cardiomyopathy. Biochem Biophys Res Commun 2015;459(1):166–71.

93. Zhu Y, Gramolini AO, Walsh MA, et al. Tbx5-dependent pathway regulating diastolic function in congenital heart disease. Proc Natl Acad Sci U S A 2008;105(14):5519–24.

94. Zhou W, Zhao L, Jiang JQ, et al. A novel TBX5 loss-of-function mutation associated with sporadic dilated cardiomyopathy. Int J Mol Med 2015; 36(1):282–8.

95. Patterson J, Coats C, McGowan R. Familial dilated cardiomyopathy associated with pathogenic TBX5 variants: expanding the cardiac phenotype associated with Holt-Oram syndrome. Am J Med Genet A 2020;182(7):1725–34.

96. Nguyen TV, Tran Vu MT, Do TNP, et al. Genetic determinants and genotype-phenotype correlations in vietnamese patients with dilated cardiomyopathy. Circ J 2021. https://doi.org/10.1253/circj.CJ-21-0077. 10.1253/circj.CJ-21-0077.

97. Chen Y, Xiao D, Zhang L, et al. The role of *Tbx20* in cardiovascular development and function. Front Cell Dev Biol 2021;9:638542.

98. Kraus F, Haenig B, Kispert A. Cloning and expression analysis of the mouse T-box gene tbx20. Mech Dev 2001;100(1):87–91.

99. Stennard FA, Harvey RP. T-box transcription factors and their roles in regulatory hierarchies in the developing heart. Development 2005;132(22): 4897–910.

100. Shen T, Aneas I, Sakabe N, et al. Tbx20 regulates a genetic program essential to adult mouse cardiomyocyte function. J Clin Invest 2011;121(12): 4640–54.

101. Fang Y, Lai KS, She P, et al. Tbx20 induction promotes zebrafish heart regeneration by inducing cardiomyocyte dedifferentiation and endocardial expansion. Front Cell Dev Biol 2020;8:738.

102. Posch MG, Gramlich M, Sunde M, et al. A gain-of-function TBX20 mutation causes congenital atrial septal defects, patent foramen ovale and cardiac valve defects. J Med Genet 2010;47(4):230–5.

103. Pan Y, Geng R, Zhou N, et al. TBX20 loss-of-function mutation contributes to double outlet right ventricle. Int J Mol Med 2015;35(4):1058–66.

104. Huang RT, Wang J, Xue S, et al. TBX20 loss-of-function mutation responsible for familial tetralogy of Fallot or sporadic persistent truncus arteriosus. Int J Med Sci 2017;14(4):323–32.

105. Luyckx I, Kumar AA, Reyniers E, et al. Copy number variation analysis in bicuspid aortic valve-related aortopathy identifies TBX20 as a contributing gene. Eur J Hum Genet 2019;27(7):1033–43.

106. Kennedy L, Kaltenbrun E, Greco TM, et al. Formation of a TBX20-CASZ1 protein complex is protective against dilated cardiomyopathy and critical for cardiac homeostasis. Plos Genet 2017;13(9): e1007011.

107. Packham EA, Brook JD. T-box genes in human disorders. Hum Mol Genet 2003;12 Spec No 1: R37–44.

108. Zhao CM, Bing-Sun, Song HM, et al. TBX20 loss-of-function mutation associated with familial dilated cardiomyopathy. Clin Chem Lab Med 2016;54(2): 325–32.

109. Zhou YM, Dai XY, Huang RT, et al. A novel TBX20 loss of function mutation contributes to adult onset dilated cardiomyopathy or congenital atrial septal defect. Mol Med Rep 2016;14(4):3307–14.

110. Vasilescu C, Ojala TH, Brilhante V, et al. Genetic basis of severe childhood-onset cardiomyopathies. J Am Coll Cardiol 2018;72(19):2324–38.

Clinical Manifestations of 22q11.2 Deletion Syndrome

Annapaola Cirillo, MD[a], Michele Lioncino, MD[a], Annachiara Maratea, MD[a], Annalisa Passariello, MD, PhD[b], Adelaide Fusco, MD[a], Fiorella Fratta, MD[b], Emanuele Monda, MD[a], Martina Caiazza, MD[a], Giovanni Signore, MD[a], Augusto Esposito, MD[a], Anwar Baban, MD, PhD[c], Paolo Versacci, MD, PhD[d], Carolina Putotto, MD, PhD[d], Bruno Marino, MD, PhD[d], Claudio Pignata, MD, PhD[e], Emilia Cirillo, MD, PhD[e], Giuliana Giardino, MD, PhD[e], Berardo Sarubbi, MD, PhD[f], Giuseppe Limongelli, MD, PhD[a], Maria Giovanna Russo, MD, PhD[b],*

KEYWORDS

- 22q11.2 deletion syndrome • Di George syndrome • Aortic arch abnormalities
- Conotruncal abnormalities

KEY POINTS

- DiGeorge syndrome (DGS), also known as "22q11.2 deletion syndrome" (22q11DS) (MIM # 192430 # 188400), is a genetic disorder caused by hemizygous microdeletion of the long arm of chromosome 22.
- Clinical phenotype is heterogeneous and may include congenital heart disease (CHD), palatal anomalies, typical facial features, and immune deficiency as a consequence of thymic aplasia/hypoplasia.
- Most of 22q11DS is sporadic with a de novo event (90%–95%) with unaffected parents and relatively low risk of recurrence for future sibling.
- The most common CHD include conotruncal defects (such as tetralogy of Fallot) (20%–45%), pulmonary atresia with ventricular septal defect (10%–25%), interrupted aortic arch (mainly type B) (5%–20%), truncus arteriosus (5%–10%), and conoventricular ventricular septal defect (10%–50%).

INTRODUCTION

DiGeorge syndrome (DGS), also known as "22q11.2 deletion syndrome" (22q11DS) (MIM # 192430 # 188400), is a genetic disorder caused by hemizygous microdeletion of the long arm of chromosome 22. It is the most frequent chromosomal microdeletion syndrome with an estimated prevalence of 1 in 3 to 6000 live births and approximately 1 in 1000 fetuses. 22q11DS is the second leading chromosomal cause of congenital heart disease (CHD), after trisomy 21.[1,2] Historically,

[a] Inherited and Rare Cardiovascular Disease Unit, Department of Translational Medical Sciences, University of Campania "Luigi Vanvitelli", Via L. Bianchi, 80131 Naples, Italy; [b] Pediatric Cardiology Unit, Department of Translational Medical Sciences, University of Campania "Luigi Vanvitelli", Via L. Bianchi, 80131 Naples, Italy; [c] Department of Pediatric Cardiology and Cardiac Surgery, Bambino Gesù Children's Hospital and Research Institute, Viale Di San Paolo, 15, 00165 Rome, Italy; [d] Department of Pediatrics, Sapienza University of Rome, Viale Regina Elena 324, 00161 Rome, Italy; [e] Department of Translational Medical Sciences - Section of Pediatrics, University of Naples Federico II, Via S. Pansini, 5, 80131 Naples, Italy; [f] Adult Congenital Heart Diseases Unit, AORN dei Colli, Monaldi Hospital, Naples
* Corresponding author. Department of Translational Medical Sciences, University of Campania "Luigi Vanvitelli", Via L. Bianchi, 80131 Naples, Italy.
E-mail address: mariagiovanna.russo@unicampania.it

Heart Failure Clin 18 (2022) 155–164
https://doi.org/10.1016/j.hfc.2021.07.009

DGS, velocardiofacial syndrome, conotruncal anomaly face syndrome (Takao syndrome), autosomal dominant Opitz G/BBB syndrome,[3] and Cayler cardiofacial syndrome[4] were identified separately. However, the development of cytogenetic and molecular analysis, particularly the widespread use of fluorescence in situ hybridization (FISH), made clear that nearly 90% of these patients shared a common genetic cause, namely a microdeletion of chromosome 22q11.2[5] (**Table 1**).

Clinical phenotype is heterogeneous and can range from mild to severe involvement, nevertheless the most common patterns of clinical manifestation may include CHD, palatal anomalies, typical facial features, and immune deficiency as a consequence of thymic aplasia/hypoplasia. Additional clinical findings may include gastrointestinal involvement and renal, dental, and skeletal anomalies. Learning difficulties and developmental delay are often present. Psychiatric illness (anxiety, depression, schizophrenia) and Parkinson disease are more prevalent than in the general population[6,7] (**Fig. 1**).

GENETIC FINDINGS IN 22q11DS

In the last decades, the introduction of FISH assays has allowed the detection of chromosomal microdeletions, which could not be previously identified using standard karyotype analysis. However, the use of FISH in clinical practice requires high index of clinical suspicion to identify the correct region for analysis. In addition, deletions and duplications whose endpoints are outside the narrow region covered by the probe used for FISH may be missed, accounting for a low sensitivity in case of small genetic loci.[7] Recently, new techniques have been introduced to overcome these limitations. These techniques include multiplex ligation-dependent probe amplification (MLPA) and chromosomal microarrays with dense, genome-wide coverage. In the last 2 decades, these methods have allowed the identification of smaller chromosomal deletions and submicroscopic duplications that were undetectable by standard karyotyping and FISH techniques. Although the use of high-resolution microarrays in infants with congenital anomalies leads, in most cases, to the identification of disease-causing genotype, the deletions of chromosome 22q11.2 are often submicroscopic and may be frequently undetected by standard FISH probes.[8] In order to overcome these limitations, MLPA, a polymerase chain reaction-based assay, provides a rapid, focused, and generally less expensive approach than microarray analysis. Nevertheless, because they do not require targeted probes, microarrays can identify other potentially disease-associated copy number variants (deletions or duplications) other than 22q11DS.[9]

The 22q11.2 region contains about 50 genes involved in tissue and organ morphogenesis. In particular, most of the 22q11DS patients carry a large deletion, approximately 2.4 to 3 Mb, usually detected by FISH or chromosomal microarray. A subgroup of patients carries smaller deletions, harbored on a 3 Mb typically deleted region (TDR) that also results in haploinsufficiency. Finally, pathogenic deletions are rarely found outside TDR.[10]

Most of 22q11DS is sporadic with a de novo event (90%–95%) with unaffected parents and relatively low risk of recurrence for future siblings.

Table 1
Clinical manifestations associated to 22q11.2 deletion syndromes

Di George syndrome	Thymus hypo/aplasia Parathyroid glands hypo/aplasia congenital heart disease Facial dysmorphism
Velocardiofacial syndrome (Shprintzen syndrome)	Palatal anomalies Congenital heart disease Facial dysmorphism
Conotruncal anomaly face syndrome (Takao syndrome)	Conotruncal congenital heart disease Facial dysmorphism
Opitz G/BBB syndrome	Ocular hypertelorism Cleft palate Hypospadias Laryngeal anomalies

Cayler cardiofacial syndrome
  (asymmetric crying face)
	Mouth asymmetry during crying
	  (for aplasia of the orbicularis muscle)
	Congenital heart disease
	Facial dysmorphism

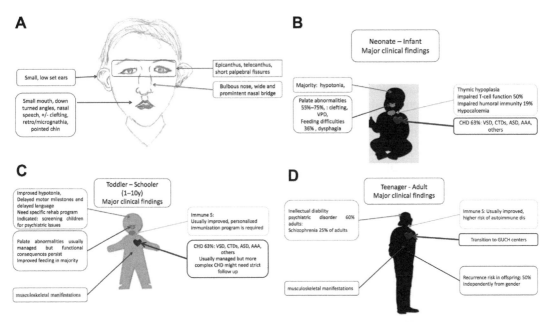

Fig. 1. (*A*) Facial features in children with 22q11.2 deletion syndrome. (*B*) Age-related major clinical findings in infants and children with 22q11.2 deletion syndrome: infants (<1 year). (*C*) Age-related major clinical findings in infants and children with 22q11.2 deletion syndrome: toddler-schooler. (*D*) Age-related major clinical findings in children with 22q11.2 deletion syndrome: teenager and adults.

However, in the remaining percentage (5%–10%), an affected individual has 50% risk of having an affected child with each offspring independently from gender following an autosomal mode of inheritance.[11] Genotype-phenotype correlations are difficult because the size of deletion is not related to the severity of clinical involvement: smaller size deletions are not associated to milder symptoms.

The instability of this *hotspot* seems to be due to the presence of several large paralogous Low copy repeats (LCRs) or segmental amplifications. LCRs may harbor sequences of genes and pseudogenes formed by duplication processes, sized 10 to 250 kbp. Each LCR is characterized by a complex modular structure with a high degree of sequence homology (>96%), therefore promoting genomic rearrangements. Misalignment and meiotic unequal nonallelic homologous recombination of LCRs represent the mechanism mediating 22q11DS, and determining as a result the deletion of the sequence located between the repeats[12] 22q11.2 locus contains 4 proximal LCRs (A–D) and 4 distal LCRs (E–H). In particular, a *DiGeorge critical region* (DGCR) (3 Mbp) contains LCR22A, LCR22B, LCR22C, and LCR22D.[2] In more than 90% of patients, the region between LCR22A-D is hemizygously deleted.

Several protein-coding genes, such as *UFD1L*, *COMT*, *TBX1*, CRKL, and DGCR8, are localized within DGCR. As shown by murine models and

human mutational analysis, *TBX1* is the most important gene for the expression of cardiovascular phenotype in 22q11.2DS. *TBX1* is part of the large family of T-box genes, which regulate tissue and organ morphogenesis during embryogenesis.[1] In particular, *TBX1* plays an important role in the development of heart outflow tract (OFT). *TBX1* is differentially expressed in the embryonic pharyngeal endoderm, where it is necessary for the separation of the aorta and pulmonary arteries (PAs), and in the "secondary heart field," where its role is crucial to adequate OFT alignment and truncal valve septation, as well as for cardiac neural crest cells migration and patterning. In addition, *TBX1* is involved in the formation of the caudal pharyngeal arches. Of note, considering that *TBX1* is expressed in the right-sided OFT, the sub-pulmonary infundibulum and proximal PAs are the most involved cardiac regions in 22q11DS and explain why tetralogy of Fallot (TOF) and pulmonary atresia (with or without interventricular septal defect) are the most common CHDs in 22q11.2DS. Furthermore, reduced levels of Tbx1 impair the development of neural crest-derived mesenchymal cells that surround the third pharyngeal pouch, leading to thymic hypoplasia.[13] Isolated *TBX1* mutations may be rarely reported in patients with DGS. Phenocopy of DGS with CHD, impaired thymus development, and hypoparathyroidism have also been observed in infants of diabetic mother or due to prenatal exposure to retinoic acid/alcohol and in patients carrying copy number variants different from 22q11.2[14]

Furthermore, studies on mouse models have demonstrated that *Tbx1* contributes to the development not only of cardiac outflow tract but also of aortic arch, left pulmonary artery, and ductus arteriosus, which are often involved in the vascular malformations typical of the syndrome.[11,15–17]

CLINICAL PRESENTATION OF 22q11DS

When the first cases were reported in the mid-1960s, 22q11DS was defined by the association between CHDs, thymic hypoplasia/aplasia, and hypoparathyroidism. Currently, the heterogeneity of the clinical presentation is well known, to such an extent that phenotypic discordance has been identified between monozygotic twins too[18] and within members of the same family.[19] The most common clinical features include facial features and palatal defects (velopharyngeal insufficiency, nasal voice, cleft palate, submucous cleft palate), CHD (particularly conotruncal defects and/or aortic arch anomalies), immunodeficiency (immune T cell defects due to thymic hypoaplasia), hypocalcemia (due to parathyroid hypoplasia), dysphagia, skeletal abnormalities, renal anomalies (absent or dysplastic kidney, vesicoureteral reflux), ophthalmologic abnormalities, developmental disabilities (speech and developmental delay during infancy and childhood), and psychiatric problems (schizophrenia).[5]

To some extent, the reported prevalence of the patterns of presentation in 22q11DS depends on the age of patient ascertainment.[9]

During gestational age, the most well-documented findings associated with 22q11.2DS are CHDs in association with cleft lip/palate and/or intrauterine growth restriction.[20] In newborns, hypocalcemia, CHD, absent thymus, and nasopharyngeal reflux are useful clinical clues ("red flags") that should raise the suspicion of an underlying 22q11DS. During infancy, facial features become more prominent, although they are not very characteristic; nevertheless, the clinical presentation is mainly characterized by delayed motor and verbal milestones. On the contrary, during adolescence the prevalence of neuropsychiatric and/or learning disabilities is significantly increased.

CONGENITAL HEART DISEASES IN 22q11DS

The prevalence of CHD in 22q11DS is debated because it varies with the population of study, the age of ascertainment, and the diagnostic setting.[7] In particular, infants and newborns will display a different range and severity of CHD compared with older children and adolescents.[20,21] Thus, it is possible that the prevalence of CHD in 22q11DS population, which most studies report to be 75% to 80%, is overestimated due to the fact that children and adults without a significant CHD may escape diagnosis of the syndrome.

The most common CHD include conotruncal defects (CTDs, such as TOF) (20%–45%), pulmonary atresia with ventricular septal defect (PA-VSD) (10%–25%), interrupted aortic arch (IAA) (mainly type B) (5%–20%), truncus arteriosus (TA) (5%–10%), and conoventricular VSD (10%–50%), a subset of VSD caused by posterior malalignment and conoseptal hypoplasia.[1,22] Albeit less frequently, other CHD have been reported in patients with 22q11DS such as hypoplastic left heart syndrome, transposition of the great arteries, double outlet right ventricle, total anomalous pulmonary venous connection, atrial septal defect, tricuspid atresia, pulmonary valve stenosis, bicuspid aortic valve or aortic stenosis, aortic origin of a pulmonary artery (hemitruncus arteriosus), and crossed PAs.

Aortic arch anomalies (AAA), both in isolated form (10%) or in association with other CHDs, have been commonly described among patients with 22q11DS, including cervical aortic arch, double aortic arch, right-sided aortic arch, and aberrant right or left subclavian artery.[23] Moreover, a progressive dilation of the aortic root in pediatric patients without major CHD has been reported, which deserves to be monitored over time.[24]

Identifying patients with AAA is particularly relevant because almost 27% of them show a symptomatic vascular ring.[25] Because respiratory symptoms including asthma and airway anomalies (ie, glottic web) are commonly diagnosed in 22q11DS, it is important to identify those with a coexistent vascular ring, who would benefit from surgical therapy.

In some 22q11DS patients, peculiar anatomic pattern of CHD are recognizable and recurrent. For instance, discontinuity, diffuse hypoplasia, and crossing of the PAs and major aortopulmonary collateral arteries (MAPCAs) are common in TOF (also in the setting of an absent pulmonary valve) and in PA-VSD. Moreover, discontinuity of the PAs may be characteristic for TA type A3 of Van Praagh, whereas hypoplasia of infundibular septum is present in both TOF and IAA.[22,26–28]

Some reports have shown that the size of the deletion region does not seem to influence the cardiac phenotype, whereas the proximal or distal location of the microdeletion is related to a slightly different prevalence of associated features.[9] Indeed, the prevalence of CHD in patients with the 3 Mb deletion and in those with proximal nested deletions (including LCR22A-LCR22B region) is about 65%. In contrast, a lower prevalence of CHD has been observed in patients carrying distal nested deletions (~32%).[25,29]

The high phenotypic variability of this genetic syndrome cannot be completely explained by the presence of the 22q11.2 deletion or the size of the deletion alone and is most likely due to the existence of additional genetic modifiers, environmental factors, or common and/or rare single nucleotide variants on the intact allele of the 22q11.2 region.[9] A recent article demonstrated that common variants located in a 350-kb region within the LCR22C-LCR22D intervals on the remaining allele were associated with an increased risk of CTDs in individuals with the typical 22q11.2 deletion. Notably, the identified variants are located in regulatory regions of the CRKL gene. This gene is involved in the embryogenetic cardiovascular development and its biallelic inactivation in mouse models, such as *TBX1*, and results in a similar spectrum of CTD[30]

Although over the past 30 years the in-depth knowledge of the specific cardiac phenotype associated with this genetic syndrome and the improvement in surgical techniques have contributed to an increase in the life expectancy of people with 22q11.2DS,[22,31] cardiovascular abnormalities still represent the leading cause of mortality (~87%) in pediatric age.[5,32]

In addition, few data in literature on adult population with 22q11DS reveal an increased risk of earlier death compared with the general population, especially from cardiovascular causes, such as sudden death or heart failure, even in the absence of CHD.[33] Recently, it has been shown that the presence of the 22q11.2 deletion and major CHD are significant independent predictors of mortality for adults with this genetic syndrome.[34]

A greater understanding of the pathogenetic mechanisms leading to the presence of CHD in patients with 22q11.2DS can also allow a better understanding of factors that may affect the clinical and surgical outcome of patients with 22q11.2DS and associated CHD.[35]

To date, with medical and surgical advances, the postoperative outcome in these patients has greatly improved. Long-term survival of patients with CTD with 22q11DS seems to be equal to that of patients with nonsyndromic CTD.[36] Some investigators, however, still report an increased mortality rate and a poorer prognosis, particularly in the subgroup of patients with TOF and PA-VSD with MAPCAs. Probably, this is due to the presence of some specific anatomic features that are worse in patients with CTD and 22q11.2DS,

pulmonary vascular reactivity, and structural airway abnormalities.[37,38]

Although 22q11.2DS does not seem to represent a surgical risk factor *per se*, a significant increase in perisurgical and postsurgical complications that may adversely affect the prognosis of these patients has been reported: heart failure, respiratory failure, longer intubation, tracheostomy, laryngeal stridor, pneumonia, and sepsis.[39]

It has been shown that in patients with TOF and 22q11.2DS there is a higher prevalence of Blalock-Taussig shunt before primary repair, longer and more complex intensive care unit, and hospital stay than those with nonsyndromic TOF.[40]

Given the clinical implications associated with the 22q11DS, clinical practice guidelines recommend genetic testing for a 22q11.2 deletion in the fetus (when an amniocentesis is to be performed), newborns, infants, children, and adults with a typical cardiac anomaly, as detailed in a recently updated AHA Scientific Statement.[41] (**Box 1**). Thanks to improvements in prenatal genetic testing, the diagnosis of 22q11DS is increasingly being made in the prenatal age. Two major studies conducted in France, investigating clinical features of fetuses with 22q11DS, both reported a very high frequency of CHD, up to 91% of fetuses, and both identified a higher prevalence of TA, up to 27% of all CHD.[21,42] These data suggest that the prevalence of CHD, especially that of the most severe CHD, may be even higher in 22q11DS. Still today, many adults with CHD remain undiagnosed, without an appropriate counseling about

---

Box 1
Current indications for the screening of patients with suspected Di George syndrome

American Heart Association Scientific Statement

Screen patients (of all ages, including fetus, if amniocentesis performed) with

- *Tetralogy of Fallot (with pulmonary valve stenosis, atresia, or absent pulmonary valve)*

- *Truncus arteriosus (all subtypes)*

- *Interrupted aortic arch (particularly type B and C)*

- *Ventricular septal defect (conoventricular, posterior malalignment, conoseptal hypoplasia) particularly with a concurrent aortic arch anomaly*

- *Isolated aortic arch anomaly (double or right-sided aortic arch, aberrant or isolated subclavian arteries)*

the reproductive risk. As the risk of recurrence for each offspring is 50% in 22q11DS, cascade screening among the first-degree relatives is critical in order to identify the previously undiagnosed adults; this is particularly true due to variable clinical expressivity of 22q11DS. In other words, a parent who is genotype positive for 22q11DS without CHD has the risk of 50% of having a child who is genotype positive who can have or not have CHD (high intrafamilial variability).

Screening patients with specific CHD is considered reasonable. For example, poor feeding and poor weight gain in an infant with VSD may reflect a significant hemodynamic burden but could instead be a consequence of the feeding disorders commonly found in the 22q11DS. In addition, genetic testing can help to identify affected patients in whom extracardiac involvement may not be detectable.

IMMUNE SYSTEM DISORDERS IN 22q11DS

The immunologic phenotype may vary widely between patients ranging from a mild reduction of T-cell number and function to a more profound defect of T cells resembling a severe combined immunodeficiency (SCID)-like phenotype.

A high percentage of patients (75%) experience impaired T-cell production: 60% of them show IgA deficit, 23% humoral defects including immunoglobulin M (IgM) deficiency and a poor response to pneumococcal polysaccharide vaccine. A significant number of patients shows recurrent sinopulmonary infections and otitis media, which may be partially attributed to other 22q11.2DS-associated comorbidities such as velopharyngeal insufficiency, gastroesophageal reflux, and asthma/rhinitis. T-cell count, which often shows a senescent or memory phenotype, tends to increase with age, and as a consequence the incidence of infections tends to decrease over time. Despite early T-cell senescence, opportunistic infections are rare, and respiratory viruses are the most common pathogen. Furthermore, patients with 22q11.2DS may show reduced T-cell receptor repertoire, decreased natural regulatory T cells, and natural killer cytotoxic activity. B-cell production and differentiation seems to be normal, except for a deficit in switched-memory B cells and decreased somatic hypermutation; this is thought to be the result of impaired activity of *helper T cells* rather than B-cell exhaustion, as evidenced by normal bone marrow B-cell output measured by kappa-deleting recombination excision circles.[43–45]

However, prophylactic treatment with broad-spectrum antibiotics and/or intravenous or subcutaneous immunoglobulin administration should rarely be continued during adulthood. In this clinical setting, immunoglobulin levels, T-cell count, and vaccine-specific antibody titers should be assessed over time and balanced with the infective risk.

Another immunologic aspect includes the higher risk of developing autoimmunity and immune dysregulation later in life, particularly autoimmune cytopenia. Notably, peculiar immunophenotypic alterations, such as decreased CD4 naive cell count and reduced antibody switch among B cells, have been identified early after diagnosis in patients who developed autoimmune sequelae. Some studies have suggested lower baseline platelet counts in patients with 22q11.2DS[46] and there are reports of 22q11DS-associated Bernard-Soulier syndrome, a severe platelet disorder caused by abnormal platelet expression of the GP1bIX-V complex.[47] Platelet abnormalities, and even bleeding predisposition, would be anticipated given the involvement of the critical platelet gene *GPIBB* by the classic deletion.[5] There are also reports of dysplastic changes in peripheral blood[48] and malignancy in certain individuals with 22q11.2DS, including atypical teratoid/rhabdoid tumors, lymphoma, neuroblastoma, acute lymphoblastic leukemia, osteosarcoma, Wilms tumor, thyroid carcinoma, and hepatoblastoma.[49]

Our knowledge about immunologic involvement in 22q11DS has been evolving over the past 50 years. Initially characterized as a pure defect in T-cell development, it is now generally accepted that immune-mediated manifestations are caused by thymic aplasia/hypoplasia. Although the severity of immunodeficiency is related with the extent of thymic hypoplasia, children who seem to have absent or small thymic shadows on chest radiograph imaging can have normal T-cell count due to ectopic thymic tissue nested within the mediastinum. Complete athymia is found in about 1.5% of patients with 22q11DS, and its clinical presentation is analogous to SCID.

B-cell dysfunction and high rates of atopy and autoimmunity require consideration for optimal clinical care and for designing an adequate monitoring approach in patients with 22q11 DS; nevertheless, there are insufficient data in current literature to recommend a specific follow-up protocol. It should be noted that atopy occurs more frequently in patients with persistently low IgM levels[50] for this very specific defect.

OTHER CLINICAL FINDINGS IN 22q11DS

Palatal abnormalities are a hallmark of 22q11DS and are often considered an indication for genetic testing.[51] They include palatal clefting and velo-pharyngeal dysfunction (VPD), even in the absence of overt clefts. There is significant hetero-geneity about the incidence and distribution of palatal abnormalities in 22q11DS patients.

Currently reported incidence of palatal abnor-malities in 22q11DS is 55% to 75%: cleft palate (2%), overt cleft palate (7.3%–11%), submucous cleft palate (SMCP) (16%–22.8%), bifid uvula (5%), and VPD (27%–42%).[52] Driscoll and col-leagues[53] reported VPD and structural palatal mal-formations to be more common in women and in Caucasian patients. VPD describes the inability of the soft palate (velum) and pharyngeal walls to close properly during speech, causing hypernasal speech.

Oksana Jackson and colleagues[54] studied a population of 1047 patients, among whom 67% were found to have a palatal abnormality. The most common finding was VPD (55.2%), whereas 28.5% had a cleft palate with coexisting VPD. Of note, 22q11DS is the most common genetic syn-drome associated with VPD.[55] Among patients with 22q11.DS, VPD is often multifactorial.

In addition, a high prevalence of submucous clefting has been described, both in its classic and "occult" form. Palatal surgery can result in sig-nificant improvements in speech and communica-tion, improving quality of life among children affected with 22q11.2DS. Repair of palatal clefts alone, both overt and submucous, is less success-ful in restoring velopharyngeal competence in pa-tients with 22q11DS, and recurrent surgery is often required.[56,57] In fact, postoperative speech out-comes are less favorable in 22q11.2DS compared with other VPD populations.[54] Additional anatomic differences include an obtuse cranial base angle with deep retropharynx resulting in relative velo-pharyngeal disproportion. Neuromuscular involve-ment also has been described, including cranial nerve abnormalities and pharyngeal muscle hypo-tonia especially in the first 1 to 2 years of life, which may contribute to velopharyngeal dysfunction.[58]

A significant number of subjects have rhinolalia/phonia, nasal regurgitation, or laryngeal penetra-tion/aspiration. Conductive (frequently bilateral) or sensorineural hearing loss are also frequently reported.[59]

Endocrinopathies are common in 22q11DS, with hypoparathyroidism being the most common clin-ical presentation. Hypocalcemia is reported in approximately 50% to 69% of patients with 22q11DS and is caused by agenesis or hypoplasia of the parathyroid glands. Hypoparathyroidism generally seems to be caused by decreased para-thyroid hormone reserve, with a predisposition to develop hypocalcemia during stress or illness.

Therefore, latent hypocalcemia symptoms, including seizures, tremors, or tetany, may occur in 22q11DS. More commonly, hypocalcemia tends to have a spontaneous resolution in newborns, with sporadic recurrence in the presence of trig-gers. Calcium levels should be monitored yearly.

Other endocrine manifestations include hypo-thyroidism, Graves disease, and growth hormone deficiency.[1]

Major *renal findings* may include renal agenesis (12%), multicystic kidney 4%, or hydronephrosis 5%.

Gastrointestinal (GI) abnormalities may include gastroesophageal reflux, esophageal dysmotility, constipation, failure to thrive, prolonged nasal tube feedings, and G-tube placement, especially in the first months of life.[60] The extent of GI involvement has been recently addressed: in particular, GI symptoms were present in up to 58% of patients. The most common complaints were abdominal pain, vomiting, gastroesophageal reflux, and chronic constipation. The evidence of sideropenic anemia, and the coexistence of hypo-proteinemia, impaired acid steatocrit, or mannitol test suggested an abnormal intestinal permeability.[61]

Among the most common *ophthalmologic ab-normalities* are tortuous retinal vessels (58%) and posterior embryotoxon (69%).

Neurologic findings may include cerebral atro-phy (1%) and cerebral hypoplasia (0.4%). *Skeletal abnormalities* are frequent among patients with 22q11DS. They include cervical spine deformities (40%–50%), vertebral dysmorphisms, (19%) and lower limbs defects (15%).[62]

Compared with other genetic syndromes, pa-tients affected by 22q11DS present variable de-gree of *dysmorphic features*, which might be overlooked when mild.

According to Human phenotype Ontology Data-base, the most common facial findings include epicanthus, bulbous nose, wide and prominent nasal bridge, telecanthus, upslanted palpebral fissure, and low-set ears. Other features include elongated face, microstomia, congenital tooth or enamel agenesis, hypertelorism, retro- and micro-gnathia, short neck, and characteristic arachnodactyly.[63,64]

Psychiatric illnesses seem to be diagnosed dur-ing adolescence. About 25% of 22q11DS patients have a diagnosis of schizophrenia, and almost 1% of patients with schizophrenia has 22q11DS.

Many studies have demonstrated the beneficial effects of omega-3 supplementation on attentional control and in transition to psychosis; therefore, it might be considered as early as possible in 22q11DS population. Pituitary dysmaturation has also been reported and could be associated with atypical neurodevelopment. Sleep and motor co-ordination abnormalities are common among patients affected by 22q11DS. An early intervention can help to provide support for affected children. Developmental milestones need to be checked at regular steps during infancy and childhood. The mean IQ of such individuals is about 70, and 22q11DS children might have impaired mathematics and other abstract reasoning.

The lifespan expectancy for adults with 22q11DS is lower than general population: the range of deaths is 18.1 to 68.6 years, with a median age of 46.4 years.[65] However, this is mainly influenced by the malformative spectrum and the need of long-term follow-up for multicentric cohorts.

The heterogeneous nature of clinical manifestations and the extent of organ involvement complicate the transition of care in this syndrome. In addition to the classic findings, the clinical phenotype may also include other manifestations, in particular dysmorphic features, which profoundly affect the self-confidence and social life. Therefore, these aspects should be taken into account in medical and psychological care of adulthood transition among patients with 22q11DS.

In conclusion, patients with 22q11DS need multidisciplinary management at all stages of their life. The clinical management and necessity for medical care and support must be both hospital and community based.

CLINICS CARE POINTS

- Clinical practice guidelines recommend genetic testing for a 22q11.2 deletion in the fetus (when an amniocentesis is to be performed), newborns, infants, children, and adults with a typical cardiac anomaly.
- A high percentage of patients (75%) experience impaired T-cell production: 60% of them show IgA deficit, 23% humoral defects including IgM deficiency and a poor response to pneumococcal polysaccharide vaccine.
- Palatal abnormalities are a hallmark of 22q11DS and are often considered an indication for genetic testing.

ACKNOWLEDGMENTS

A special acknowledgment to Michela Piscopo, Daniela Lafera, and Ciro De Prisco.

DISCLOSURE

The authors have nothing to disclose.

REFERENCES

1. Campbell IM, Sheppard SE, Crowley TB, et al. What is new with 22q? An update from the 22q and You Center at the Children's Hospital of Philadelphia. Am J Med Genet A 2018;176A:2058–69.
2. Hou HT, Chen HX, Wang XL, et al. Genetic characterisation of 22q11.2 variations and prevalence in patients with congenital heart disease [published correction appears in Arch Dis Child. 2020 May 28;:]. Arch Dis Child 2020;105(4):367–74.
3. McDonald-McGinn DM. Autosomal dominant "Opitz" GBBB syndrome due to a 22q11.2 deletion. Am J Med Genet 1996;64(3):525–6.
4. Giannotti A, Digilio MC, Marino B, et al. Cayler cardiofacial syndrome and del 22q11: part of the CATCH22 phenotype. Am J Med Genet 1994;53(3):303–4.
5. McDonald-McGinn DM, Sullivan KE, Marino B, et al. 22q11.2 deletion syndrome. Nat Rev Dis Primers 2015;1:15071.
6. Kobrynski L, Sullivan KE. Velocardiofacial syndrome, DiGeorge syndrome: the chromosome 22q11.2 deletion syndromes. Lancet 2018;370:1443–52.
7. Morrow BE, McDonald-McGinn DM, Emanuel BS, et al. Molecular genetics of 22q11.2 deletion syndrome. Am J Med Genet A 2018;176(10):2070–81.
8. Kuo1 C, Signer R, Saitta S. Immune and Genetic Features of the Chromosome 22q11.2 Deletion (DiGeorge Syndrome). Curr Allergy Asthma Rep 2018;18:75.
9. Goldmuntz E. 22q11.2 deletion syndrome and congenital heart disease. Am J Med Genet C: Semin Med Genet 2020. https://doi.org/10.1002/ajmg.c.31774.
10. Babcock M, Pavlicek A, Spiteri E, et al. Shuffling of Genes Within Low-Copy Repeats on 22q11 (LCR22) by Alu-Mediated Recombination Events During Evolution. Genome Res 2003;13:2519–32.
11. Xu H, Morishima M, Wylie JN, et al. Tbx1 has a dual role in the morphogenesis of the cardiac outflow tract. Development 2004;131(13):3217–27.
12. Maeda J, Yamagishi H, McAnally J, et al. Tbx1 is regulated by forkhead proteins in the secondary heart field. Developmental Dyn 2006. https://doi.org/10.1002/dvdy.20686.
13. Giardino G, Borzacchiello C, De Luca M, et al. T-Cell Immunodeficiencies With Congenital Alterations of Thymic Development: Genes Implicated and Differential Immunological and Clinical Features. Front Immunol 2020;11:1837.
14. Cirillo E, Prencipe MR, Giardino G, et al. Clinical Phenotype, Immunological Abnormalities, and

Genomic Findings in Patients with DiGeorge Spectrum Phenotype without 22q11.2 Deletion. J Allergy Clin Immunol Pract 2020;8(9):3112–20.

15. Merscher S, Funke B, Epstein JA, et al. TBX1 is Responsible for Cardiovascular Defects in Velo-Cardio-Facial/DiGeorge Syndrome. Cell 2001;104: 619–29.

16. Lindsay EA, Vitelli F, Su H, et al. Tbx1 Haploinsufficieny in the DiGeorge Syndrome Region Causes Aortic Arch Defects in Mice. Nature 2001;410:97–101.

17. Mastromoro G, Calcagni G, Versacci P, et al. Left Pulmonary Artery in 22q11.2 Deletion Syndrome. Echocardiographic Evaluation in Patients without Cardiac Defects and Role of Tbx1 in Mice. PLoS One 2019;14:e0211170.

18. Halder A, Jain M, Chaudhary I, et al. Chromosome 22q11.2 microdeletion in monozygotic twins with discordant phenotype and deletion size. Mol Cytogenet 2012. https://doi.org/10.1186/1755-8166-5-13.

19. Cirillo E, Giardino G, Gallo V, et al. Intergenerational and intrafamilial phenotypic variability in 22q11.2 deletion syndrome subjects. BMC Med Genet 2014;15:1.

20. Schindewolf E, Khalek N, Johnson MP, et al. Expanding the fetal phenotype: Prenatal sonographic findings and perinatal outcomes in a cohort of patients with a confirmed 22q11.2 deletion syndrome. Am J Med Genet 2018;1–7. https://doi.org/10.1002/ajmg.a.38665.

21. Besseau-Ayasse J, Violle-Poirsier C, Bazin A, et al. A French collaborative survey of 272 fetuses with 22q11.2 deletion: Ultrasound findings, fetal autopsies and pregnancy outcomes. Prenatal Diagn 2014;34(5):424–30.

22. Marino B, Digilio MC, Toscano A, et al. Anatomic patterns of conotruncal defects associated with deletion 22q11. Genet Med 2001;3(1):45–8.

23. Momma K, Matsuoka R, Takao A. Aortic arch anomalies associated with chromosome 22q11 deletion (CATCH 22). Pediatr Cardiol 1999;20(2):97–102.

24. John AS, McDonald-McGinn DM, Zackai EH, et al. Aortic root dilation in patients with 22q11.2 deletion syndrome. Am J Med Genet A 2009;149A(5): 939–42.

25. Unolt M, Versacci P, Anaclerio S, et al. Congenital heart diseases and cardiovascular abnormalities in 22q11.2 deletion syndrome: From well-established knowledge to new frontiers. Am J Med Genet A 2018;176(10):2087–98.

26. Momma K, Ando M, Matsuoka R. Truncus arteriosus communis associated with chromosome 22q11 deletion. J Am Coll Cardiol 1997;30(4):1067–71.

27. Marino B, Digilio MC, Persiani M, et al. Deletion 22q11 in patients with interrupted aortic arch. Am J Cardiol 1999;84(3):360–1. A9.

28. Marino B, Digilio MC, Toscano A, et al. Deficiency of the infundibular septum in patients with interrupted aortic arch and del 22q11. Cardiol Young 2000; 10(4):428–9.

29. Rump P, de Leeuw N, van Essen AJ, et al. Central 22q11.2 Deletions. Am J Med Genet A 2014;164A: 2707–23.

30. Zhao Y, Diacou A, Johnston HR, et al. Complete Sequence of the 22q11.2 Allele in 1,053 Subjects with 22q11.2 Deletion Syndrome Reveals Modifiers of Conotruncal Heart Defects. Am J Hum.Genet 2020;106:26–40.

31. Momma K. Cardiovascular anomalies associated with chromosome 22q11.2 deletion syndrome. Am J Cardiol 2010;105:1617–24.

32. Repetto GM, Guzman ML, Delgado I, et al. Case fatality rate and associated factors in patients with 22q11 microdeletion syndrome: a retrospective cohort study. BMJ Open 2014;4:e005041.

33. Bassett AS, Chow EW, Husted J, et al. Premature death in adults with 22q11.2 deletion syndrome. J Med Genet 2009;46:324–30.

34. Van L, Heung T, Graffi J, et al. All-cause mortality and survival in adults with 22q11.2 deletion syndrome. Genet Med 2019;21:2328–35.

35. Marino B, Digilio MC. Congenital Heart Disease and Genetic Syndromes: Specific Correlation between Cardiac Phenotype and Genotype. Cardiovasc Pathol 2000;9:303–15.

36. Michielon G, Marino B, Oricchio G, et al. Impact of DEL22q11, trisomy 21, and other genetic syndromes on surgical outcome of conotruncal heart defects. J Thorac Cardiovasc Surg 2009;138(3):565–70.e2.

37. Anaclerio S, Di Ciommo V, Michielon G, et al. Conotruncal heart defects: impact of genetic syndromes on immediate operative mortality. Ital Heart J 2004; 5(8):624–8.

38. Carotti A, Albanese SB, Filippelli S, et al. Determinants of Outcome After Surgical Treatment of Pulmonary Atresia with Ventricular Septal Defect and Major Aortopulmonary Collateral Arteries. J Thorac Cardiovasc Surg 2010;140:1092–103.

39. Ziolkowska L, Kawalec W, Turska-Kmiec A, et al. Chromosome 22q11.2 Microdeletion in Children with Conotruncal Heart Defects:Frequency, Associated Cardiovascular Anomalies, and Outcome Following Cardiac Surgery. Eur J Pediatr 2008;167: 1135–40.

40. Mercer-Rosa L, Pinto N, Yang W, et al. 22q11.2 Deletion syndrome is associated with perioperative outcome in tetralogy of Fallot. J Thorac Cardiovasc Surg 2013;146(4):868–73.

41. Pierpont ME, Brueckner M, Chung WK, et al. Genetic Basis for Congenital Heart Disease: Revisited: A Scientific Statement From the American Heart Association. Circulation 2018;138:e653–711.

42. Noël AC, Pelluard F, Delezoide AL, et al. Fetal phenotype associated with the 22q11 deletion. Am J Med Genet A 2014;164A(11):2724–31.

43. McDonald-McGinn DM, Tonnesen MK, Laufer-Cahana A, et al. Phenotype of the 22q11.2 deletion in individuals identified through an affected relative: Casta wide FISHing net! Genet Med 2001;3:23–9.

44. Cancrini C, Puliafito P, Digilio MC, et al. Italian Network for primary immunodeficiencies. J Pediatr 2014;164(6):1475–80.

45. Gennery AR. Immunological aspects of 22q11.2 deletion syndrome. Cell. Mol. Life Sci. 2011;69:17–27.

46. Lawrence, McDonald-McGinn DM, Zackai E, et al. Thrombocytopenia in patients with chromosome 22q11.2 deletion syndrome. J Pediatr 2003;143:277–8.

47. Budarf ML, Konkle BA, Ludlow LB, et al. identification of patients with Bernard Soulier Syndrome and a delection in the D George-VeloCardioFacial chromosomal region in 22q11.2. Hum Mol Genet 1995;4:763–6.

48. Ozbek D, Olcay Y, Tokel. Dysplastic changes in the peripheral blood of children with microdelection 22q11.2. Am J Hematol 2004;77:126–31.

49. Bosse KR, Shukla AR, Pawel B, et al. Malignant Rhabdoid tumor of the blood and ganglioglioma in 14 y.o male with a germline 22q11.2 deletion. Cancer Genet 2014;207:415–9.

50. Giardino G, Radwan N, Koletsi P, et al. Clinical and immunological features in a cohort of patients with partial DiGeorge syndrome followed at a single center. Blood 2019;133(24):2586–96.

51. Stevens CA, Carey JC, Shigeoka AO. Di George anomaly and velocardiofacial syndrome. Pediatrics 1990 Apr;85(4):526–30.

52. Widdershoven JC, Bowser M, Sheridan MB, et al. A candidate gene approach to identify modifiers of the palatal phenotype in 22q11.2 deletion syndrome patients. Int J Pediatr Otorhinol 2013;77:123–7.

53. McDonald-McGinn & Sullivan. Chomosome 22q11.2 deletion syndrome. Medicine 2011;90:1–18.

54. Driscoll DA, Boland T, Emanuel BS, et al. Evaluation of potential modifiers of the palatal phenotype in the 22q11.2 deletion syndrome. Cleft Palate cranio Facial J 2006;43:435–41.

55. Jackson O, Crowley TB, Sharkus R, et al. Palatal evaluation and treatment in 22q11.2 deletion syndrome. Am J Med Genet 2019;179:1184–95.

56. Gart MS, Gosain AK. Surgical management of velopharyngeal insufficiency. Clin Plast Surg 2014;41:253–70.

57. Bezuhly M, Fischbach S, Klaiman P, et al. Impact of 22q deletion syndrome on speech outcomes following primary surgery for submocous cleft palate. Plast Reconstr Surg 2012;129:502–10.

58. Basta MN, Silvestre J, Stransky C, et al. A 35 year experience with syndromic cleft palate repair operative outcomes and long-term speech function. Ann Plast Surg 2014;73(Suppl 2):S130–5.

59. Grasso F, Cirillo E, Quaremba G, et al. Otolaryngological features in a cohort of patients affected with 22q11.2 deletion syndrome: A monocentric survey. Am J Med Genet A 2018;176(10):2128–34.

60. Baylis W, Watson PJ, Moller KT. Structural and functional causes of hypernasality in velocardiofacial syndrome. A pilot Study. Folia Phoniatr Logop 2009;61:93–6.

61. Cheung ENM. Prevalence of Hypocaemia and it's associated features in 22q11.2 dletion syndrome. Clin Endocr 2014;81:190–6.

62. Giuliana G, Cirillo E, Maio F. Gastrointestinal involvement in patients affected with 22q11.2 deletion syndrome. Scand J Gastroenterol 2014;49(3):274–9.

63. Binenbaum G, McDonald-McGinn DM, Zackai EH, et al. Sclerocornea associated with the chromosome 22q11.2 deletion syndorme. Am J Med Genet 2008;146:904–9.

64. Cancrini C, Puliafito P, Digilio MC, et al. Clinical Features and Follow-Up in Patients with 22q11.2 Deletion Syndrome. J Pediatr 2014;164(6):1475–80.e2.

65. Vorstman JA, Breetvelt EJ, Duijff SN, et al. Cognitive decline preceding the onset of psychosis in patient with 22q11.2 deletion syndrome. JAMA psychiatry 2015;72:377–85.

The Heart Muscle and Valve Involvement in Marfan Syndrome, Loeys-Dietz Syndromes, and Collagenopathies

Adelaide Fusco, MD[a], Alfredo Mauriello, MD[a], Michele Lioncino, MD[a],
Giuseppe Palmiero, MD[a], Fiorella Fratta, MD[a], Chiara Granato, MD, PhD[b],
Annapaola Cirillo, MD, PhD[a], Martina Caiazza, MD[a], Emanuele Monda, MD[a],
Antonello Credendino, MD[c], Giovanni Signore, MD[a],
Francesco Natale, MD, PhD[a], Flavia Chiosi, MD[d], Gioacchino Scarano, MD[a],
Alessandro Della Corte, MD, PhD[a], Stefano Nistri, MD, PhD[e],
Maria Giovanna Russo, MD, PhD[a], Giuseppe Limongelli, MD, PhD[a],
Guglielmina Pepe, MD, PhD[f],*

KEYWORDS

- Marfan syndrome • Ehlers-Danlos syndrome • Loeys-Dietz syndrome • Fibrillinopathies
- Collagenophaties • TGFbetapathies • Cardiomyopathy: mitral valve prolapse

KEY POINTS

- Thoracic aortic syndromes are hereditary diseases that directly or indirectly affect the genesis of various organs mostly after a mutation of the TGF-β pathway.
- Cardiac involvement is typical of several inherited connective tissue disorders including Marfan syndrome, vascular Ehlers-Danlos syndrome, and Loeys-Dietz syndromes.
- The main cardiovascular anomalies involve the mitral and aortic valves as well as the aorta.
- The involvement of the heart muscle can present itself as primitive in Marfan syndrome.

INTRODUCTION

To date, about 200 heritable connective tissue disorders (CTDs) have been described. The heritable connective tissue disorders are multisystemic diseases displaying manifestations in the heart, blood vessels, eyes, bone, skin, joints, and lungs. After their discovery, casual mutations in wide range of genes encoding structural proteins, modifying enzymes, or components of signaling pathway were detected.[1]

Part of the ICTDs belong also to the hereditary thoracic aortic aneurysms and dissections (HTAADs). Marfan syndrome (MFS), vascular Ehlers-Danlos syndrome (vEDS), and Loeys-Dietz syndromes (LDSs), with cardiac and valve involvement, are the most representative and severe of the HTAADs group. These three disorders belong

[a] Department of Translational Medical Sciences, University of Campania "Luigi Vanvitelli", Naples 80131, Italy;
[b] Grupo de Enfermedades Cardiovasculares, Vall d'Hebron Institut de Recerca (VHIR), Barcelona, Spain;
[c] Department of Orthopaedics, AORN dei Colli, Monaldi Hospital; [d] Department of Ophthalmology, Azienda Ospedaliera dei Colli AORN Monaldi, Naples 80100, Italy; [e] Cardiology Service, CMSR Veneto Medica, Altavilla Vicentina, Italy; [f] Department of Experimental and Clinical Medicine, University of Florence, CRR Tuscany Marfan Center, Florence, Italy
* Corresponding author.
E-mail address: guglielmina.pepe@unifi.it

Heart Failure Clin 18 (2022) 165–175
https://doi.org/10.1016/j.hfc.2021.07.007
1551-7136/22/© 2021 Elsevier Inc. All rights reserved.

to both ICTDs and syndromic HTAADs categories. They are rare inherited autosomal dominant disorders, and MFS, LDS, and vEDS display an incidence of approximately 1 in 5000, 1 in 10,000, and 1 in 50,000, respectively.

DISCUSSION

MFS was described for the first time in 1896 by the French pediatrician Antoine Marfan, who identified in some subjects a phenotype characterized by dolichostenomelia, arachnodactyly, and dolichocephaly (**Fig. 1**).

The characterizing manifestations of MFS involve cardiovascular, ocular, and systemic features (SFs) (**Table 1**) (which display skeletal, ocular, and cardiovascular manifestations and involve also skin, the lungs, and central nervous system) that have to reach a score = greater than 7 to be positive. The clinical diagnosis is based on the presence of two of the three clinical features or one clinical stigma together with the presence of a first-degree relative affected by MFS or a pathogenic mutation in FBN1 gene (**Box 1**).

It is caused, in more than 90% of cases, by heterozygous mutations in FBN1, coding for the extracellular matrix (ECM) protein fibrillin-1. FBN1 gene is located on chromosome 15q21.1. The cardiovascular phenotype is represented by thoracic aortic aneurysm at the sinuses of Valsalva and dissection.[2] About 75% of patients with MFS has a familiar history; therefore, approximately 25% of Marfans present as sporadic cases. LDS is caused by mutations in genes encoding TGBR1/2, SMAD2/3, or TGFB2/3. The aforementioned genes code for components of the TGF-β-signaling pathway. Here, we will limit our description to the two most severe types, LDS type 1/TGFBR1 and LDS type 2/TGFBR2, which can be distinguished from MFS by the unique presence of hypertelorism, bifid uvula or cleft palate, aortic and arterial aneurysm, and tortuosity. Besides, LDS type 2/TGFBR2 may display features overlapping with vEDS such as translucent skin with easily visible underlying veins, easy bruising, and dystrophic scars.

Since the initial description of LDS, families with aortic aneurysms without significant outward features have also been described. LDS is an autosomal dominant disorder. De novo mutations cover about two-third of cases, whereas the other one-third are familial.[3]

LDS type 1 and 2 represent the most severe and common covering 20%-25% and 55%-60%, respectively, of the syndrome. LDS1 and LDS2 are 100% associated to TGFBR1 and TGFBR2, respectively. It is characterized by vascular findings (cerebral, thoracic [ectasia in Valsalva is present in 95% of patients], 50% of LDS patients present thoracic aneurysm undetectable by echocardiography, and abdominal arterial aneurysms and/or dissections tortuosity affect more cerebral and sovra-aortic vessels), skeletal manifestations (pectus excavatum or pectus carinatum, scoliosis, joint laxity, arachnodactyly, talipes equinovarus, cervical spine malformation, and/or instability), craniofacial features (widely spaced eyes, strabismus, bifid uvula/cleft palate, and craniosynostosis [>in LDS1, <in LDS2] that can involve any suture), and cutaneous findings (velvety and translucent skin, easy bruising, and dystrophic scars, milia, prominently on the face); eyes: individuals with LDS are predisposed to widespread and aggressive arterial aneurysms and pregnancy-related complications including uterine rupture and death. Individuals with LDS can show a strong predisposition for allergic/inflammatory diseases

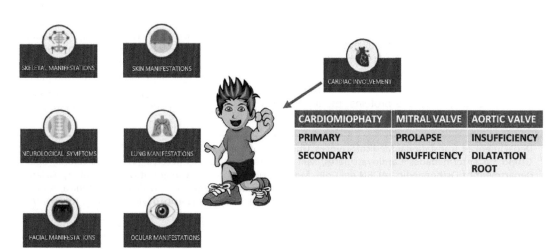

CARDIOMIOPHATY	MITRAL VALVE	AORTIC VALVE
PRIMARY	PROLAPSE	INSUFFICIENCY
SECONDARY	INSUFFICIENCY	DILATATION ROOT

Fig. 1. Central image of clinical features of Marfan syndrome.

Table 1	
Systemic score of Ghent criteria	
Systemic Involvement	**Points**
Wrist and thumb sign	3
Wrist or thumb sign	1
Pectus carinatum deformity	2
Pectus excavatum or chest asymmetry	1
Hindfoot deformity	2
Plain flat foot	1
Spontaneous pneumothorax	2
Dural ectasia	2
Protrusio acetabuli	2
Scoliosis or thoracolumbar kyphosis	1
Reduced elbow extension	1
3 of 5 facial features	1
Skin striae	1
Severe myopia (>3 diopters)	1
Mitral valve prolapse	1
Reduced upper segment/ lower segment (UL/LS) and increased arm span/height	1

Box 1
Ghent criteria for clinical diagnosis

In the absence of family history: 1

1. Ao ($Z \geq 2$) and EL = MFS
2. Ao ($Z \geq 2$) and FBN1 = MFS
3. Ao ($Z \geq 2$) and Syst (≥ 7 pts) = MFS
4. EL and FBN1 with known Ao = MFS

   EL with or without Syst and with FBN1 not known with Ao or no FBN1 = ELS

   Ao ($Z < 2$) and Syst (≥ 5 with at least one skeletal feature) without EL = MASS

   MVP and Ao ($Z < 2$) and Syst (<5) without EL = MVPS

In the presence of family history:

5. EL and FH of MFS (as defined above) = MFS
6. Syst (≥ 7) and FH of MFS (as defined above) = MFS
7. Ao ($Z \geq 2$ above 20 year old, ≥ 3 below 20 years) + FH of MFS = MFS

including asthma, eczema, and reactions to food or environmental allergens. There is also an increased incidence of gastrointestinal inflammation including eosinophilic esophagitis and gastritis or inflammatory bowel disease.

Arterial aneurysms have been observed in almost all side branches of the aorta including, but not limited to, the subclavian, renal, superior mesenteric, hepatic, and coronary arteries. Aortic dissection has been observed in early childhood (age ≥ 6 months) and/or at aortic dimensions that do not confer risk in other connective tissue disorders such as MFS. Arterial tortuosity can be generalized but most commonly involves the head and neck vessels.

There are no formal diagnostic criteria for diagnosis of LDS. However, TGFBR1/2 genetic testing should be considered in the following scenarios:

1. Patients with the typical clinical triad of hypertelorism, cleft palate, and arterial aneurysm.
2. Early-onset aortic aneurysm with variable combination of other features including manifestations related to collagen alterations.
3. Families with autosomal dominant thoracic aortic aneurysms, especially those families with precocious aortic/arterial dissection.
4. Patients with an MFS-like phenotype.
5. Patients clinically similar to vascular EDS (thin skin with atrophic scars, easy bruising, joint

hypermobility) and normal type III collagen biochemistry.
6. Isolated young probands with aortic root dilatation/dissection. If patients present with premature onset of osteoarthritis in addition to any of the aforementioned clinical scenarios, SMAD3 may be prioritized as the causal gene. Mutation in TGFB2 may also be considered, when the clinical presentation is rather mild. It should be remembered that the clinical overlap is so large that it is not possible to predict the correct causal gene on the basis of clinical signs alone. If craniosynostosis and intellectual disability are associated characteristics, SKI may be the first gene to be analyzed.

Compared to MFS, LDS cardiovascular manifestations tend to be more severe. In contrast, no association is reported between LDS and the presence of ectopia lentis, a key distinguishing feature of MFS[1] with only one exception at present regarding a patient with LDS type 4.[4]

Ehlers-Danlos syndrome is a broad term that describes a group of heritable connective tissue disorders that are classified together because of shared phenotypic and genotypic features. The phenotypic features are tissue fragility, joint hypermobility, and skin hyperextensibility. These characteristics can vary in degree across all subtypes. The different involvement of the various organs and systems helps to differentiate Ehlers-Danlos syndrome from other disorders of joint hypermobility. Genetically, Ehlers-Danlos syndrome results from defects in genes involved in collagen biosynthesis or structure. Since the discovery of Ehlers-Danlos syndrome, five different classification systems have been used by clinicians. The Villefranche Nosology, which was the most recent nosology used until 2017, recognized six Ehlers-Danlos syndrome subtypes according to major and minor clinical criteria. Since the introduction of the Villefranche Nosology, research on Ehlers-Danlos syndrome has expanded, and new subtypes were discovered. Therefore, an updated classification system for Ehlers-Danlos syndrome was proposed. The International Consortium on Ehlers-Danlos syndrome, formed in 2012, devised the 2017 International Classification of the Ehlers-Danlos Syndromes, which delineated clinical subtypes according to their clinical manifestations. The 13 clinical subtypes reported by the 2017 International Classification of the Ehlers-Danlos Syndromes are Classical EDS, vEDS, Kyphoscoliotic EDS, Arthrochalasia EDS, Dermatosparaxis EDS, Brittle cornea syndrome, Classical-like EDS, Spondylodysplastic EDS, Musculocontractural EDS, Myopathic EDS, Periodontal EDS, Cardiac-valvular EDS (cvEDS), Hypermobile EDS. Each subtype has a set of major and minor criteria to guide clinicians evaluating patients with suspected EDS. EDS is associated with an increased incidence of cardiovascular abnormalities, such as mitral valve prolapse and aortic dissection.[5]

Ehlers-Danlos syndromes are typically diagnosed based on clinical findings and family history. Nevertheless, genetic consultation should be considered in certain patients:

i. Patients with a family history positive for EDS.
ii. Beighton score greater than or equal to 5.
iii. History of recurrent dislocations with minor trauma, recurrent postoperative instability, and personal or family history of arterial or visceral rupture.

Geneticists will make the diagnosis and subtype classification (**Table 2**). Timely diagnosis of Ehlers-Danlos syndrome is essential before initiating the appropriate care of these patients, including genetic counseling for patients and families, musculoskeletal treatment, cardiovascular screening (for valvular and vascular abnormalities), and optimizing perioperative treatment.

SUMMARY
Cardiovascular Features in Marfan Syndrome

The cardiovascular manifestations of MFS account for a large percentage of the morbidity and mortality of the disease. The most prominent cardiovascular feature is a dilation of the aortic root (**Figs. 2** and **3**), at the level of the sinus of Valsalva, which is present in the vast majority of patients. However, great variability in rate of ectasia is observed between affected individuals. As a consequence of the dilatation at the aortic root, aortic regurgitation might develop.[6] The ectasia might evolve toward an aneurysm. The aneurysm might lead to a type A dissection or rupture.[4]

A minority of MFS patients (10%–20%) show an ectasia of the descended and abdominal aorta, which can lead to a type B dissection.[7,8]

Another important common manifestation of MFS is mitral valve prolapse (MVP).[9,10] Although, only a minority of MFS patients will meet surgery as a consequence of MVP. MVP leads to complications such as severe mitral valve regurgitation, especially in adolescent women, and can result in heart failure and pulmonary hypertension.[8] In addition, calcification of the mitral valve can already be present at a young age.[9] However, the same clinical determinants (echocardiographic criteria, age, body mass index, and body surface area) that predict outcomes in idiopathic mitral valve prolapse also predict outcomes in mitral valve prolapse associated with MFS.[11] Incidence of aortic dilatation and mitral prolapse in patients with MFS is comparable in children and adults of the same sex.[12]

The other heart valves are also involved, including tricuspid valve prolapse and regurgitation and aortic valve insufficiency.[8] Although the bicuspid aortic valve (BAV) has been suggested to be more common,[13,14] congenital heart malformations occur far less frequent in MFS than LDS.[15] Moreover a more recent article shows no preferential association of BAV with MFS.[16] Further investigation will be required to investigate if there are differences among populations.

Dilatation of the main pulmonary artery is also commonly observed in patients with MFS, but dissections or ruptures are rare.

Dilated cardiomyopathy is an underestimated clinical feature of the syndrome. Myocardial dysfunction is often considered to be the consequence of valvular involvement and ventricular volume overload.[8] However, in a subgroup of patients without significant valvular dysfunction, subclinical cardiac dysfunction has been described. A combination of increased aortic wall stiffness and ECM abnormalities might explain these features.[15]

In one study, it was observed that the reduction in aortic elasticity (of which flow wave velocity [FWV] is a measurable derivative) was associated with an increase in afterload with subsequent cardiac involvement. However, there is no significant relation between LVEF and FWV, suggesting that the impairment of ventricular function was not

Table 2
Summary of the characteristics of the main types of Ehlers Danlos syndrome

Major Subtype	Inheritance	Major Diagnostic Criteria (and Other Clinical Features)	Genes
Classic	AD (or AR)	Significant skin hyperextensibility and velvety skin. Significant tissue fragility and widened atrophic scars: and/or Significant joint hypermobility.	COL5A1, COL5A2
Hypermobile	AD	Significant joint hypermobility. Moderate skin hyperextensibility and/or velvety skin. (no significant tissue fragility or wound healing abnormalities)	TNXB
Vascular (more serious)	AD	Fragility or spontaneous rupture of vasculature or visceral organs. Significant bruising. Thin, translucent skin. Characteristic facies of prominent eyes, thin face, nose, and lobeless ears. (No significant skin hyperextensibility. Joint hypermobility restricted to minor joints.)	COL3A1
Kyphoscoliotic	AR	Significant joint hypermobility. Severe muscular hypotonia at birth. Progressive kyphoscoliosis. Globe rupture.	PLOD1
Arthrochalasic	AD	Severe joint hypermobility with recurrent subluxations. Congenital bilateral hip dislocation, (moderate skin hyperextensibility and tissue fragility)	COL1Al, COL1A2
Dermatosparactic	AR	Severe skin fragility. Sagging and redundant skin. (Easy bruising and soft, doughy skin)	ADAMTS2
Progeroid	AR	Wrinkled face. Frizzy and thin hair. Sparse eyelashes and eyebrows.	B4GALT7
Cardiac valve	AR	Hyperextensible skin. Joint hypermobility. Heart valve defects.	COL1A2

due to reduced aortic elasticity. Probably, the altered fibrillin-1 causes impairment of myocardial contraction. Furthermore, fibrillin-1 mutation leads to an altered TGF-β expression in the ECM of the myocardium. Excess of TGF-β in the ECM of the myocardium possibly leads to altered genetic expression through activation of the SMAD pathway and, consequently, to myocardial structural changes. TGF-β is also known to be involved in fibrosis in pressure-loaded heart failure and to be overexpressed in the myocardium of patients with idiopathic hypertrophic cardiomyopathy.[17]

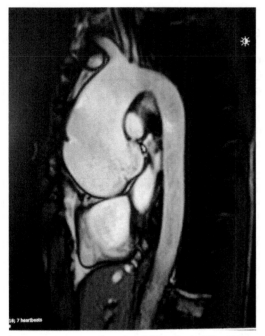

Fig. 2. TC Image. Dilatation of aortic root in patient with Marfan syndrome.

Worsening of regional myocardial deformation may be the first sign of reduction of the left ventricular systolic function. Significant decrease of the

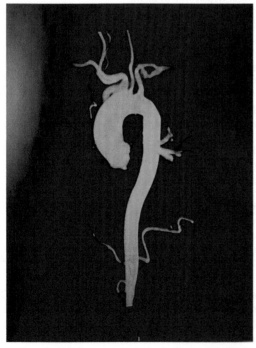

Fig. 3. Dilatation of aortic root in patient with Marfan syndrome. TC image.

circumferential strain is founded in the interventricular septum and inferior wall[18] (**Figs. 4–6**).

In particular, a uniform reduction in regional deformation of the RV-free lateral wall was demonstrated. Biventricular ejection fraction was impaired in patients with MFS, and the involvement was independent of aortic elasticity and β-blocker usage. A strong correlation between LVEF and RVEF has been observed regarding the heart deterioration.[17]

The biventricular dilatation and dysfunction are usually mild, asymptomatic, and independent from other cardiovascular manifestations.

Additionally, a minority of patients can present arrhythmias regardless of the presence of ventricular dysfunction.[8,9]

Recently, it was thought to use sacubitril/valsartan for the treatment of heart failure associated with cardiomyopathy associated to MFS. There is a case report describing the use of the drug in a young patient. Sacubitril/valsartan has been added to optimal medical therapy after hemodynamic stabilization. The patients have had a progressive clinical, laboratory, and echocardiographic improvement. After 9-month follow-up, the patient maintained a free survival from heart failure and a good quality of life.[19]

Neonatal MFS is typically more serious. It is characterized by early onset severe tricuspid and mitral valve regurgitation, which can lead them to death because of the development of the heart fealure.[20]

Furthermore, a study based on a cohort of 30 young people showed that the absence of family history and the presence of BAV were associated to severe aortic phenotype and worse prognosis.[2]

The valve insufficiencies are independent from aortic dilation.

A higher incidence of pregnancy-related complications, particularly aortic dissection, has been observed in patients with MFS.[21]

Cardiovascular Features in Loeys-Dietz Syndrome

The main cardiovascular feature in LDS is dilatation of the aortic root at the level of the sinus of Valsalva. This complication is present in the vast majority of patients,[22] similar to MFS. Dilatation of the aortic root can be associated with aortic valve involvement. Impaired left ventricular systolic function could be the consequence of coronary artery involvement.[8]

LDS has a high association with many congenital heart diseases (CHDs). For example, the prevalence of patent ductus arteriosus (PDA) and atrial septal defects (ASDs) is much higher in individuals

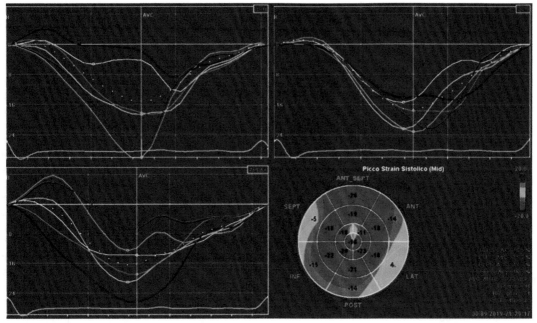

Fig. 4. Global longitudinal in patient with Marfan syndrome.

with LDS types 1 and 2 than in the general population. The reported prevalence of PDA and ASD in these populations are 35%–54% and 22%–31%, respectively.[23–25] Prevalence of mitral valve prolapse, left ventricular hypertrophy, and aneurysmal disease is higher in individuals with LDS than in the general population.[23,26] The link between CHD and LDS suggests the importance to perform periodic and frequent echocardiography to monitor patients for possible cardiac complications.[26]

In LDS, pulmonary valve stenosis that could also develop over time has been observed.[22]

As in MFS, MVP and mitral valve insufficiency are more frequently observed in LDS than in general population,[26,27] but they appear to be somewhat less common in LDS than in MFS.[28]

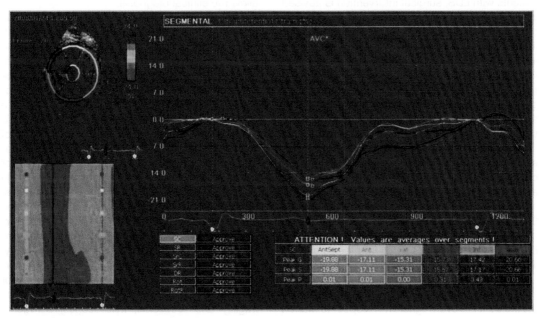

Fig. 5. Radial strain in patient with Marfan syndrome.

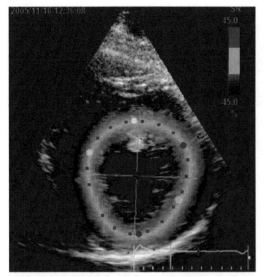

Fig. 6. Radial strain in patient with Marfan syndrome.

Owing to the aggressive nature of the aortic disease associated with LDS and the low rate of complications associated with valve-sparing aortic root replacement surgery, prophylactic surgery of the aortic root is recommended at smaller aortic dimensions compared with the aortic size required for the surgical replacement of other inherited aortopathies.[26,29]

In addition, the size threshold for surgery is lower than that advised by the American College of Cardiology Foundation and the American Heart Association for surgical repair in cases of atherosclerotic ascending aortic aneurysms (5.5 cm). In patients with LDS, surgical intervention is advised when the absolute aortic root diameter is greater than 4.4 cm at angiography.[29] In a recently published series,[30] the investigators suggested lowering the aortic root diameter threshold to 4 cm for a subgroup with a higher risk for dissection at this smaller diameter: females with TGFBR2 gene mutations and severe phenotypic features such as aortic tortuosity, hypertelorism, and bifid uvula.

Another group[26] recommended considering earlier intervention in patients who have severe craniofacial features and a family history of severe aortic disease and particularly when there is an increment of rate of aortic diameter greater than 0.5 cm per year.[26]

Left ventricular hypertrophy and atrial fibrillation may develop,[22,31] especially in older patients. These aspects are both uncommon in MFS.

A high incidence of pregnancy-related complications has been observed. However, in LDS, the incidence is even higher with respect to Marfan patients. Underlying the increased risk, there are probably several factors, including hemodynamic changes, hormonal influences, and the change of elastic fiber organization during pregnancy.[22]

Cardiovascular Features in Ehlers-Danlos Syndrome

vEDS, cvEDS, and hypermobile Ehlers-Danlos display cardiovascular involvement.

The cvEDS is caused by rare recessive loss-of-function mutations in COL1A2. When no mutations are detected in these diseases, a copy number variation analysis searching for duplications or large deletions is required as a second step. Deep intronic mutations may go undetected. The cvEDS is an infrequent subtype of Ehlers-Danlos syndrome with classical mitral or aortic valve involvement. The compromise of all cardiac valves is rare. The occurrence of symptoms or the presence of right ventricular dysfunction with increased volumes in asymptomatic patients determines indications of valvular replacement to avoid the appearance of heart failure. Strict testing follow-up can help to determine the optimal time of intervention in patients with a high rate of intraoperative and postoperative complications.[32]

Major criteria are represented by severe and progressive aortic and mitral valve problems, skin involvement with hyperextensibility, thin and easy bruising skin, and joint hypermobility of small joints. Minor criteria display pectus excavatum, pes planus, planovalgus, and Hallux valgus, joint dislocations, inguinal hernia. Two major criteria or one major criterion and 2 or more minor criteria allow the clinical diagnosis.[33]

The vascular form of Ehlers-Danlos syndrome is caused by dominant mutations in COL3A1 with few cases of mutations in COL1A1 involving Arg312Cys, Arg574Cys, and Arg1093Cys substitutions causing vascular fragility.[34] Concordance between mitral valve prolapse and abnormal production of type III collagen in patients suggests a pathogenetic link between the characteristic biochemical abnormality of vascular form of Ehlers-Danlos syndrome and mitral valve prolapse. Major criteria are positive familiarity for vEDS in the presence of pathogenic mutation in COL3A1 gene, arterial rupture in young adults, and a positive history for sigmoid colon perforation in absence of other bowel diseases and diverticula. Uterine rupture often during the third trimester of pregnancy but also after delivery, spontaneous carotid-cavernous sinus fistula formation also appear among major criteria. Minor criteria include characteristic facies, gingival fragility and recession, keratoconus, acrogeria, thin translucent skin with evident subcutaneous venous and spontaneous bruising, early-onset varicose veins, spontaneous pneumothorax, congenital hip dislocation, hypermobility of small joints, tendon and muscle rupture, and talipes equinovarus. The presence of 2 or 3 major criteria or 1 major criterion with more minor criterion requires genetic analysis.

The hypermobile form of Ehlers-Danlos syndrome, the only one without known associated genes at present, includes MPV.

Medical Drug Therapy

Although no reduction in mortality or dissection rate has been observed in any trial, beta-blockers, in particular atenolol, remain the mainstay for medical treatment in Marfan/heritable thoracic aortic disease patients, reducing wall shear stress and aortic growth rate. Rigid antihypertensive medical treatment aimed at a 24-hour ambulatory systolic blood pressure less than 130 mm Hg (110 mm Hg in patients with aortic dissection) is important, although there are no data to establish outright blood pressure thresholds. Angiotensin receptor antagonists did not prove to have a superior effect when compared with beta-blockers or in addition to beta-blockers in several trials but are considered in patients with bradycardia and/or asthma and may be considered as an alternative in patients intolerant to beta-blockers. Medical treatment should be continued after surgery. The risk of complications is not reduced after surgery. Ongoing meta-analyses of medical treatment trials may help define subgroups based on genetic and clinical data who benefit from specific treatment. As no medical trials have been conducted in non-Marfan HTAD, they are all treated as Marfan patients.[22]

Surgical Treatment

Prophylactic aortic root surgery is the only definitive treatment for the prevention of aortic dissection in MFS and related HTADs. In patients with anatomically normal aortic valves and low-grade regurgitation, a valve-sparing aortic root replacement by a Dacron prosthesis and reimplantation of the coronary arteries into the prosthesis (David procedure) has become the preferred surgical procedure with good long-term outcome, in HTADs. Composite graft replacement, usually with a mechanical valve, is a more durable alternative but does require lifelong anticoagulation. The decision on which technique to use should be made on an individual basis, and patient preferences and surgical experience should be taken into account. Marfan and related HTADs are associated with a risk of redissection and recurrent aneurysm in the distal aorta, especially in patients with previous dissection. With improved life expectancy, these complications now occur more frequently. Open aortic surgery remains the main method for treatment of distal aortic disease, although hybrid procedures with endovascular stenting where proximal and distal landing is possible that Dacron tube may be considered in selected cases are also preferred.[35]

Follow-up Recommendations

Lifelong and regular multidisciplinary follow-up at an expert center is required. Echocardiography and CCT/CMR (these last every 4 years) are the principal examinations.[22]

Cardiovascular surgery in children with MFS is uncommonly performed, and consequently, no physician, surgeon, or even institution has gained extensive experience. The most important predictors are age and size of the children in determining the outcomes of these surgical interventions. By the time children with MFS reach the age of 10 or 12 years, the operations in the aortic root and mitral valve can be performed as safely as they are in young adults. However, the prognosis is usually poor if surgery is needed during infancy. The outcome of aortic surgery in neonates is likely worse than mitral valve surgery.[35]

- The characterizing manifestations of MFS involve cardiovascular, ocular, and systemic features (SF).
- Almost 50% of LDS patients present thoracic aneurysm previously undetectable by echocardiography and abdominal arterial aneurysms and/or dissections tortuosity affecting cerebral and sovra-aortic vessels.
- LDS type1/TGFBR1 and LDS type2/TGFBR2 can usually be distinguished from MFS by the unique presence of hypertelorism, bifid uvula, and/or cleft palate.

CLINICS CARE POINTS

DISCLOSURE

The authors have nothing to disclose.

REFERENCES

1. Meester JAN, Verstraeten A, Schepers D, et al. Differences in manifestations of Marfan syndrome,

Ehlers-Danlos syndrome, and Loeys-Dietz syndrome. Ann Cardiothorac Surg 2017;6(6):582–94.

2. Monda E, Fusco A, Melis D, et al. Clinical significance of family history and bicuspid aortic valve in children and young adult patients with Marfan syndrome. Cardiol Young 2020;30(5):663–7.

3. Van Laer L, Dietz H, Loeys B. Loeys-Dietz syndrome. Adv Exp Med Biol 2014;802:95–105.

4. Braverman AC, Blinder KJ, Khanna S, et al. Ectopia lentis in Loeys-Dietz syndrome type 4. Am J Med Genet A 2020;182(8):1957–9.

5. Miller E, Grosel JM. A review of Ehlers-Danlos syndrome. J Am Acad Physician Assist 2020;33(4):23–8.

6. Attias D, Stheneur C, Roy C, et al. Comparison of clinical presentations and outcomes between patients with TGFBR2 and FBN1 mutations in Marfan syndrome and related disorders. Circulation 2009;120:2541–9.

7. Verstraeten A, Alaerts M, Van Laer L, et al. Marfan Syndrome and Related Disorders: 25 Years of Gene Discovery. Hum Mutat 2016;37:524–31.

8. Bradley TJ, Bowdin SC, Morel CF, et al. The Expanding Clinical Spectrum of Extracardiovascular and Cardiovascular Manifestations of Heritable Thoracic Aortic Aneurysm and Dissection. Can J Cardiol 2016;32:86–99.

9. De Backer J, Loeys B, Devos D, et al. A critical analysis of minor cardiovascular criteria in the diagnostic evaluation of patients with Marfan syndrome. Genet Med 2006;8:401–8.

10. Faivre L, Collod-Beroud G, Loeys BL, et al. Effect of mutation type and location on clinical outcome in 1,013 probands with Marfan syndrome or related phenotypes and FBN1 mutations: an international study. Am J Hum Genet 2007;81:454–66.

11. Rybczynski M, Treede H, Sheikhzadeh S, et al. Predictors of outcome of mitral valve prolapse in patients with the Marfan syndrome. Am J Cardiol 2011;107(2):268–74.

12. Brown OR, Henry D, Kloster FE, et al. Aortic Root Dilatation and Mitral Valve Prolapse in Marfan's Syndrome - An Echocardiographic Study. Circulation 1975;52(4):651–7.

13. Amezcua-Guerra L, Santiago C, Espinola-Zavaleta N, et al. Bicuspid aortic valve: a synergistic factor for aortic dilation and dissection in Marfan syndrome? Rev Invest Clin 2010;62:39–43.

14. Nistri S, Porciani MC, Attanasio M, et al. Association of Marfan syndrome and bicuspid aortic valve: frequency and outcome. Int J Cardiol 2012;155(2):324–5.

15. Attias D, Mansencal N, Auvert B, et al. Prevalence, characteristics, and outcomes of patients presenting with cardiogenic unilateral pulmonary edema. Circulation 2010;122:1109–15.

16. Milleron O, Ropers J, Arnoult F, et al. Clinical Significance of Aortic Root Modification Associated With Bicuspid Aortic Valve in Marfan Syndrome. Circ Cardiovasc Imaging 2019;12(3):e008129.

17. de Witte P, Aalberts JJ, Radonic T, et al. Intrinsic biventricular dysfunction in Marfan syndrome. Heart 2011;97(24):2063–8.

18. Lunev E, Malev E, Korshunova A, et al. Cardiomyopathy in patients with Marfan syndrome and marfanoid habitus. Curr Res Cardiol 2017;4(1):138–42.

19. Spoto S, Valeriani E, Locorriere L, et al. Use of sacubitril/valsartan in Marfan syndrome-related cardiomyopathy: The first case report. Medicine (Baltimore) 2019;98(47):e17978.

20. Takeda N, Yagi H, Hara H, et al. Pathophysiology and Management of Cardiovascular Manifestations in Marfan and Loeys-Dietz Syndromes. Int Heart J 2016;57:271–7.

21. Maeda J, Kosaki K, Shiono J, et al. Variable severity of cardiovascular phenotypes in patients with an early-onset form of Marfan syndrome harboring FBN1 mutations in exons 24-32. Heart Vessels 2016;31:1717–23.

22. Smith K, Gros B. Pregnancy-related acute aortic dissection in Marfan syndrome: A review of the literature. Congenit Heart Dis 2017;12:251–60.

23. Tirone D. Cardiovascular Operations in Children With Marfan Syndrome. Semin Thorac Cardiovasc Surg 2019. https://doi.org/10.1053/j.semtcvs.2019.07.009.

24. Loeys BL, Chen J, Neptune ER, et al. A syndrome of altered cardiovascular, craniofacial, neurocognitive and skeletal development caused by mutations in TGFBR1 or TGFBR2. Nat Genet 2005;37(3):275–81.

25. Loeys BL, Schwarze U, Holm T, et al. Aneurysm syndromes caused by mutations in the TGF-beta receptor. N Engl J Med 2006;355(8):788–98.

26. MacCarrick G, Black JH 3rd, Bowdin S, et al. Loeys-Dietz syndrome: a primer for diagnosis and management. Genet Med 2014;16(8):576–87.

27. Van de Laar IM, van der Linde D, Oei EH, et al. Phenotypic spectrum of the SMAD3-related aneurysms-osteoarthritis syndrome. J Med Genet 2012;49:47–57.

28. Renard M, Callewaert B, Malfait F, et al. Thoracic aortic-aneurysm and dissection in association with significant mitral valve disease caused by mutations in TGFB2. Int J Cardiol 2013;165:584–7.

29. Hiratzka LF, Bakris GL, Beckman JA, et al. 2010 ACCF/AHA/AATS/ACR/ASA/SCA/SCAI/SIR/STS/SVM guidelines for the diagnosis and management of patients with thoracic aortic disease: a report of the American College of Cardiology Foundation/American Heart Association Task Force on Practice Guidelines, American Association for Thoracic Surgery, American College of Radiology, American Stroke Association, Society of Cardiovascular Anesthesiologists, Society for Cardiovascular Angiography and Interventions, Society of Interventional Radiology, Society of Thoracic Surgeons, and

Society for Vascular Medicine. J Am Coll Cardiol 2010;55(14):e27–129.

30. Jondeau G, Ropers J, Regalado E, et al. International registry of patients carrying TGFBR1 or TGFBR2 mutations: results of the MAC (Montalcino Aortic Consortium). Circ Cardiovasc Genet 2016; 9(6):548–58.

31. van der Linde D, van de Laar IM, Bertoli-Avella AM, et al. Aggressive cardiovascular phenotype of aneurysms-osteoarthritis syndrome caused by pathogenic SMAD3 variants. J Am Coll Cardiol 2012;60: 397–403.

32. Chango Azanza DX, Munín MA, Sánchez GA, et al. Prolapse and regurgitation of the four heart valves in a patient with Ehlers-Danlos Syndrome: a case report. Eur Heart J Case Rep 2019;3(2): ytz052.

33. Jaffe AS, Geltman EM, Rodey GE, et al. Mitral valve prolapse: a consistent manifestation of type IV Ehlers-Danlos syndrome. The pathogenetic role of the abnormal production of type III collagen. Circulation 1981;64:121–5.

34. Malfait F, Francomano C, Byers P, et al. The 2017 international classification of the Ehlers-Danlos syndromes. Am J Med Genet C Semin Med Genet 2017;175(1):8–26.

35. Baumgartner H, De Backer Je, Babu-Narayan SV, et al, ESC Scientific Document Group. 2020 ESC Guidelines for the management of adult congenital heart disease: The Task Force for the management of adult congenital heart disease of the European Society of Cardiology (ESC). Endorsed by: Association for European Paediatric and Congenital Cardiology (AEPC), International Society for Adult Congenital Heart Disease (ISACHD). Eur Heart J 2021;42(Issue 6):563–645.

New Frontiers in the Treatment of Homozygous Familial Hypercholesterolemia

Arturo Cesaro, MD[a,b], Fabio Fimiani, BSc[c], Felice Gragnano, MD[a,b], Elisabetta Moscarella, MD[a,b], Alessandra Schiavo, MD[a,b], Andrea Vergara, MD[a,b], Leo Akioyamen, MD[d], Laura D'Erasmo, MD, PhD[e], Maurizio Averna, MD[f], Marcello Arca, MD[e], Paolo Calabrò, MD, PhD[a,b],*

KEYWORDS

- Homozygous familial hypercholesterolemia • PCSK9 • Lomitapide • Inclisiran • Gene therapy
- Gene-editing • Angiopoietin-like 3 • Low-density lipoprotein cholesterol

KEY POINTS

- Homozygous familial hypercholesterolemia (HoFH) is a rare genetic disorder.
- Extreme elevations in low-density lipoprotein cholesterol and early-onset, progressive atherosclerotic cardiovascular disease are the most frequent clinical manifestations in affected patients.
- To date, the treatment of HoFH represents a challenge in the real-life clinical scenario.
- Low-density lipoprotein receptor (LDLR) residual activity is the major determinant of phenotype in patients with HoFH and standard lipid-lowering therapy works primarily on an LDLR-mediated pathway.
- Novel medications targeting non-LDLR pathways and strategies that involve gene-editing are innovative approaches for HoFH treatments.

INTRODUCTION

Homozygous familial hypercholesterolemia (HoFH) is a rare and life-threatening genetic disease that affects approximately 1 in 160,000 to 320,000 people.[1–4] It is clinically characterized by plasma total cholesterol levels greater than 13 mmol/L (>500 mg/dL), extensive xanthomas, and early and progressive atherosclerotic cardiovascular disease (ASCVD).[1,5–7] The most common cause is a mutation in both alleles of the gene encoding for the low-density lipoprotein cholesterol (LDL-C) receptor (LDLR). Yet, other disease-causing mutations may be present in alleles of other genes, which include apolipoprotein B (ApoB), proprotein convertase subtilisin/kexin type 9 (PCSK9), and LDLR adaptor protein (LDLRAP1). Pathogenic variants of LDLR, ApoB, and PCSK9 are responsible for autosomal dominant hypercholesterolemia, and mutations in

[a] Department of Translational Medical Sciences, University of Campania "Luigi Vanvitelli", Naples, Italy; [b] Division of Cardiology, A.O.R.N. "Sant'Anna e San Sebastiano", Edificio C – Cardiologia Universitaria, Via Ferdinando Palasciano 1, Caserta 81100, Italy; [c] Unit of Inherited and Rare Cardiovascular Diseases, A.O.R.N. Dei Colli "V. Monaldi", Via Leonardo Bianchi snc, Naples 80131, Italy; [d] Faculty of Medicine, University of Toronto, 200 Elizabeth Street, Toronto, Ontario M5G 2C4, Canada; [e] Department of Translational and Precision Medicine "Sapienza" University of Rome, Azienda Ospedaliero-Universitaria Policlinico Umberto I, Ex III Clinica Medica, Viale dell'Università, 37, Rome 00185, Italy; [f] Department of Health Promotion Sciences Maternal and Infantile Care, University of Palermo, A.O.U.P 'Paolo Giaccone' Padiglione n. 10, Via del Vespro 129, Palermo 90127, Italy
* Corresponding author. Division of Cardiology, A.O.R.N. "Sant'Anna e San Sebastiano", Edificio C – Cardiologia Universitaria, Via Ferdinando Palasciano 1, Caserta 81100, Italy.
E-mail address: paolo.calabro@unicampania.it
Twitter: @arturocesaro (A.C.); @FeliceGragnano (F.G.); @paolocalabro1 (P.C.)

Heart Failure Clin 18 (2022) 177–188
https://doi.org/10.1016/j.hfc.2021.07.008

LDLRAP1 are responsible for autosomal recessive hypercholesterolemia.[8,9]

The most severe phenotype is typically found in patients with mutations that lead to complete loss of LDLR function in both copies of the gene (receptor-negative/null mutations).[1,10] Given the complications of ASCVD associated with HoFH, reducing the impact of elevated LDL-C levels is critical.

Based on the evidence that lowering LDL-C levels can mitigate atherosclerosis progression and delay the onset of clinically evident ASCVD, lipid-lowering therapy (LLT) should be initiated as soon as possible.[11–13] The 2013 Consensus Statement of the European Atherosclerosis Society (EAS) established primary prevention LDL-C targets in adults with HoFH of less than 2.5 mmol/L (<100 mg/dL; <3.5 mmol/L [<135 mg/dL]) in children or less than 1.8 mmol/L (<70 mg/dL) in adults with established ASCVD.[1] The 2019 European Society of Cardiology (ESC)/EAS Guidelines for the management of dyslipidemias highlighted the impact of genetic hypercholesterolemia on the development of CV, recommending very ambitious LDL-C targets.[2] In FH patients with ASCVD (very high risk), they recommend (class I, level C) to achieve ≥50% reduction of LDL-C from baseline and a target LDL-C less than 1.4 mmol/L (<55 mg/dL). Furthermore, for primary prevention, patients with FH who are at very high risk should achieve an LDL-C reduction of ≥50% from baseline, and an LDL-C goal of less than 1.4 mmol/L (<55 mg/dL).[2]

Management of patients with HoFH presents a notable challenge in clinical practice, with most available therapies failing to provide effective treatment responses. The aim of this review is to provide a comprehensive overview of currently available treatments and emerging therapeutic strategies for HoFH patients.

TRADITIONAL THERAPIES FOR HOMOZYGOUS FAMILIAL HYPERCHOLESTEROLEMIA PATIENTS

Statins are the first-line therapy for the management of hypercholesterolemia in HoFH patients. Current guidelines recommend the use of a high potency statin at the maximum tolerated dose as the first approach.[1,2] Statins work by increasing LDLRs on the surface of hepatocytes; therefore, patients with mutations in the LDLR gene should not theoretically benefit. Yet, statins do have an effect (albeit smaller than in other forms of FH) on reducing LDL-C levels by acting on alternative pathways of cholesterol production.[14] LDL-C reduction observed in these patients is approximately 20%.[1] Of note, statins have been shown

to delay the onset of cardiovascular events and to prolong survival in patients with HoFH.[12] The 2019 ESC/EAS Guidelines suggest that children with FH should be treated with a proper diet, according to the same guidelines and low-dose statins from the age of 6 to 10 years, and doses should be increased to achieve the goal LDL-C: in children older than 10 years, the goal is an LDL-C less than 3.5 mmol/L (less than 135 mg/dL), and in younger children, the goal is a ≥50% reduction.[2]

Ezetimibe is a selective cholesterol absorption inhibitor that works by binding to the Niemann-Pick C1 Like 1 (NPC1L1) protein.[15] Polymorphisms in NPC1L1 are associated with lower serum LCL-C and lower rate of cardiovascular events. In particular, ezetimibe inhibits the intestinal dietary and biliary cholesterol absorption by affecting its enterocyte uptake.[15] The use of ezetimibe in combination therapy with statins has shown to offer an additional reduction in LDL-C levels of about 10% to 15%.[16–19] Therefore, ezetimibe may be the first non-statin lipid-lowering drug for the management of hypercholesterolemia in HoFH patients. A summary of the available and developing drugs is shown in **Fig. 1**.

Extracorporeal removal of LDL-C is an effective but costly and time-consuming adjunctive treatment for HoFH.[20–22] A single treatment can reduce plasma LDL-C levels by 55%–70% from baseline, which enables patients to achieve near-normal values with a weekly regimen of apheresis. Side effects of apheresis include more frequent hypotension, but other reactions like abdominal pain, nausea, hypocalcemia, and iron deficiency anemia should not be overlooked. These are rarely serious but can be debilitating and impact patients' quality of life.

There is clinical evidence that long-term apheresis of lipoproteins may contribute to plaque regression and/or stabilization and improved prognosis among patients affected by HoFH.[23,24] The European Consensus Document[1] suggests that treatment should be started as early as possible in patients with very severe homozygous phenotypes, ideally within 5 years and no later than 8 years of age. However, age and frequency of treatment can present challenges because of the availability of specialized centers, severity of disease, and choice of the patient and their families.

Liver transplantation corrects molecular defects in the organ that is most responsible for LDL clearance, which leads to a marked improvement in LDL-C levels. Although it is an effective therapeutic strategy, either alone or in combination with a heart transplant,[25–27] there are obvious

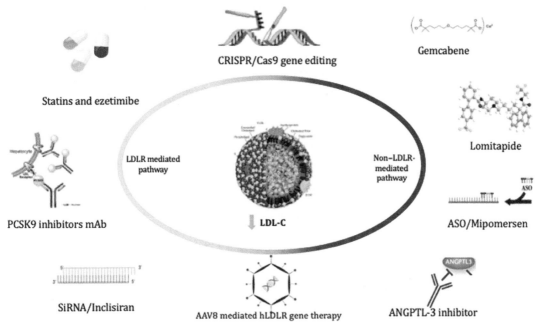

Fig. 1. Current and future medications for the treatment of homozygous familial hypercholesterolemia. AAV8, adeno-associated virus8; ANGPTL-3, angiopoietin-like protein 3; ASO; antisense oligonucleotides; CRISPR/Cas9, clustered regularly interspaced short palindromic repeats (CRISPR)–CRISPR-associated gene 9; LDL-C, low-density lipoprotein cholesterol; LDLR, low-density lipoprotein receptor; mAb, monoclonal antibody; MTP, microsomal triglyceride transport protein; PCSK9, proprotein convertase subtilisin/kexin type 9; SiRNA, small interfering RNA.

drawbacks, such as the high risk of post-transplant surgical complications and mortality, scarcity of donors, and the need for lifelong treatment with immunosuppressive therapy.[28]

PCSK9 INHIBITION
Monoclonal Antibodies PSCK9 Inhibitors

HoFH is associated with markedly elevated PCSK9 levels, with or without statin treatment.[29–31] Thus, the use of PCSK9 inhibitors as adjunctive therapy in patients with defective mutations in the LDLR gene or those with gain-of-function mutations of PCSK9 offers an additional therapeutic approach toward optimizing LDL-C reduction.[29] PCSK9 inhibitors inhibit the interaction of PCSK9 with LDLR and increase its recycling to the cell surface of hepatocytes.[32,33] Two agents have been approved for the treatment of FH as an add-on therapy to standard LLT[2,34,35]: evolocumab, which is a fully human immunoglobin (Ig) G2, and alirocumab, a fully human IgG1 anti-PCSK9 monoclonal antibody. Both evolocumab and alirocumab have been approved for the treatment of FH as an add-on therapy to standard LLT.[2,34,35] PCSK9 inhibitors have been shown to dramatically reduce LDL-C levels and improve prognoses of patients with established CV disease or heterozygous FH.[36–38] Moreover, they have

become part of routine clinical practice in the management of dyslipidemias, and they are currently recommended for lowering LDL-C in patients who cannot achieve target levels with a combination therapy of statin and ezetimibe.[2]

PCSK9 inhibitors have been shown to be safe and effective in the treatment of HoFH (**Table 1**). In inhibiting the functioning of PCSK9, they work to increase the expression of endogenous LDLRs. The Trial Evaluating PCSK9 Antibody in Subjects with LDLR Abnormalities (TESLA) study[39] was a two-part (parts A and B) phase II/III multicenter trial that was designed to evaluate the safety, tolerability, and efficacy of evolocumab compared with placebo in patients with HoFH. The third phase, a randomized controlled double-blind study, involved 49 adult and adolescent (aged ≥12 years) patients with HoFH who were being treated with a stable dose of statins. Participants were randomly assigned in a 2:1 ratio to treatment with 420 mg of evolocumab or placebo subcutaneously every 4 weeks for 12 weeks. The primary endpoint was percentage change in LDL-C from baseline to week 12. Secondary efficacy endpoints were absolute change in LDL-C from baseline to week 12 and percentage change in HDL cholesterol, triglycerides, ApoB, lipoprotein (a) [Lp(a)], and PCSK9 from baseline to week 12. Compared with placebo, evolocumab significantly

Table 1
Major medications in the treatment of HoFH and their effect in reducing LDL-C

Drug Name	Mechanism of Action	Administration Route and Dosage	Efficacy in HoFH Patients	Adverse Events
PCSK9 Inhibitors	Inhibition of PCSK9 by mAb	*Subcutaneous* Evolocumab 420 mg monthly/every 2 wk Alirocumab 150 mg every 2 wk	LDL-C reduction (20%-30%)	Injection site reactions and Flu-like symptoms
Inclisiran	Inhibition of PCSK9 by siRNA	*Subcutaneous* 300 mg (every 3 mo)	LDL-C reduction (12%-37%)	Injection site reactions
Lomitapide	Reduced secretion of ApoB-containing lipoproteins by the liver via inhibition of MTP	*Oral* 5–60 mg daily	Reduction in: LDL-C (50%) ApoB (49%) TG (45%)	• Hepatic steatosis • Gastrointestinal disorders • Impaired liver function
Mipomersen	Inhibition of ApoB synthesis	*Subcutaneous* 200 mg – weekly (160 mg in subjects < 50 kg [110 lbs])	Reduction in: LDL-C (20%-50%) Lp(a) (30%)	• Injection site reactions • Flu-like symptoms • Impaired liver function • Liver steatosis
Evinacumab	Inhibition of ANGPTL-3	*Intravenous* 15 mg/kg every 4 wk	Reduction in: LDL-C (~47%) TG (~50%)	Flu-like symptoms

Abbreviations: ANGPTL-3, angiopoietin-like protein 3; ApoB, apolipoprotein B; HoFH, homozygous familial hypercholesterolemia; LDL-C, low-density lipoprotein cholesterol; Lp(a), lipoprotein (a); mAb, monoclonal antibody; MTP, microsomal triglyceride transport protein; PCSK9, proprotein convertase subtilisin/kexin type 9; SiRNA, small interfering RNA; TG, triglycerides.

reduced LDL-C levels at 12 weeks by 30.9% (95% confidence interval [CI], −43.9% to −18.0%; P<.0001). Overall, participants in the evolocumab group showed a significant reduction in ApoB levels at 12 weeks compared with those in the placebo group. However, evolocumab did not significantly reduce Lp(a) levels.[39,40] In patients with at least one defective LDLR mutation, evolocumab reduced LDL-C by 41% (95% CI, −53 to −28, P<.0001) compared with placebo. The open-label Trial Assessing Long Term Use of PCSK9 Inhibition in Subjects With Genetic LDL Disorders (TAUSSIG)[41,42] evaluated the safety and efficacy of evolocumab for LDL-C reduction. A once or twice monthly 420-mg dose was administered to 106 patients with HoFH at least 4 weeks alongside standard LLT. All patients received 420 mg of evolocumab subcutaneously each month or every 2 weeks if the patient was on apheresis. Most patients participated in the TESLA study part A, and part B participants were eligible to enter the TAUSSIG directly. All patients in the treatment arms of the TESLA trials continued with monthly 420-mg doses of evolocumab, whereas those in the placebo group changed to the active drug. An interim

subset analysis with a median follow-up of 1.7 years included 72 patients who were on drug therapy only and 34 who were on apheresis, and 14 patients were younger than 18 years. In this analysis, evolocumab significantly reduced mean LDL-C by 20.6% at week 12% and 23.3% at week 48 (P<.0001 for both).[41] Furthermore, at a median follow-up of 4.1 years, mean change in LDL-C from baseline to week 12 was −21.2% (−59.8 mg/dL) in patients with HoFH. In patients with HoFH who were up-titrated by 420 mg every 2 weeks (even those who were not undergoing apheresis), mean LDL-C improved from −19.6% at week 12 to −29.7% after 12 weeks.[42]

The Study in Participants With Homozygous Familial Hypercholesterolemia (ODYSSEY HoFH study) was a randomized, double-blind, placebo-controlled, parallel-group, phase III study that evaluated the efficacy and safety of 150-mg of alirocumab administered every 2 weeks in adult patients with HoFH.[43] Participants were randomized in a 2:1 ratio to receive either 150 mg of alirocumab or placebo every 2 weeks, and randomization was stratified by apheresis treatment status. The primary efficacy endpoint was percent change in LDL-C from baseline to week 12 and the key secondary efficacy endpoints were percent change in non-HDL, ApoB, total cholesterol, Lp(a), triglycerides, and ApoA1 from baseline to week 12. At week 12, the mean difference in LDL-C percent change from baseline was −35.6% (P<.0001). Decreases in all other atherogenic lipoproteins were approximately 30%, which including Lp (a) (all P<.0001).[43]

Inclisiran

Inclisiran is a synthetic double-stranded RNA oligonucleotide designed to selectively silence PCSK9 gene in hepatocytes.[44] It is a chemically synthesized small interfering RNA (siRNA) molecule that reduces the production of PCSK9. It consists of 2 nucleotide strands conjugated to the ligand, triantennary N-acetylgalactosamine (GalNAc).[44,45] The last one targets inclisiran to the liver by binding specifically to the asialoglycoprotein receptors (ASGPR), which are expressed on hepatocytes. Inclisiran is taken in by the cell where it then binds to the RNA-induced silencing complex as well as the messenger RNA (mRNA) encoding PCSK9. The siRNA complex cleaves the PCSK9 mRNA, preventing the synthesis of the PCSK9 protein.[44,45] Phase I studies conducted in healthy volunteers with plasma LDL-C levels ≥100 mg/dL showed that inclisiran for 3 months significantly reduces PCSK9 (by approximately 70% with doses of >300 mg) and LDL-C (by approximately 50% with doses of >100 mg) levels.[44] No clinically relevant adverse events were reported during the treatment period. The ORION-2 study (multicenter, phase II, open-label, single-arm pilot study) evaluated the efficacy and safety of inclisiran in HoFH patients, in addition to the maximum tolerated dose of LLT (statin/ezetimibe) and found an average LDL-C reduction of approximately 30%.[46] The Study of Inclisiran in Participants with Homozygous Familial Hypercholesterolemia (ORION-5 study) is an ongoing phase III, two-part (double-blind placebo-controlled/open-label) multicenter study (NCT03851705) to evaluate the safety, tolerability, and efficacy of inclisiran in subjects with HoFH (**Table 2**).

ARE DRUGS THAT DO NOT TARGET THE LOW-DENSITY LIPOPROTEIN RECEPTOR PATHWAY THE SOLUTION FOR TREATING PATIENTS WITH HOMOZYGOUS FAMILIAL HYPERCHOLESTEROLEMIA?
Lomitapide

Lomitapide is a first-in-class agent approved by the United States Food and Drug Administration (US FDA) in 2012 and the European Medicines

Agency (EMA) in 2013 for the treatment of HoFH and is currently the most potent available drug. Lomitapide is an oral inhibitor of the microsomal triglyceride transport protein (MTP), which is responsible for the transfer of triglycerides and phospholipids to chylomicrons and very-low-density lipoproteins (VLDL) during their assembly in the endoplasmic reticulum of enterocytes and hepatocytes.[47] Inhibition of MTP leads to reduced secretion of these lipoproteins, and the mechanism of action is independent of LDLR activity. Thus, this drug is also active in "receptor-negative" patients.

In an open-label study of patients with HoFH, lomitapide at maximally tolerated doses, in addition to standard therapy (including LDL apheresis), was shown to reduce LDL-C and ApoB by approximately 50% and Lp (a) by 15% at 26 weeks, with persistent LDL-C reduction at 12 months.[48] The most frequently observed adverse events were gastrointestinal symptoms and hepatic steatosis (see **Table 1**). Elevation of liver enzymes was also observed, but this resolved with dose reduction or temporary drug interruption. Gastrointestinal adverse events (eg, nausea, flatulence, and diarrhea) were reduced through the implementation of gradual dose escalation combined with a low-fat diet (<20% fat energy) and administration of the drug without food.[48] The recommended starting dose is 5 mg once daily, followed by dose escalation (up to 60 mg) depending on efficacy and tolerability. Lomitapide is not recommended during pregnancy and therefore, contraception is recommended for use in HoFH patients who are of childbearing age. A multicenter study of an Italian cohort of patients with HoFH showed that the use of lomitapide as an add-on to standard therapy, at an average daily dose of 19 mg, lowered LDL-C levels by 68.2%; moreover, response variability in LDL-C reduction was not associated to HoFH genotype.[49] Some case or case series reports showed greater efficacy, with LDL-C reductions of more than 75%, which in some cases, enabled the cessation of apheresis.[50] Although the efficacy and safety of lomitapide are well documented, there is limited data on long-term cardiovascular outcomes. A recent simulation model study of 149 South African HoFH patients demonstrated the benefits of lomitapide therapy, in addition to conventional LLT, in terms of survival and reduced risk of major cardiovascular events (MACEs).[51] Notably, in the survival benefit analysis, starting lomitapide at age 18 years and reducing LDL-C by 3.3 mmol/L (127.6 mg/dL) from baseline would increase life expectancy by 11.2 years and might be able to delay the first MACE by 5.7 years.[51] The Lomitapide

Table 2
Ongoing clinical trials for gene therapy for HoFH

Drug	Administration Route	NCT Trial Number	Study Design	Patients	Primary Endpoint
AAV8.TBG. hLDLR	Intravenous injection	NCT02651675	Phase I/II—Open Label	12	Number of participants experiencing investigational product-related adverse events (up to 52 wk). Clinical laboratory parameters; and adverse event reporting
IONIS ANGPTL3-LRx	Subcutaneous injection	NCT02709850	Phase I— Randomized	61	Safety and tolerability of single and multiple doses of IONIS ANGPTL3-LRx (incidence, severity, and dose-relationship of adverse effects and changes in the laboratory parameters; up to day 127)
Inclisiran (ALN-PCSsc)	Subcutaneous injection	NCT03851705	Phase III— Randomized	56	Percent change in LDL-C levels from baseline to day 150

Abbreviations: AAV, adeno-associated virus; ANGPTL-3, angiopoietin-like protein 3; hLDLR, human low-density lipoprotein receptor; HoFH, homozygous familial hypercholesterolemia; LDL-C, low-density lipoprotein cholesterol.

Observational Worldwide Evaluation Registry (LOWER; NCT02135705) has been established and is making available long-term efficacy and safety data of lomitapide in clinical practice. Analysis of the first 5 years since the registry was established has shown that the efficacy and safety of lomitapide are consistent with phase III trial data despite using a much lower median dose of 10 mg versus 40 mg in phase III.[52]

Mipomersen

Mipomersen is a second-generation antisense oligonucleotide (ASO) that is delivered by subcutaneous injection, which targets mRNA of ApoB, the major protein of LDL-C, and its precursor VLDL. Mipomersen reduces ApoB mRNA transduction and ApoB synthesis from the ribosome, which results in reduced VLDL secretion.[53] The drug was approved by the FDA in January 2013 for the treatment of HoFH for doses of 200 mg/wk subcutaneously. In a double-blind placebo-controlled study in patients with HoFH,

mipomersen (200 mg weekly, in addition to standard LLT) led to reductions from baseline to 26 weeks in plasma levels of LDL-C (mean 25%), ApoB (27%), and Lp(a) (31%) versus placebo.[54] The most frequently reported adverse events were injection site reactions (76% of patients) and flu-like symptoms. Increases in liver enzymes have also been reported during treatment with mipomersen; in 12% of patients, increases of more than 3 times the ULN were observed, with and without concomitant increases in liver fat. However, in most cases, there was a subsequent decrease during treatment.

Possible Drawbacks of Lomitapide and Mipomersen Therapy

Because of the risk of hepatic toxicity, both lomitapide and mipomersen have been approved for limited use. Although the potential cardiovascular benefits, which are associated with a substantial reduction in LDL-C, outweigh the theoretic risk of steatohepatitis and fibrosis in very-high-risk patients, a systematic evaluation of long-term efficacy and hepatic safety is needed. In addition, both drugs have side effects that may limit their long-term use. Lomitapide is contraindicated for patients taking moderate to strong CYP3A4 inhibitors. Furthermore, because the safety of lomitapide and mipomersen has not been evaluated in patients with HoFH aged less than 18 and less than 12 years, respectively, or in those treated with apheresis, therapy in these patients should be considered via a special access system or only if all other options have been explored to avoid rapid progression of atherosclerosis.

An important criticism of these drugs is their cost. Although the high cost of these approaches may be a concern, the overall cost of adequate treatment for HoFH remains low because of its rarity. Moreover, costs may be offset by the savings achievable through the prevention of associated cardiovascular complications.

Angiopoietin-like 3 Inhibitor

In recent years, the angiopoietin-like 3 (ANGPTL-3) protein has emerged as a target for HoFH patients because it is involved in lipid metabolism and LDL-C reduction.[55–58] The role of ANGPTL-3 in humans has emerged from 2 sets of observations: genome-wide studies that have demonstrated an association between genomic polymorphisms located near or within the ANGPTL-3 gene and triglyceride and HDL levels, and the finding that some individuals with combined familial hypolipidemia (reduced levels of all lipoproteins) are in fact homozygous carriers (or compound heterozygotes) of ANGPTL-3 gene mutations, which results in a complete loss of function of the ANGPTL-3 protein.[56–59] Furthermore, individuals who were heterozygous carriers of ANGPTL-3 gene mutations with loss of function had lower plasma lipoprotein levels than those of control subjects.[57,60] ANGPTL-3 inhibits 2 intravascular lipases: lipoprotein lipase (LPL) and endothelial lipase (EL). LPL is responsible for hydrolysis of triglycerides contained in chylomicrons and VLDLs, whereas EL functions predominantly as a phospholipase and hydrolyzes phospholipids from HDLs. The lack of inhibition of these 2 enzymes, which occurs in patients with the ANGPTL-3 genetic defect, results in increased activity of the 2 lipolytic enzymes.

Individuals with complete genetic ANGPTL-3 deficiency (ie, homozygotes/heterozygotes compounded by mutations in the ANGPTL-3 gene) show a conspicuous reduction in plasma LDL-C levels. A possible strategy to deactivate ANGPTL-3 is based on the use of a specific monoclonal antibody, which was successfully achieved for anti-PCSK9 antibodies. In fact, an antihuman ANGPTL-3 antibody (REGN1500 antibody) has been generated and tested in animal models. The monoclonal REGN1500 (evinacumab) antibody is a fully-humanized antihuman ANGPTL-3 antibody that is capable of binding with high affinity, even with ANGPTL-3 from other species. The mechanism of this reduction has been explored in normal mice and mice with hypercholesterolemia due to genetic defects in plasma clearance of ApoB-containing lipoproteins (ie, mice with inactivation of the ApoE [ApoE−/−], LDLR [LDLR−/−], or LRP1 chylomicron receptor gene [LRP1−/−]).[61] Animals were treated with the anti-ANGPTL-3 antibody, REGN1500, to deactivate endogenous ANGPTL-3. Antibody treatment reduced plasma triglyceride and cholesterol levels by 40% in VLDL and LDL, and concomitantly reduced plasma ApoB-100 levels in both normal and hypercholesterolemic mice. A 60% reduction in hepatic triglyceride production in VLDL (VLDL-TG) was observed in REGN1500-treated mice, which suggested that reduced hepatic secretion of VLDL-TG contributes to the reduction of plasma triglycerides. However, in REGN1500-treated mice, no reduction in hepatic secretion of ApoB-100 into VLDL (VLDL-ApoB100) was observed to account for the reduced plasma ApoB-100 levels, which indicated that treated animals were undergoing an increased removal of ApoB-containing lipoproteins from circulation. However, there was no increase in receptor-mediated plasma clearance of lipoproteins containing ApoE (β-VLDL) or ApoB-100 (LDL) in normal mice treated with REGN1500. Reduction in plasma levels of LDL-C and ApoB-100 induced by REGN1500 treatment was also observed in ApoE−/−, LDLR−/−, and LRP1−/− mice, which suggested that antibody-mediated ANGPTL-3 deactivation induces the accelerated removal of ApoB-containing lipoproteins from plasma via a different pathway to that of the receptor-mediated pathway.[61] The Evinacumab Lipid Studies in Patients with Homozygous Familial Hypercholesterolemia (ELIPSE HoFH trial) trial is a phase III, double-blind, placebo-controlled pilot study on the efficacy and safety of evinacumab in patients with HoFH.[62] A total of 65 patients were randomized to receive either evinacumab 15 mg/kg intravenously every 4 weeks (n = 43) alongside standard LLT or LLT alone (placebo, n = 22). Evinacumab was shown to reduce LDL-C levels by 47.1% after 24 weeks of treatment and had a good safety profile, which resulted in a between-group difference of 49.0%. Significant reductions were also observed in other key secondary endpoints, which included ApoB, non-HDL-C, and total cholesterol levels, compared with placebo ($P<.0001$ for all measures).[62] Similar levels of LDL-C reduction have also been observed in the most difficult-to-treat patients, who often do not respond to other therapies because of limited LDLR function, which are described as null/null (<15% LDLR function on in vitro assays) or negative/negative (genetic variants that likely result in minimal or no LDLR function by mutation analysis) patients. The most common adverse reactions (>3% of patients) from the combined safety analysis of placebo-controlled studies after 24 weeks that occurred more frequently in the evinacumab group (n = 81) compared with the placebo group (n = 54) were nasopharyngitis (16% vs 13%), influenza-like illness (7% vs 6%), dizziness (6% vs 0%), rhinorrhea (5% vs 0%), nausea (5% vs 2%), extremity pain (4% vs 0% placebo), and asthenia (4% vs 0%).[62]

Gemcabene

Gemcabene is a dialkyl ether dicarboxylic acid, which has been shown to be a lipid-lowering agent. It is a peroxisome proliferation-activated receptor (PPARα) agonist. It acts by improving the clearance of VLDLs in the plasma and inhibiting the hepatic biosynthesis of fatty acids and cholesterol; with LDL-C reduction achieved in an LDLR-independent manner. The Efficacy and Safety of Gemcabene in Patients With Homozygous Familial Hypercholesterolemia on Stable, Lipid-Lowering Therapy (COBALT-1) study is a phase II, open-label trial that aimed to investigate efficacy, tolerability, and safety of gemcabene as add-on therapy to current LLT for HoFH patients.[63] For this purpose, 8 patients with a clinical or genetic diagnosis of HoFH on stable standard LLT, including statins, ezetimibe, and PCSK9 inhibitors, were enrolled. Patients were followed up for 12 weeks and they received 300 mg of gemcabene, orally once daily for 4 weeks, followed by 600 mg of the drug, orally once daily for 4 weeks, followed by 900 mg once daily for further 4 weeks. Mean change from baseline in LDL-C was −26% (P = .004), −30% (P = .001), and −29% (P = .001) at weeks 4, 8, and 12, respectively.[63] To date, it is not yet approved for use in clinical practice and further studies are needed to determine safety.

IS GENE THERAPY A STEP INTO THE FUTURE?

A nonoptimal response to standard therapy in HoFH patients is primarily related to residual LDLR activity. Notably, patients with null/null or negative/null mutations have a poor response to therapy. In this context, gene therapy could play a crucial role by enabling the replacement of the defective gene with a functional LDLR gene, which would allow restoration of normal LDL metabolism and, in turn, a significant reduction in plasma LDL-C (see **Table 2**).

A pilot study of liver-directed gene therapy included 5 patients with HoFH who ranged in age from 7 to 41 years.[64] In these patients, cells treated with a recombinant retrovirus that expressed the normal human LDLR cDNA were infused into the liver. Significant and prolonged reduction in LDL-C was observed in 3 of the 5 patients, and in vivo LDL catabolism was increased by 53%.[64]

Adeno-Associated Virus-Mediated Human Low-Density Lipoprotein Receptor Gene Therapy

Adeno-associated virus (AAV) is a member of the *Parvoviridae* family. AAV vectors are safe platforms for gene therapy delivery because they are not pathogenic for humans and have low immunogenicity. There are several AAV serotypes with different organ-specific tropism. Notably, in mouse models, AAV8 has been shown to be more effective in hepatocyte transduction (81.2% vs 4.2%) and gene transfer (2.1 vs 52 genome copies/cell) compared with AAV2, with a significant reduction in total cholesterol profile (227 mg/dL vs 1032 mg/dL, $P<.001$).[65] The first clinical trial (phases I and II) designed to evaluate the safety and effectiveness of AAV-based liver-directed gene therapy, RGX-501 (Regenxbio, Inc), for the treatment of HoFH is currently ongoing (NCT02651675; AAV8-mediated Low Density Lipoprotein Receptor Gene Replacement in Subjects With Homozygous Familial Hypercholesterolemia). The study aims to assess the effectiveness of a single intravenous dose of human LDLR gene therapy using plasma LDL-C levels as a surrogate biomarker for human LDLR transgene expression. The primary safety endpoint is the number of participants who experience investigational product-related adverse events.

To date, only 2 AAV-mediated therapies have been approved by the FDA: AAV2-mediated delivery of the RPE65 gene for biallelic RPE65 mutation-associated retinal dystrophy and AAV9-mediated delivery of the SMN1 gene for the treatment of spinal muscular atrophy type I in children younger than 2 years of age. Additional studies in this area will enable the development of further applications of therapy, and the results of the trials in patients with HoFH will change the entire picture of the disease.

Antisense Oligonucleotides

ASOs are short single-stranded sequences of DNA that hybridize with complementary mRNAs. For

HoFH therapy, mipomersen, which targets the mRNA of ApoB, has already been approved and is being used in the treatment of HoFH in the United States. The aim of a randomized, double-blind, placebo-controlled phase I trial of ASO targeting hepatic ANGPTL-3 mRNA (NCT02709850) was to evaluate the safety and tolerability of single and multiple doses of IONIS-ANGPTL-3-LRx in healthy volunteers with elevated triglycerides and patients with familial hypercholesterolemia.[66] IONIS-ANGPTL-3-LRx is a second-generation ligand GalNAc-conjugated ASO drug that is targeted toward the human ANGPTL-3 mRNA coding sequence. After 6 weeks of treatment, patients in the multiple-dose treatment group showed a reduction in ANGPTL-3 levels (46.6%–84.5%, $P<.01$ for all doses), triglycerides (33.2%–63.1%), and LDL-C (1.3%–32.9%).[66] Although the study did not include patients with HoFH, researchers hypothesized that ASO would be useful in treating HoFH by reducing levels of ANGPTL-3.

Clustered Regularly Interspaced Short Palindromic Repeats/Cas9 Gene-Editing

The clustered regularly interspaced short palindromic repeats (CRISPR)–CRISPR-associated gene 9 (Cas9) system has shown to be an efficient gene-editing complex.[67] DNA strands at the target site are cleaved by an RNA-guided nuclease.[67] When the standard DNA repair system of the cell attempts to repair the DNA, the engineered donor DNA provided by the CRISPR-Cas9 system is inserted into the target site. A recent preclinical study showed that AAV-CRISPR/Cas9 treatment corrected LDLR mutations in a subset of hepatocytes in an LDLR mutant mouse model. Compared with the control groups (n = 6 in each group), the AAV-CRISPR/Cas9 treatment group (n = 6) had greater reductions in cholesterol, triglycerides, and LDL-C levels.[68] Thus, the CRISPR-Cas9 system could play a crucial role in the repair of LDLR mutations or multiple genes defects, such as PCSK9, ApoB, and ANGPTL-3, and may become a valuable therapeutic strategy for the treatment of HoFH.

A recent application of the CRISPR-Cas9 system has been shown to be effective in reprogramming T-cells that are isolated from HoFH patients into induced pluripotent stem cells.[69] Results have been promising and have shown the presence of LDLRs in the cell membrane, which offers interesting opportunities for future treatments.

SUMMARY

Conventional LLT for the treatment of HoFH presents challenges in clinical practice. Recent developments of new therapeutic strategies have enabled unimaginable LDL-C levels in patients with HoFH. Although residual LDL-C receptor activity is crucial for response to therapy, drugs with mechanisms of action that are independent of this pathway have been developed. Promising prospects come from monoclonal antibodies and gene-editing drugs. In this regard, gene therapy appears to be the most innovative approach toward improving therapeutic algorithms for HoFH.

CLINICS CARE POINTS

- The presence of plasma total cholesterol values >500 mg/dL, extensive xanthomas, and premature atherosclerotic cardiovascular disease raises the clinical suspicion of homozygous familial hypercholesterolemia (HoFH).
- Genetic test to assess the involved mutation and dysfunctional pathway is helpful in determining risk and selecting appropriate treatment strategies.
- A genetic study of the family members of patients with HoFH could be informative in the early identification of relatives with homozygous or heterozygous disease.
- Orphan drugs for the treatment of HoFH are very effective but can be burdened by some side effects. Accurate and careful management of adverse effects may increase adherence and persistence of therapy with benefits in terms of cardiovascular outcomes.

DISCLOSURE

M. Averna has served as a consultant for Akcea, Amgen, Amryt, Daiichi-Sankio, Novartis, Piam, Sanofi/Genzyme, Shire, and SOBI. L. D'Erasmo has received personal fees for public speaking, consultancy, or grant support from Amryt Pharmaceuticals, Akcea Therapeutics, Pfizer, Amgen, and Sanofi. M. Arca has received research grant support from Amryt Pharmaceutical, Amgen, IONIS, Akcea Therapeutics, Pfizer, and Sanofi; has served as a consultant for Amgen, Aegerion, Akcea Therapeutics, Regeneron, Sanofi, and Alfasigma and received lecturing fees from Amgen, Amryth Pharmaceutical, Pfizer, Sanofi, and AlfaSigma.

REFERENCES

1. Cuchel M, Bruckert E, Ginsberg HN, et al. Homozygous familial hypercholesterolaemia: new insights

and guidance for clinicians to improve detection and clinical management. A position paper from the Consensus Panel on Familial Hypercholesterolaemia of the European Atherosclerosis Society. Eur Heart J 2014;35(32):2146–57.

2. Mach F, Baigent C, Catapano AL, et al. 2019 ESC/ EAS guidelines for the management of dyslipidaemias: lipid modification to reduce cardiovascular risk. Eur Heart J 2020;41(1):111–88.

3. Sjouke B, Kusters DM, Kindt I, et al. Homozygous autosomal dominant hypercholesterolaemia in the Netherlands: prevalence, genotype–phenotype relationship, and clinical outcome. Eur Heart J 2015; 36(9):560–5.

4. Austin MA. Genetic causes of monogenic heterozygous familial hypercholesterolemia: a HuGE prevalence review. Am J Epidemiol 2004;160(5):407–20.

5. Sjouke B, Hovingh GK, Kastelein JJP, et al. Homozygous autosomal dominant hypercholesterolaemia. Curr Opin Lipidol 2015;26(3):200–9.

6. Bertolini S, Calandra S, Arca M, et al. Homozygous familial hypercholesterolemia in Italy: clinical and molecular features. Atherosclerosis 2020;312:72–8.

7. D'Erasmo L, Minicocci I, Nicolucci A, et al. Autosomal recessive hypercholesterolemia. J Am Coll Cardiol 2018;71(3):279–88.

8. Rader DJ, Cohen J, Hobbs HH. Monogenic hypercholesterolemia: new insights in pathogenesis and treatment. J Clin Invest 2003;111(12):1795–803.

9. Varret M, Abifadel M, Rabès J-P, et al. Genetic heterogeneity of autosomal dominant hypercholesterolemia. Clin Genet 2007;73(1):1–13.

10. Sniderman AD, Tsimikas S, Fazio S. The Severe hypercholesterolemia phenotype. J Am Coll Cardiol 2014;63(19):1935–47.

11. Kolansky DM, Cuchel M, Clark BJ, et al. Longitudinal evaluation and assessment of cardiovascular disease in patients with homozygous familial hypercholesterolemia. Am J Cardiol 2008;102(11):1438–43.

12. Raal FJ, Pilcher GJ, Panz VR, et al. Reduction in mortality in subjects with homozygous familial hypercholesterolemia associated with advances in lipid-lowering therapy. Circulation 2011;124(20):2202–7.

13. Bélanger AM, Akioyamen L, Alothman L, et al. Evidence for improved survival with treatment of homozygous familial hypercholesterolemia. Curr Opin Lipidol 2020;31(4):176–81.

14. Raal FJ, Pappu AS, Illingworth DR, et al. Inhibition of cholesterol synthesis by atorvastatin in homozygous familial hypercholesterolaemia. Atherosclerosis 2000;150(2):421–8.

15. Altmann SW, Davis HR, Zhu L-J, et al. Niemann-Pick C1 Like 1 protein is critical for intestinal cholesterol absorption. Science 2004;303(5661):1201–4.

16. Cannon CP, Blazing MA, Giugliano RP, et al. Ezetimibe added to statin therapy after acute coronary syndromes. N Engl J Med 2015;372(25):2387–97.

17. Kastelein JJP, Akdim F, Stroes ESG, et al. Simvastatin with or without ezetimibe in familial hypercholesterolemia. N Engl J Med 2008;358(14):1431–43.

18. Pisciotta L, Fasano T, Bellocchio A, et al. Effect of ezetimibe coadministered with statins in genotype-confirmed heterozygous FH patients. Atherosclerosis 2007;194(2):e116–22.

19. Gagné C, Gaudet D, Bruckert E. Efficacy and safety of ezetimibe coadministered with atorvastatin or simvastatin in patients with homozygous familial hypercholesterolemia. Circulation 2002;105(21):2469–75.

20. Thompson GR. Recommendations for the use of LDL apheresis. Atherosclerosis 2008;198(2):247–55.

21. Harada-Shiba M, Arai H, Oikawa S, et al. Guidelines for the management of familial hypercholesterolemia. J Atheroscler Thromb 2012;19(12):1043–60.

22. Goldberg AC, Hopkins PN, Toth PP, et al. Familial hypercholesterolemia: screening, diagnosis and management of pediatric and adult patients. J Clin Lipidol 2011;5(3):S1–8.

23. Schuff-Werner P, Fenger S, Kohlschein P. Role of lipid apheresis in changing times. Clin Res Cardiol Suppl 2012;7(S1):7–14.

24. Gragnano F, Calabrò P. Role of dual lipid-lowering therapy in coronary atherosclerosis regression: evidence from recent studies. Atherosclerosis 2018; 269:219–28.

25. Maiorana A, Nobili V, Calandra S, et al. Preemptive liver transplantation in a child with familial hypercholesterolemia. Pediatr Transplant 2011;15(2):E25–9.

26. Ibrahim M, El-Hamamsy I, Barbir M, et al. Translational lessons from a case of combined heart and liver transplantation for familial hypercholesterolemia 20 years post-operatively. J Cardiovasc Transl Res 2012;5(3):351–8.

27. Tevfik K, Yucel Y, Turan K, et al. Liver transplantation as a treatment option for three siblings with homozygous familial hypercholesterolemia. Pediatr Transplant 2011;15(3):281–4.

28. Malatack MD. Liver transplantation as treatment for familial homozygous hypercholesterolemia: too early or too late. Pediatr Transplant 2011;15(2):123–5.

29. Raal F, Panz V, Immelman A, et al. Elevated PCSK9 levels in untreated patients with heterozygous or homozygous familial hypercholesterolemia and the response to high-dose statin therapy. J Am Heart Assoc 2013;2(2):e000028.

30. Cao Y-X, Jin J-L, Sun D, et al. Circulating PCSK9 and cardiovascular events in FH patients with standard lipid-lowering therapy. J Transl Med 2019;17(1):367.

31. Guo Q, Feng X, Zhou Y. PCSK9 variants in familial hypercholesterolemia: a comprehensive synopsis. Front Genet 2020;11.

32. Seidah NG, Awan Z, Chretien M, et al. PCSK9: a key modulator of cardiovascular health. Circ Res 2014; 114(6):1022–36.

33. Cesaro A, Bianconi V, Gragnano F, et al. Beyond cholesterol metabolism: The pleiotropic effects of proprotein convertase subtilisin/kexin type 9 (PCSK9). Genetics, mutations, expression, and perspective for long-term inhibition. Biofactors 2020;46(3):367–80.

34. Gragnano F, Natale F, Concilio C, et al. Adherence to proprotein convertase subtilisin/kexin 9 inhibitors in high cardiovascular risk patients: an Italian single-center experience. J Cardiovasc Med 2018;19(2):75–7.

35. Cesaro A, Gragnano F, Fimiani F, et al. Impact of PCSK9 inhibitors on the quality of life of patients at high cardiovascular risk. Eur J Prev Cardiol 2019;4–6.

36. Sabatine MS, Giugliano RP, Keech AC, et al. Evolocumab and clinical outcomes in patients with cardiovascular disease. N Engl J Med 2017;376(18):1713–22.

37. Schwartz GG, Steg PG, Szarek M, et al. Alirocumab and cardiovascular outcomes after acute coronary syndrome. N Engl J Med 2018;379(22):2097–107.

38. Calabrò P, Gragnano F, Pirro M. Cognitive function in a randomized trial of evolocumab. N Engl J Med 2017;377(20):1996–7.

39. Raal FJ, Honarpour N, Blom DJ, et al. Inhibition of PCSK9 with evolocumab in homozygous familial hypercholesterolaemia (TESLA Part B): a randomised, double-blind, placebo-controlled trial. Lancet 2015;385(9965):341–50.

40. Cesaro A, Schiavo A, Moscarella E, et al. Lipoprotein(a): a genetic marker for cardiovascular disease and target for emerging therapies. J Cardiovasc Med 2021;22(3):151–61.

41. Raal FJ, Hovingh GK, Blom D, et al. Long-term treatment with evolocumab added to conventional drug therapy, with or without apheresis, in patients with homozygous familial hypercholesterolaemia: an interim subset analysis of the open-label TAUSSIG study. Lancet Diabetes Endocrinol 2017;5(4):280–90.

42. Santos RD, Stein EA, Hovingh GK, et al. Long-term evolocumab in patients with familial hypercholesterolemia. J Am Coll Cardiol 2020;75(6):565–74.

43. Blom DJ, Harada-Shiba M, Rubba P, et al. Efficacy and safety of alirocumab in adults with homozygous familial hypercholesterolemia. J Am Coll Cardiol 2020;76(2):131–42.

44. Fitzgerald K, White S, Borodovsky A, et al. A highly durable RNAi therapeutic inhibitor of PCSK9. N Engl J Med 2017;376(1):41–51.

45. Nişhikido T, Ray KK. Inclisiran for the treatment of dyslipidemia. Expert Opin Investig Drugs 2018;27(3):287–94.

46. Hovingh GK, Lepor NE, Kallend D, et al. Inclisiran durably lowers low-density lipoprotein cholesterol and proprotein convertase subtilisin/kexin type 9 expression in homozygous familial hypercholesterolemia. Circulation 2020;141(22):1829–31.

47. Hussain MM, Rava P, Walsh M, et al. Multiple functions of microsomal triglyceride transfer protein. Nutr Metab (Lond) 2012;9(1):14.

48. Cuchel M, Meagher EA, du Toit Theron H, et al. Efficacy and safety of a microsomal triglyceride transfer protein inhibitor in patients with homozygous familial hypercholesterolaemia: a single-arm, open-label, phase 3 study. Lancet 2013;381(9860):40–6.

49. D'Erasmo L, Cefalù AB, Noto D, et al. Efficacy of lomitapide in the treatment of familial homozygous hypercholesterolemia: results of a real-world clinical experience in Italy. Adv Ther 2017;34(5):1200–10.

50. Sperlongano S, Gragnano F, Natale F, et al. Lomitapide in homozygous familial hypercholesterolemia. J Cardiovasc Med 2018;19(3):83–90.

51. Leipold R, Raal F, Ishak J, et al. The effect of lomitapide on cardiovascular outcome measures in homozygous familial hypercholesterolemia: a modelling analysis. Eur J Prev Cardiol 2017;24(17):1843–50.

52. Underberg JA, Cannon CP, Larrey D, et al. Long-term safety and efficacy of lomitapide in patients with homozygous familial hypercholesterolemia: five-year data from the Lomitapide Observational Worldwide Evaluation Registry (LOWER). J Clin Lipidol 2020;14(6):807–17.

53. Crooke ST, Geary RS. Clinical pharmacological properties of mipomersen (Kynamro), a second generation antisense inhibitor of apolipoprotein B. Br J Clin Pharmacol 2013;76(2):269–76.

54. Raal FJ, Santos RD, Blom DJ, et al. Mipomersen, an apolipoprotein B synthesis inhibitor, for lowering of LDL cholesterol concentrations in patients with homozygous familial hypercholesterolaemia: a randomised, double-blind, placebo-controlled trial. Lancet 2010;375(9719):998–1006.

55. Kersten S. Angiopoietin-like 3 in lipoprotein metabolism. Nat Rev Endocrinol 2017;13(12):731–9.

56. Minicocci I, Montali A, Robciuc MR, et al. Mutations in the ANGPTL3 gene and familial combined hypolipidemia: a clinical and biochemical characterization. J Clin Endocrinol Metab 2012;97(7):E1266–75.

57. Arca M, D'Erasmo L, Minicocci I. Familial combined hypolipidemia. Curr Opin Lipidol 2020;31(2):41–8.

58. Calandra S, Tarugi P, Averna M, et al. Familial combined hypolipidemia due to mutations in the ANGPTL3 gene. Clin Lipidol 2013;8(1):81–95.

59. Ruhanen H, Haridas PAN, Minicocci I, et al. ANGPTL3 deficiency alters the lipid profile and metabolism of cultured hepatocytes and human lipoproteins. Biochim Biophys Acta Mol Cell Biol Lipids 2020;1865(7):158679.

60. Minicocci I, Santini S, Cantisani V, et al. Clinical characteristics and plasma lipids in subjects with familial combined hypolipidemia: a pooled analysis. J Lipid Res 2013;54(12):3481–90.

61. Wang Y, Gusarova V, Banfi S, et al. Inactivation of ANGPTL3 reduces hepatic VLDL-triglyceride secretion. J Lipid Res 2015;56(7):1296–307.

62. Raal FJ, Rosenson RS, Reeskamp LF, et al. Evinacumab for homozygous familial hypercholesterolemia. N Engl J Med 2020;383(8):711–20.

63. Gaudet D, Durst R, Lepor N, et al. Usefulness of gemcabene in homozygous familial hypercholesterolemia (from COBALT-1). Am J Cardiol 2019; 124(12):1876–80.

64. Grossman M, Rader DJ, Muller DWM, et al. A pilot study of ex vivo gene therapy for homozygous familial hypercholesterolaemia. Nat Med 1995;1(11): 1148–54.

65. Lebherz C, Gao G, Louboutin J-P, et al. Gene therapy with novel adeno-associated virus vectors substantially diminishes atherosclerosis in a murine model of familial hypercholesterolemia. J Gene Med 2004;6(6):663–72.

66. Graham MJ, Lee RG, Brandt TA, et al. Cardiovascular and metabolic effects of ANGPTL3 antisense oligonucleotides. N Engl J Med 2017;377(3):222–32.

67. Sander JD, Joung JK. CRISPR-Cas systems for editing, regulating and targeting genomes. Nat Biotechnol 2014;32(4):347–55.

68. Zhao H, Li Y, He L, et al. In vivo AAV-CRISPR/Cas9–mediated gene editing ameliorates atherosclerosis in familial hypercholesterolemia. Circulation 2020; 141(1):67–79.

69. Okada H, Nakanishi C, Yoshida S, et al. Function and immunogenicity of gene-corrected iPSC-derived hepatocyte-like cells in restoring low density lipoprotein uptake in homozygous familial hypercholesterolemia. Sci Rep 2019;9(1):4695.

Spontaneous Coronary Artery Dissection
A Rare Event?

Michael Würdinger, MD[a], Victoria L. Cammann, MD[a],
Jelena R. Ghadri, MD[a], Christian Templin, MD, PhD, FESC[b],*

KEYWORDS

• Spontaneous coronary artery dissection • SCAD • Epidemiology • Outcome

KEY POINTS

• Spontaneous coronary artery dissection describes the spontaneous separation of the coronary artery wall, leading to myocardial ischemia.
• Previously considered a rare disease, spontaneous coronary artery dissection has emerged an important cause of acute coronary syndrome, especially in young women.
• Recent scientific interest, with most clinical studies published within the past 5 years, has shed light on many aspects of this underestimated disease.
• There are still many uncertainties regarding pathophysiology, risk factors, acute treatment, and optimal long-term management.

INTRODUCTION

Spontaneous coronary artery dissection (SCAD) is an occasional cause of acute coronary syndrome (ACS) predominantly affecting younger women. It arises from the spontaneous separation of an epicardial coronary artery wall. The concomitant formation of an intramural hematoma (IMH) leads to compression of the true lumen, resulting in myocardial ischemia.[1,2] The underlying pathophysiologic mechanism is still unidentified. There are 2 theories on the formation of SCAD. The first theory proposes an intimal tear as the primary event enabling blood entering and generation of a false lumen and secondary leading to the IMH[1] (inside-out hypothesis). However, there is evidence that IMH is the primary event leading to consecutive intimal rupture, because IMH without an intimal tear has been found in a proportion of patients in optical coherence tomography studies.[3–5] Therefore, a further theory proposes a primary disruption of vasa vasorum leading to hemorrhage into the vessel wall with formation of an IMH without an intimal tear.[6] The increased pressure within the vessel wall might cause a rupture into the true lumen, resulting in an intimal rupture in certain patients (outside-in hypothesis).

Since its initial description by H.C. Pretty in 1931,[7] SCAD had been considered a very rare cause of ACS that is frequently related with pregnancy.[8] However, it has been found that pregnancy-related SCAD only makes up a minority of cases. Contrary to previous assumptions, SCAD has evolved into an essential entity of ACS and sudden cardiac death, especially in young females and patients lacking classic cardiovascular risk factors.[9] Even if cases have been increasingly reported over time, SCAD can be assumed to be an underdiagnosed and under-reported disease.

In this article, the authors assess the evolution of scientific literature on SCAD and the changes of epidemiologic conceptions over the last decades. Furthermore, a comprehensive review of recent findings about clinical presentation, predisposing factors, treatment, and outcome is presented.

[a] Department of Cardiology, University Heart Center, University Hospital Zurich, Raemistrasse 100, Zurich 8091, Switzerland; [b] Andreas Grüntzig Heart Catheterization Laboratories, Department of Cardiology, University Heart Center, University Hospital Zurich, Raemistrasse 100, Zurich 8091, Switzerland
* Corresponding author.
E-mail address: Christian.Templin@usz.ch

Heart Failure Clin 18 (2022) 189–199
https://doi.org/10.1016/j.hfc.2021.07.015
1551-7136/22/© 2021 The Author(s). Published by Elsevier Inc. This is an open access article under the CC BY-NC-ND license (http://creativecommons.org/licenses/by-nc-nd/4.0/).

INCREASE OF SCIENTIFIC INTEREST

Since its initial description in 1931,[7] publications in the scientific literature have been scarce. However, this fact has considerably changed within the last decade. We have reviewed the PubMed (National Library of Medicine) database for literature on "spontaneous coronary artery dissection" from 1975 to April 2021 and further analyzed the articles concerning the type of publication. We have found a total of 1527 articles on SCAD in this period. Of those, two-thirds have been case reports (1047 publications), and 157 publications have been clinical studies. The remaining have been reviews, systematic reviews and meta-analyses, letters, comments, and notes. There has been a distinct increase in scientific literature within the last years (**Fig. 1**). Until 10 years ago, published articles have almost exclusively consisted of case reports, and 72% of overall literature come from the last 10 years. Eighty percent of clinical studies originate from the most recent 5 years.

This dramatic increase in scientific interest may be due to the introduction of an angiographic classification by Saw in 2014,[2] and position papers from the European Society of Cardiology and the American Heart Association in 2018[10,11] that might have led to a greater degree of familiarity and awareness among physicians. Furthermore, SCAD has been classified as a type 2 acute myocardial infarction (MI) in the Fourth Universal Definition of Myocardial Infarction[12] and has been considered as an entity of MI with nonobstructive coronary arteries in current scientific statements from the American Heart Association and the European Society of Cardiology.[13,14] However, clinical studies still represent a minority of all publications. Further research purposes are needed to overcome current lack of knowledge about SCAD.

EPIDEMIOLOGY

Historically, SCAD had been assumed to be a rare cardiovascular disease almost exclusively occurring in pregnant women.[8] Indeed, the population predominantly affected by SCAD are young and middle-aged females and individuals lacking classic cardiovascular risk factors.[9] This aspect may be contributing to the underdiagnosis of SCAD, because the index of suspicion of MI is low in this population. The true incidence and prevalence remain unknown, but seem to be substantially higher than previously assumed.

Table 1 gives an overview of prevalences of SCAD in published ACS and angiography cohorts. These reports have demonstrated SCAD being accountable for up to 4% of all ACS[15–23] and occurring in 0.02% to 1.10% of all coronary angiographies.[24–31] Even if SCAD still seems to be an infrequent cause of MI in the general population, the rates are significantly higher when looking at ACS cohorts of younger age. SCAD prevalence is as high as 3.1% to 9.7% in patients with premature MI at an age of less than 45 years.[32–34] The highest prevalence of SCAD can be found in younger females with SCAD accounting for 8.8% to 11.1% of ACS events in female patients less than 60 years of age[35–37] and for 8.7% to 45.0% of ACS in women less than 50 years of age.[20,29,33,38] SCAD is the most common cause of pregnancy-associated MI (43%), with most cases occurring in the third trimester or the early postpartum phase.[39] It has been found in 2 of

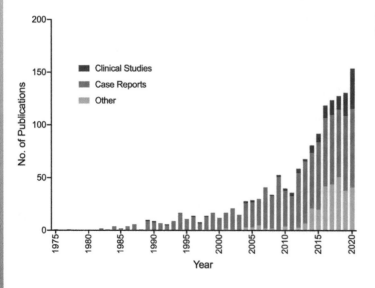

Fig. 1. Scientific publications on SCAD from 1975 to 2020.

Table 1
Prevalence of SCAD in ACS and coronary angiography cohorts

Author, Year	Cohort	N Cohort	N SCAD	% SCAD
SCAD in coronary angiography cohorts				
Liu et al,[31] 2019	Coronary angiographies	76,359	118	0.15
Rigatelli et al,[30] 2018	Coronary angiographies	10,954	37	0.25
Vanzetto et al,[29] 2009	Coronary angiographies	11,605	23	0.02
Mortensen et al,[28] 2009	Coronary angiographies	32,869	22	0.07
Unal et al,[27] 2008	Coronary angiographies	5000	6	0.12
Maeder et al,[26] 2005	Coronary angiographies	5054	5	0.1
Hering et al,[25] 1998	Coronary angiographies	3803	42	1.1
Hiasa et al,[24] 1990	Coronary angiographies	5400	23	0.43
SCAD in ACS cohorts				
Daoula et al,[23] 2020	ACS	198000	83	0.04
Lobo et al,.[22] 2019	STEMI	5208	53	1
Clare et al,[21] 2019	MI	26,598	208	0.78
Nakashima et al,[20] 2016	MI	20,195	63	0.31
Nishiguchi et al,[19] 2016	ACS	326	13	4
Saia et al,[18] 2015	STEMI	140	2	2.1
Tokura et al,[17] 2014	ACS	1159	10	0.86
Hendiri et al,[16] 2005	MI	1100	6	0.5
Rigatelli et al,[15] 2004	ACS	941	2	0.2
SCAD in premature ACS				
Lorca et al,[37] 2021	Males <55 y/ females <60 y with STEMI	366	7	1.9
Yang et al,[34] 2020	<40 y with MI	431	13	3.1
Vautrin et al,[33] 2020	<45 y with STEMI	144	14	9.7
Lim et al,[32] 1996	<40 y with MI	29	2	6.9
SCAD in young females with ACS				
Lorca et al,[37] 2021	Females <60 y with STEMI	63	7	11.1
Kim et al,[36] 2021	Females <60 y with ACS	148	13	8.8
Inoue et al,[35] 2021	Females <60 y with PCI	187	19	10.2
Meng et al,[38] 2017	Females <50 y with MI	60	21	35
Nakashima et al,[20] 2016	Females <50 y with MI	100	45	45
Vanzetto et al,[29] 2009	Females <50 y with ACS	264	23	8.7
Vautrin et al,[33] 2020	Females <45 y with STEMI	51	11	22

Abbreviations: MI, myocardial infarction; PCI, percutaneous coronary intervention; STEMI, ST-elevation myocardial infarction.

100,000 pregnancies in a nationwide health care database in Canada.[40] However, pregnancy-associated SCAD seems to be less common than previously considered and accounts for 4.7% to 16.7% of SCAD cases.[9,41–43] The number of SCAD cases among patients who died of sudden cardiac death seems to be underestimated, because postmortem data are mostly based on case reports. However, a prevalence of 2% has been found in an autopsy cohort of patients who died from sudden death in 1992.[44]

Although SCAD predominantly affects younger women with 81% to 98% female patients and a reported mean age ranging from 45 to 54 years,[21,43,45–52] data have shown SCAD as a significant cause of MI in older women. Therefore, there is a need for its consideration as a cause of MI in older patient groups as well.[53,54]

SPONTANEOUS CORONARY ARTERY DISSECTION CLASSIFICATION

In 2014, an angiographic classification of SCAD has been introduced and widely accepted to describe the different types depending on its angiographic appearance[2] (**Fig. 2**): type 1 is characterized by the pathognomonic appearance of contrast dye staining of the arterial wall with multiple radiolucent lumens. However, it only accounts for 29% to 52% of cases.[9,55] Type 2 is more common (42%–60%)[9,55] and characterized by a long diffuse (>20 mm) and smooth stenosis with varying severity in coronary angiography. There are normal vessel segments proximal and distal to the stenosis in type 2A, whereas diffuse narrowing extends to the distal tip of the affected artery in type 2B. Type 3 lesions mimic atherosclerotic stenoses and are defined as a focal or tubular stenosis (<20 mm). They account for 3.6% to 10.8% of SCAD.[9,55] Type 3 lesions are angiographically indistinguishable from atherosclerosis and require intravascular imaging to confirm the diagnosis. SCAD can affect any coronary artery, but the left anterior descending artery is the most frequently affected vessel (43%–60%). Less commonly involved are the circumflex artery (16%–38%), the right coronary artery (10%–29%), and the left main coronary artery (0%–12%).[9,55] Dissections tend to affect the mid to distal segments,[2] and multivessel dissections are reported in 4% to 20% of cases.[46,55,56]

Predisposing Factors and Triggering Events

SCAD frequently occurs on the basis of underlying predisposing conditions with or without an optional triggering event (**Table 2**). Potential triggering factors have been found in more than one-half of patients, with up to 50.3% experiencing emotional stress and 28.9% physical triggers before the SCAD event.[9] Interestingly, intense physical activity was more often identified as a potential trigger among men and emotional stress has been reported to be more frequent in women.[53] Both emotional and physical triggers are supposed to increase shear stress within the coronary artery wall as the common mechanism leading to SCAD.[57]

A large proportion of patients have predisposing conditions that seem to increase the vulnerability for SCAD. The most commonly found predisposing conditions are arteriopathies. These conditions can be divided into atherosclerotic and nonatherosclerotic arteriopathies that lead to a weakening of the vessel wall. The most frequently identified nonatherosclerotic arteriopathy is fibromuscular dysplasia with a prevalence of 31.1% to 45.0% in patients with SCAD.[9,46,48] Owing to this high coincidence, all patients with SCAD should be

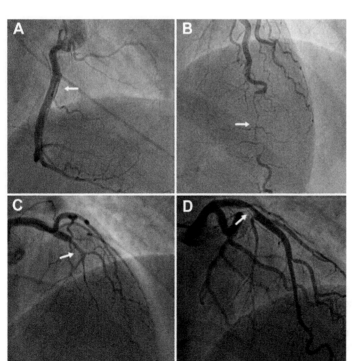

Fig. 2. Types of SCAD. (A) Type 1: contrast dye staining of the arterial wall with multiple radiolucent lumens. (B) Type 2A: long diffuse stenosis without involvement of the distal end of the artery. (C) Type 2B: long diffuse stenosis that extends to the distal tip of the artery. (D) Type 3: focal or tubular stenosis. Arrows: site of SCAD.

Table 2
Predisposing conditions and triggering events

Predisposing Conditions	Prevalence (%)
Fibromuscular dysplasia	31.1–45
Connective tissue disorders	2.6–3.6
Marfan syndrome, Loeys–Dietz syndrome, Ehlers–Danlos syndrome, polycystic kidney disease	
Multiparity (≥4 pregnancies)	8.9–10
Hormonal therapy	10–20
Hormonal contraception, postmenopausal hormonal substitution, infertility treatment	
Systemic inflammatory diseases	4.7–11
Rheumatoid arthritis, lupus erythematosus, vasculitides, inflammatory bowel diseases, sarcoidosis	
Psychiatric diseases	
Depression	9–19.5
Anxiety disorder	11.7–27.8
Migraine	32.5–52
Hypothyroidism	11.3–26

Triggering events (overall prevalence >50%)	Prevalence (%)
Intense physical labor	
Isometric exercise or endurance	10–29
Valsalva maneuver	
Vomiting, defecation, coughing, weightlifting	12
Pregnancy or postpartum period	4.7–16.7
Emotional stress	10–50
Drugs	
Cocaine, methamphetamine	0.3–2.5

Data from Refs.[9,20,41–43,46,48,49,53,58–60,64,69]

screened for arteriopathies. Other associated conditions are connective tissue disorders (2.6%–3.6%) such as Marfan syndrome, Ehlers–Danlos syndrome, or Loeys–Dietz syndrome,[9,46,49] and systemic inflammatory diseases (4.7%–11%).[9,49,58] However, systemic inflammatory diseases have not been found significantly more often than in a control group without SCAD.[58] Further disorders with an increased prevalence in patients

with SCAD are migraine (32.5%–52.0%),[9,46,49] depression (9.0%–19.5%), anxiety disorder (11.7%–27.8%),[9,49,59] and hypothyroidism (11.3%–26.0%).[9,49,60]

A subgroup of SCAD is associated with pregnancy or postpartum period (4.7%–16.7%)[9,41–43] and the administration of female sex hormones (10%–20%).[9,49] The exact mechanism behind pregnancy-related SCAD has yet to be determined. Acute pregnancy-related hemodynamic stress and chronic hormonal and hemodynamic-related vascular degeneration might lead to a higher susceptibility to SCAD during and after pregnancy. Multiple pregnancy, treatment for infertility, and multiparity have been shown to increase the risk for pregnancy-related SCAD.[61]

CLINICAL PRESENTATION

The clinical presentation of SCAD is variable, but the majority of patients present with an ACS. Patients frequently report typical symptoms such as acute chest pain (96%), often radiating to the left arm (52%) or to the neck (22%). Other encountered symptoms are back pain (14%), shortness of breath (20%) and unspecific symptoms such as nausea and vomiting (24%), diaphoresis (21%), or dizziness (9%).[62]

An electrocardiogram (ECG) at admission frequently shows ischemic changes in patients with SCAD. 30% to 49% of patients present with ST-segment elevation MI and 47% to 70% present with non–ST-segment elevation MI.[9,50,63,64] In patients with non–ST-segment elevation MI, the most frequent ECG changes are T-wave inversions. ST-segment depressions and normal ECGs are less typical.[65] Even if SCAD results in MI with elevated cardiac biomarkers in most cases, 0.4% to 4.0% of patients present with normal cardiac biomarkers.[9,63] This proportion might represent patients with unstable angina owing to relative coronary ischemia or patients not evaluated in the correct timeframe after the SCAD event.

A minority of patients initially presents with complications of SCAD such as ventricular arrhythmias, cardiac arrest, or cardiogenic shock (3%–14%).[53,64] Sudden cardiac death is estimated to occur in 3% to 11% of cases; of note, the rate of sudden cardiac death in SCAD is likely to be underestimated because of little investigation and postmortem cases.[57]

DIAGNOSIS

Because the clinical presentation, ECG findings, and elevation of classic cardiac biomarkers in SCAD are comparable with those in atherosclerotic ACS, invasive testing using coronary angiography remains the current standard for SCAD. Of note, fibrillin-1 has recently been identified as a potential biomarker for the diagnosis and prediction of unfavorable outcomes[66] and might help with noninvasive diagnosis in the future.

SCAD is likely underdiagnosed owing to a low index of suspicion of ACS in this young patient group. Clinical features that increase the probability for SCAD in patients presenting with chest pain are female patients less than 50 years of age, no evidence of coronary atherosclerosis, pregnancy or peripartum state, history of fibromuscular dysplasia or other arteriopathies related to SCAD, and recent intense emotional or physical stress.[2] Parallel with ACS guidelines, urgent coronary angiography should be performed in all patients with ST-segment elevation. Otherwise, it might be postponed in patients with non–ST-segment elevation MI, and further stratification by echocardiography and other noninvasive imaging techniques might be performed in the meantime. However, coronary angiography is recommended for all patients with a high index of suspicion of SCAD, because it has the greatest sensitivity owing to its high spatial and temporal resolution.[2]

Almost all cases of SCAD type 1 and most cases of SCAD type 2 can be diagnosed directly by coronary angiography. However, even types 1 and 2 might be missed owing to a lack of familiarity with the angiographic appearance of SCAD.[1] In patients with long and smooth stenoses, the intravenous administration of nitroglycerin should be performed to rule out coronary vasospasm.[2] SCAD type 3 lesions cannot be distinguished from atherosclerotic stenosis by coronary angiography.[2] Intracoronary imaging, that is, optical coherence tomography and intravascular ultrasound examination, is proposed as and additional tool in unclear cases and SCAD type 3. Many patients with negative angiographic findings are later positively diagnosed with SCAD, when intracoronary imaging is performed.[3] Here, the dissection membrane and the IMH can be visualized.[1] Of these techniques, optical coherence tomography is recommended as the preferred tool owing to its greater spatial resolution, even if intravascular ultrasound examination has a deeper penetration level.[2] Intracoronary imaging should be considered in diagnostic uncertainty or if PCI is needed. However, it should be used with caution, because it implements the risk of propagation of the dissection and of negative effects on coronary arterial flow.

Noninvasive cardiac imaging modalities have not yet an established role in the diagnosis of SCAD. Cardiac computed tomography angiography has several shortcomings with a lower spatial and temporal resolution compared with coronary angiography. Even though key features of SCAD in cardiac computed tomography angiography have been described recently, sensitivity and specificity are inferior to that of coronary angiography. IMH appears like noncalcified atherosclerotic plaque on cardiac computed tomography angiography, emphasizing the importance of invasive coronary angiography for correct diagnosis.[67] However, cardiac computed tomography angiography might be useful for the noninvasive follow-up of SCAD in large-caliber vessels. Data on the value of cardiac MRI in SCAD are very rare. It could help to clarify the diagnosis in uncertain cases by visualization of late gadolinium enhancement at the site of SCAD[50] and might have a prognostic role by evaluation of the extent of myocardial damage.[68]

INITIAL MANAGEMENT

Owing to the low prevalence of SCAD, present recommendations for management of patients with SCAD are based on observational studies and expert opinion. The main therapeutic objective is the preservation of thrombolysis in myocardial infarction (TIMI) residual flow rather than restoring the coronary artery architecture. Conservative treatment is favored in stable patients without ongoing ischemia because interventional treatment has been shown to have low success and high complication rates.[9] Furthermore, most SCAD lesions completely heal over time. Follow-up coronary angiographies have shown complete recovery in 91% to 100% of patients treated conservatively within 30 days.[53,69,70] The reasons for absent healing in some cases are not known. In one exemplary series, only 2.3% of conservatively treated patients needed subsequent revascularization.[9]

As mentioned elsewhere in this article, percutaneous coronary intervention in patients with SCAD has been shown to be associated with an increased risk of complications compared with percutaneous coronary intervention in atherosclerotic ACS. Successful procedures have been reported in 29% to 78% of patients in larger SCAD cohorts.[9,71,72] Thus, interventional treatment of SCAD is reserved for high-risk situations such as ongoing ischemia, hemodynamic instability, or high-risk anatomy (left main or proximal 2-vessel SCAD).[54] Revascularization should be attempted through conservative stenting to minimize the risk of further dissection extension and to allow spontaneous healing of the residual dissection. If residual distal dissection occurs after revascularization with normal arterial flow and no significant lumen narrowing, no further interventional treatment is advised.[3] Nevertheless, there are several reports on more innovative interventional approaches such as bioresorbable scaffolds[73–75] and cutting balloon angioplasty[76–79] with better results than traditional stenting methods.

Coronary artery bypass grafting has rarely been performed in patients with SCAD and is reserved for cases with hemodynamic instability or ongoing ischemia and impossible or unsuccessful interventional revascularization.[9,43,71]

MEDICAL AND SUPPORTIVE THERAPY

Data on the optimal medical management of SCAD are scarce, and it is frequently based on clinical judgment of physicians. Some experts recommend a dual antiplatelet therapy based on its advance in atherosclerotic ACS. However, with IMH as the central pathophysiology in SCAD, its use is controversial, and the optimal duration of treatment is unclear. The use of statins in nonatherosclerotic arteries is discussed controversially, as well. One observational study has shown that beta blockers and optimal control of hypertension decrease the risk of recurrence.[65] However, these results are hypothesis generating and need to be confirmed in prospective randomized-controlled trials.

Follow-up of patients should be performed by an interdisciplinary team and offer further supportive therapy consisting of psychiatric support, obstetric counseling, and cardiac rehabilitation. A distinct proportion of patients suffer from psychiatric comorbidities after the SCAD event. A recent study has found post-traumatic stress disorder in 28%, anxiety disorder in 41%, and depression in 32% of patients after SCAD.[80] Therefore, psychiatric assessment and, if needed, medical or nonmedical therapy is recommended for all patients with SCAD. Furthermore, many patients are of childbearing age and some might have the desire to have children. The risk of further pregnancies after SCAD is controversial. However, a recent study has demonstrated no increase in recurrence of SCAD during and after pregnancy.[81] It must be mentioned that this study was limited by a small sample size. Patients, therefore, should be counseled regarding the potential risks of recurrence and severe course of pregnancy-associated SCAD. The usefulness of cardiac rehab has been under debate in the past because physical labor is known to trigger SCAD events. However, rehabilitation has been shown to be safe in patients with SCAD and has led to physical and emotional benefits and lower rates of major adverse cardiac events.[82,83]

COMPLICATIONS AND PROGNOSIS

Wide discrepancies have been reported regarding the prognosis for SCAD, but recent publications show more consistent findings about the outcomes. The rate of overall major adverse cardiac events during the index hospitalization is reported to range from 6.0% to 8.8%. Acute complications mostly consist of recurrent ischemia owing to progression of SCAD and arrhythmias. Cardiogenic shock, cardiac arrest, and death are rare[9,51] (**Table 3**).

Patients who survive the acute phase present with a low long-term mortality,[47] and the 10-year survival rate in SCAD is reported to be 92%.[64] The long-term mortality rate is low both in patients managed conservatively and with revascularization.[71] Survival rates are significantly higher in patients with SCAD compared with patients with atherosclerotic ACS. However, the rates of major adverse cardiac events are significant and comparable with those in atherosclerotic ACS.[64] Studies have reported major adverse cardiac events in 6.0% to 19.9% of patients at 2 to 3 years of follow-up[54,65] and in 7.8% to 12.6% at 4 to 5 years of follow-up.[47,69] Recurrence is reported in 6% to 17% of cases and represents the major part of long-term complications.[46,47] No significant difference has been found in recurrence rates between conservatively managed patients and patients treated with revascularization, most likely

Table 3 In-hospital complications	
Complications (6.0%–8.8%)	**Prevalence (%)**
Death	0.1–1.0
Recurrent MI	3.0–6.1
SCAD progression	3.0
Iatrogenic dissection	1.0
De novo SCAD	<0.1
Other	<1.0
Cardiogenic shock or arrest	2.0
Heart failure	0.4–1.0
Ventricular arrhythmia	3.0–4.0
Atrial fibrillation	1.0
Stroke/TIA	1.0
Pericarditis	2.0

Abbreviations: TIA, transient ischemic attack.
Data from Refs.[9,51]

because almost all recurrent SCAD events occur in other coronary arteries than the initial event.[71]

SUMMARY

SCAD seems to be much more frequent than previously assumed. It is not only a disease of young women during pregnancy or the postpartum state, but affects all sexes and age groups. Scientific interest has clearly increased over the last decade, being reflected by a rising number of scientific publications over time. However, SCAD is still an underdiagnosed entity of ACS, clinicians are rather unfamiliar with this disease, and suspicion might be low within the typical patient collective.

CLINICS CARE POINTS

- SCAD is an infrequent cause of ACS with comparable clinical features.
- It should be considered especially in young women, during pregnancy or the postpartum period, in patients with fibromuscular dysplasia or other arteriopathies, and after physical or emotional stress.
- Coronary angiography is the standard in diagnosis, and conservative treatment is preferred.
- Outcomes are characterized by significant recurrence rates, and periodic follow-up with an interdisciplinary approach is recommended.

DISCLOSURE

The research has been funded by the Swiss Heart Foundation and the Iten-Kohaut Foundation.

REFERENCES

1. Saw J, Mancini GB, Humphries K, et al. Angiographic appearance of spontaneous coronary artery dissection with intramural hematoma proven on intracoronary imaging. Catheter Cardiovasc Interv 2016;87(2):E54–61.
2. Saw J. Coronary angiogram classification of spontaneous coronary artery dissection. Catheter Cardiovasc Interv 2014;84(7):1115–22.
3. Alfonso F, Paulo M, Gonzalo N, et al. Diagnosis of spontaneous coronary artery dissection by optical coherence tomography. J Am Coll Cardiol 2012; 59(12):1073–9.
4. Jackson R, Al-Hussaini A, Joseph S, et al. Spontaneous coronary artery dissection: pathophysiological insights from optical coherence tomography. JACC Cardiovasc Imaging 2019;12(12):2475–88.
5. Motreff P, Malcles G, Combaret N, et al. How and when to suspect spontaneous coronary artery dissection: novel insights from a single-centre series on prevalence and angiographic appearance. EuroIntervention 2017;12(18):e2236–43.
6. Kwon TG, Gulati R, Matsuzawa Y, et al. Proliferation of coronary adventitial vasa vasorum in patients with spontaneous coronary artery dissection. JACC Cardiovasc Imaging 2016;9(7):891–2.
7. Pretty HC. Dissecting aneurysm of coronary artery in a woman aged 42: rupture. Br Med J 1931;1:667.
8. Bac DJ, Lotgering FK, Verkaaik AP, et al. Spontaneous coronary artery dissection during pregnancy and post partum. Eur Heart J 1995;16(1):136–8.
9. Saw J, Starovoytov A, Humphries K, et al. Canadian spontaneous coronary artery dissection cohort study: in-hospital and 30-day outcomes. Eur Heart J 2019;40(15):1188–97.
10. Adlam D, Alfonso F, Maas A, et al. European Society of Cardiology, Acute Cardiovascular Care Association, SCAD study group: a position paper on spontaneous coronary artery dissection. Eur Heart J 2018; 39(36):3353–68.
11. Hayes SN, Kim ESH, Saw J, et al. Spontaneous coronary artery dissection: current state of the science: a scientific statement from the American Heart Association. Circulation 2018;137(19):e523–57.
12. Thygesen K, Alpert JS, Jaffe AS, et al. Fourth universal definition of myocardial infarction (2018). J Am Coll Cardiol 2018;72(18):2231–64.
13. Tamis-Holland JE, Jneid H, Reynolds HR, et al. Contemporary diagnosis and management of patients with myocardial infarction in the absence of obstructive coronary artery disease: a scientific statement from the American Heart Association. Circulation 2019;139(18):e891–908.
14. Agewall S, Beltrame JF, Reynolds HR, et al. ESC working group position paper on myocardial infarction with non-obstructive coronary arteries. Eur Heart J 2017;38(3):143–53.
15. Rigatelli G, Rigatelli G, Rossi P, et al. Normal angiogram in acute coronary syndromes: the underestimated role of alternative substrates of myocardial ischemia. Int J Cardiovasc Imaging 2004;20(6):471–5.
16. Hendiri T, Bonvini RF, Martin W, et al. [Acute myocardial infarction due to spontaneous coronary artery dissection]. Arch Mal Coeur Vaiss 2005;98(10):974–8.
17. Tokura M, Taguchi I, Kageyama M, et al. Clinical features of spontaneous coronary artery dissection. J Cardiol 2014;63(2):119–22.
18. Saia F, Komukai K, Capodanno D, et al. Eroded versus ruptured plaques at the culprit site of STEMI:

in vivo pathophysiological features and response to primary PCI. JACC Cardiovasc Imaging 2015;8(5): 566–75.

19. Nishiguchi T, Tanaka A, Ozaki Y, et al. Prevalence of spontaneous coronary artery dissection in patients with acute coronary syndrome. Eur Heart J Acute Cardiovasc Care 2016;5(3):263–70.

20. Nakashima T, Noguchi T, Haruta S, et al. Prognostic impact of spontaneous coronary artery dissection in young female patients with acute myocardial infarction: a report from the Angina Pectoris-Myocardial Infarction Multicenter Investigators in Japan. Int J Cardiol 2016;207:341–8.

21. Clare R, Duan L, Phan D, et al. Characteristics and clinical outcomes of patients with spontaneous coronary artery dissection. J Am Heart Assoc 2019; 8(10):e012570.

22. Lobo AS, Cantu SM, Sharkey SW, et al. Revascularization in patients with spontaneous coronary artery dissection and ST-segment elevation myocardial infarction. J Am Coll Cardiol 2019;74(10):1290–300.

23. Daoulah A, Al-Faifi SM, Hurley WT, et al. Spontaneous Coronary Artery Dissection: Does Being Unemployed Matter? Insights from the GSCAD Registry. Curr Cardiol Rev 2021;17(3):328–39.

24. Hiasa Y, Otani R, Wada T, et al. [Primary coronary artery dissection: its incidence and genesis studied by clinical and coronary angiographic findings]. Kokyu To Junkan 1990;38(11):1127–31.

25. Hering D, Piper C, Hohmann C, et al. [Prospective study of the incidence, pathogenesis and therapy of spontaneous, by coronary angiography diagnosed coronary artery dissection]. Z Kardiol 1998; 87(12):961–70.

26. Maeder M, Ammann P, Angehrn W, et al. Idiopathic spontaneous coronary artery dissection: incidence, diagnosis and treatment. Int J Cardiol 2005;101(3): 363–9.

27. Unal M, Korkut AK, Kosem M, et al. Surgical management of spontaneous coronary artery dissection. Tex Heart Inst J 2008;35(4):402–5.

28. Mortensen KH, Thuesen L, Kristensen IB, et al. Spontaneous coronary artery dissection: a Western Denmark Heart Registry study. Catheter Cardiovasc Interv 2009;74(5):710–7.

29. Vanzetto G, Berger-Coz E, Barone-Rochette G, et al. Prevalence, therapeutic management and medium-term prognosis of spontaneous coronary artery dissection: results from a database of 11,605 patients. Eur J Cardiothorac Surg 2009;35(2):250–4.

30. Rigatelli G, Dell'Avvocata F, Picariello C, et al. Characterization of single vs. recurrent spontaneous coronary artery dissection. Asian Cardiovasc Thorac Ann 2018;26(2):89–93.

31. Liu X, Xu C, Liu C, et al. Clinical characteristics and long-term prognosis of spontaneous coronary artery dissection: A single-center Chinese experience. Pak J Med Sci 2019;35(1):106–12.

32. Lim YT, Ling LH, Tambyah PA, et al. Myocardial infarction in patients aged 40 years and below: an angiographic review. Singapore Med J 1996;37(4): 352–5.

33. Vautrin E, Jean ABP, Fourny M, et al. Sex differences in coronary artery lesions and in-hospital outcomes for patients with ST-segment elevation myocardial infarction under the age of 45. Catheter Cardiovasc Interv 2020;96(6):1222–30.

34. Yang J, Biery DW, Singh A, et al. Risk factors and outcomes of very young adults who experience myocardial infarction: the partners YOUNG-MI Registry. Am J Med 2020;133(5):605–12. e601.

35. Inoue Y, Tanaka A, Asano H, et al. Clinical characteristics and treatment of spontaneous coronary artery dissection in young women undergoing percutaneous coronary intervention. J Cardiovasc Med (Hagerstown) 2021;22(1):14–9.

36. Kim Y, Han X, Ahn Y, et al. Clinical characteristics of spontaneous coronary artery dissection in young female patients with acute myocardial infarction in Korea. Korean J Intern Med 2021;36(1):106–13.

37. Lorca R, Pascual I, Aparicio A, et al. Premature STEMI in Men and Women: Current Clinical Features and Improvements in Management and Prognosis. J Clin Med 2021;10(6):1314.

38. Meng PN, Xu C, You W, et al. Spontaneous coronary artery dissection as a cause of acute myocardial infarction in young female population: a single-center study. Chin Med J (Engl) 2017;130(13): 1534–9.

39. Elkayam U, Jalnapurkar S, Barakkat MN, et al. Pregnancy-associated acute myocardial infarction: a review of contemporary experience in 150 cases between 2006 and 2011. Circulation 2014;129(16): 1695–702.

40. Faden MS, Bottega N, Benjamin A, et al. A nationwide evaluation of spontaneous coronary artery dissection in pregnancy and the puerperium. Heart 2016;102(24):1974–9.

41. McGrath-Cadell L, McKenzie P, Emmanuel S, et al. Outcomes of patients with spontaneous coronary artery dissection. Open Heart 2016;3(2):e000491.

42. Tweet MS, Hayes SN, Codsi E, et al. Spontaneous coronary artery dissection associated with pregnancy. J Am Coll Cardiol 2017;70(4):426–35.

43. Chen S, Merchant M, Mahrer KN, et al. Spontaneous Coronary Artery Dissection: Clinical Characteristics, Management, and Outcomes in a Racially and Ethnically Diverse Community-Based Cohort. Perm J 2019;23(18):278.

44. Corrado D, Thiene G, Cocco P, et al. Non-atherosclerotic coronary artery disease and sudden death in the young. Br Heart J 1992;68(6):601–7.

45. Lettieri C, Zavalloni D, Rossini R, et al. Management and long-term prognosis of spontaneous coronary artery dissection. Am J Cardiol 2015;116(1):66–73.

46. Kok SN, Hayes SN, Cutrer FM, et al. Prevalence and clinical factors of migraine in patients with spontaneous coronary artery dissection. J Am Heart Assoc 2018;7(24):e010140.

47. Cheung CC, Starovoytov A, Parsa A, et al. In-hospital and long-term outcomes among patients with spontaneous coronary artery dissection presenting with ventricular tachycardia/fibrillation. Heart Rhythm 2020;17(11):1864–9.

48. Combaret N, Gerbaud E, Dérimay F, et al. National French registry of spontaneous coronary artery dissections: prevalence of fibromuscular dysplasia and genetic analyses. EuroIntervention 2020;17(6):508–15.

49. Smaardijk VR, Mommersteeg PMC, Kop WJ, et al. Psychological and clinical characteristics of female patients with spontaneous coronary artery dissection. Neth Heart J 2020;28(9):485–91.

50. Al-Hussaini A, Abdelaty A, Gulsin GS, et al. Chronic infarct size after spontaneous coronary artery dissection: implications for pathophysiology and clinical management. Eur Heart J 2020;41(23):2197–205.

51. García-Guimaraes M, Bastante T, Macaya F, et al. Spontaneous coronary artery dissection in Spain: clinical and angiographic characteristics, management, and in-hospital events. Rev Esp Cardiol (Engl Ed) 2021;74(1):15–23.

52. McAlister CP, Yi M, Adamson PD, et al. Trends in the detection, management and 30-day outcomes of spontaneous coronary artery dissection: a six-year, New Zealand centre experience. Heart Lung Circ 2021;30(1):78–85.

53. Saw J, Aymong E, Sedlak T, et al. Spontaneous coronary artery dissection: association with predisposing arteriopathies and precipitating stressors and cardiovascular outcomes. Circ Cardiovasc Interv 2014;7(5):645–55.

54. Alfonso F, Paulo M, Lennie V, et al. Spontaneous coronary artery dissection: long-term follow-up of a large series of patients prospectively managed with a "conservative" therapeutic strategy. JACC Cardiovasc Interv 2012;5(10):1062–70.

55. Daoulah A, Al-Faifi SM, Alhamid S, et al. Spontaneous coronary artery dissection in the gulf: G-SCAD registry. Angiology 2021;72(1):32–43.

56. Fahey JK, Chew A, Ihdayhid AR, et al. Women with spontaneous coronary artery dissection are at increased risk of iatrogenic coronary artery dissection. Heart Lung Circ 2021;30(1):e23–8.

57. Saw J, Mancini GBJ, Humphries KH. Contemporary review on spontaneous coronary artery dissection. J Am Coll Cardiol 2016;68(3):297–312.

58. Kronzer VL, Tarabochia AD, Lobo Romero AS, et al. Lack of association of spontaneous coronary artery dissection with autoimmune disease. J Am Coll Cardiol 2020;76(19):2226–34.

59. Sharma S, Kaadan MI, Duran JM, et al. Risk factors, imaging findings, and sex differences in spontaneous coronary artery dissection. Am J Cardiol 2019;123(11):1783–7.

60. Camacho Freire SJ, Díaz Fernández JF, Gheorghe LL, et al. Spontaneous coronary artery dissection and hypothyroidism. Rev Esp Cardiol (Engl Ed) 2019;72(8):625–33.

61. Vijayaraghavan R, Verma S, Gupta N, et al. Pregnancy-related spontaneous coronary artery dissection. Circulation 2014;130(21):1915–20.

62. Luong C, Starovoytov A, Heydari M, et al. Clinical presentation of patients with spontaneous coronary artery dissection. Catheter Cardiovasc Interv 2017;89(7):1149–54.

63. Daoulah A, Al-Faifi SM, Madan M, et al. Clinical presentation and outcome of patients with spontaneous coronary artery dissection versus atherosclerotic coronary plaque dissection. Crit Pathw Cardiol 2021;20(1):36–43.

64. Tweet MS, Hayes SN, Pitta SR, et al. Clinical features, management, and prognosis of spontaneous coronary artery dissection. Circulation 2012;126(5):579–88.

65. Saw J, Humphries K, Aymong E, et al. Spontaneous coronary artery dissection: clinical outcomes and risk of recurrence. J Am Coll Cardiol 2017;70(9):1148–58.

66. Hui P, Bai Y, Su X, et al. The value of plasma fibrillin-1 level in patients with spontaneous coronary artery dissection. Int J Cardiol 2020;302:150–6.

67. Tweet MS, Akhtar NJ, Hayes SN, et al. Spontaneous coronary artery dissection: acute findings on coronary computed tomography angiography. Eur Heart J Acute Cardiovasc Care 2019;8(5):467–75.

68. Tan NY, Hayes SN, Young PM, et al. Usefulness of cardiac magnetic resonance imaging in patients with acute spontaneous coronary artery dissection. Am J Cardiol 2018;122(10):1624–9.

69. Rogowski S, Maeder MT, Weilenmann D, et al. Spontaneous coronary artery dissection: angiographic follow-up and long-term clinical outcome in a predominantly medically treated population. Catheter Cardiovasc Interv 2017;89(1):59–68.

70. Hassan S, Prakash R, Starovoytov A, et al. Natural history of spontaneous coronary artery dissection with spontaneous angiographic healing. JACC Cardiovasc Interv 2019;12(6):518–27.

71. Tweet MS, Eleid MF, Best PJ, et al. Spontaneous coronary artery dissection: revascularization versus conservative therapy. Circ Cardiovasc Interv 2014;7(6):777–86.

72. Conrotto F, D'Ascenzo F, Cerrato E, et al. Safety and efficacy of drug eluting stents in patients with spontaneous coronary artery dissection. Int J Cardiol 2017;238:105–9.

73. Watt J, Egred M, Khurana A, et al. 1-Year follow-up optical frequency domain imaging of multiple bioresorbable vascular scaffolds for the treatment of spontaneous coronary artery dissection. JACC Cardiovasc Interv 2016;9(4):389–91.

74. Sengottuvelu G, Rajendran R. Full polymer jacketing for long-segment spontaneous coronary artery dissection using bioresorbable vascular scaffolds. JACC Cardiovasc Interv 2014;7(7):820–1.

75. Panoulas VF, Ielasi A. Bioresorbable scaffolds and drug-eluting balloons for the management of spontaneous coronary artery dissections. J Thorac Dis 2016;8(10):E1328–30.

76. Ito T, Shintani Y, Ichihashi T, et al. Non-atherosclerotic spontaneous coronary artery dissection revascularized by intravascular ultrasonography-guided fenestration with cutting balloon angioplasty. Cardiovasc Interv Ther 2017;32(3):241–3.

77. Alkhouli M, Cole M, Ling FS. Coronary artery fenestration prior to stenting in spontaneous coronary artery dissection. Catheter Cardiovasc Interv 2016; 88(1):E23–7.

78. Motreff P, Barber-Chamoux N, Combaret N, et al. Coronary artery fenestration guided by optical coherence tomography before stenting: new interventional option in rescue management of compressive spontaneous intramural hematoma. Circ Cardiovasc Interv 2015;8(4):e002266.

79. Yumoto K, Sasaki H, Aoki H, et al. Successful treatment of spontaneous coronary artery dissection with cutting balloon angioplasty as evaluated with optical coherence tomography. JACC Cardiovasc Interv 2014;7(7):817–9.

80. Johnson AK, Hayes SN, Sawchuk C, et al. Analysis of posttraumatic stress disorder, depression, anxiety, and resiliency within the unique population of spontaneous coronary artery dissection survivors. J Am Heart Assoc 2020;9(9):e014372.

81. Tweet MS, Young KA, Best PJM, et al. Association of pregnancy with recurrence of spontaneous coronary artery dissection among women with prior coronary artery dissection. JAMA Netw Open 2020;3(9): e2018170.

82. Chou AY, Prakash R, Rajala J, et al. The first dedicated cardiac rehabilitation program for patients with spontaneous coronary artery dissection: description and initial results. Can J Cardiol 2016; 32(4):554–60.

83. Krittanawong C, Tweet MS, Hayes SE, et al. Usefulness of cardiac rehabilitation after spontaneous coronary artery dissection. Am J Cardiol 2016;117(10): 1604–9.

Moving?

Make sure your subscription moves with you!

To notify us of your new address, find your **Clinics Account Number** (located on your mailing label above your name), and contact customer service at:

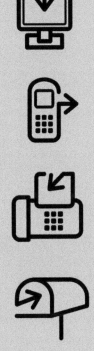

Email: journalscustomerservice-usa@elsevier.com

800-654-2452 (subscribers in the U.S. & Canada)
314-447-8871 (subscribers outside of the U.S. & Canada)

Fax number: 314-447-8029

**Elsevier Health Sciences Division
Subscription Customer Service
3251 Riverport Lane
Maryland Heights, MO 63043**

*To ensure uninterrupted delivery of your subscription, please notify us at least 4 weeks in advance of move.

Printed and bound by CPI Group (UK) Ltd, Croydon, CR0 4YY

03/10/2024

01040363-0004